Equine Pharmacology

Editor

K. GARY MAGDESIAN

VETERINARY CLINICS OF NORTH AMERICA: EQUINE PRACTICE

www.vetequine.theclinics.com

Consulting Editor
THOMAS J. DIVERS

April 2017 • Volume 33 • Number 1

ELSEVIER

1600 John F. Kennedy Boulevard • Suite 1800 • Philadelphia, Pennsylvania, 19103-2899

http://www.vetequine.theclinics.com

VETERINARY CLINICS OF NORTH AMERICA: EQUINE PRACTICE Volume 33, Number 1
April 2017 ISSN 0749-0739, ISBN-13: 978-0-323-52437-7

Editor: Katie Pfaff
Developmental Editor: Donald Mumford

Veterinary Clinics of North America: Equine Practice (ISSN 0749-0739) is published in April, August, and December by Elsevier Inc., 360 Park Avenue South, New York, NY 10010-1710. Business and Editorial Offices: 1600 John F. Kennedy Blvd., Suite 1800, Philadelphia, PA 19103-2899. Subscription prices are $270.00 per year (domestic individuals), $506.00 per year (domestic institutions), $100.00 per year (domestic students/residents), $315.00 per year (Canadian individuals), $637.00 per year (Canadian institutions), $365.00 per year (international individuals), $637.00 per year (international institutions), and $180.00 per year (international and Canadian students/residents). To receive student/resident rate, orders must be accompanied by name of affiliated institution, date of term, and the signature of program/residency coordinator on institution letterhead. Orders will be billed at individual rate until proof of status is received. Foreign air speed delivery is included in all *Clinics* subscription prices. All prices are subject to change without notice. **POSTMASTER:** Send address changes to *Veterinary Clinics of North America: Equine Practice*, 3251 Riverport Lane, Maryland Heights, MO 63043. Customer Service (orders, claims, online, change of address): Elsevier Health Sciences Division, Subscription **Customer Service, 3251 Riverport Lane, Maryland Heights, MO 63043. Tel: 1-800-654-2452 (U.S. and Canada); 314-447-8871 (outside U.S. and Canada). Fax: 314-447-8029. E-mail: journalscustomerservice-usa@elsevier.com (for print support);** E-mail: **journalsonlinesupport-usa@elsevier. com (for online support)**.

Reprints. For copies of 100 or more of articles in this publication, please contact the Commercial Reprints Department, Elsevier Inc., 360 Park Avenue South, New York, NY 10010-1710. Tel.: 212-633-3874; Fax: 212-633-3820; E-mail: reprints@elsevier.com.

Veterinary Clinics of North America: Equine Practice is covered in *MEDLINE/PubMed (Index Medicus), Excerpta Medica, Current Contents/Agriculture, Biology and Environmental Sciences,* and *ISI.*

Contributors

CONSULTING EDITOR

THOMAS J. DIVERS, DVM
Diplomate, American College of Veterinary Internal Medicine; Diplomate, American College of Veterinary Emergency and Critical Care; Steffen Professor of Veterinary Medicine, Section of Large Animal Medicine, College of Veterinary Medicine, Cornell University, Ithaca, New York

EDITOR

K. GARY MAGDESIAN, DVM
Diplomate, American College of Veterinary Internal Medicine; Diplomate, American College of Veterinary Emergency and Critical Care; Diplomate, American College of Veterinary Clinical Pharmacology; Henry Endowed Chair of Emergency Medicine and Critical Care, Department of Medicine and Epidemiology, School of Veterinary Medicine, University of California, Davis, Davis, California

AUTHORS

FRANK M. ANDREWS, DVM, MS
Equine Health Studies Program, Department of Veterinary Clinical Sciences, School of Veterinary Medicine, Louisiana State University, Baton Rouge, Louisiana

MANDY L. CHA, BS, BVSc
Kulshan Veterinary Hospital, Lynden, Washington

LAIS R.R. COSTA, MV, MS, PhD
Diplomate, American College of Veterinary Internal Medicine - Large Animal; Diplomate, American Board of Veterinary Practitioners–Equine; William R. Pritchard Veterinary Medical Teaching Hospital, University of California, Davis, Davis, California

THOMAS J. DIVERS, DVM
Diplomate, American College of Veterinary Internal Medicine; Diplomate, American College of Veterinary Emergency and Critical Care; Steffen Professor of Veterinary Medicine, Section of Large Animal Medicine, College of Veterinary Medicine, Cornell University, Ithaca, New York

ANDY E. DURHAM, BSc, BVSc, CertEP, DEIM, MRCVS
Diplomate, European College of Equine Internal Medicine; Professor, Liphook Equine Hospital, Liphook, Hampshire, United Kingdom

STEEVE GIGUÈRE, DVM, PhD
Diplomate, American College of Veterinary Internal Medicine, Department of Large Animal Medicine, Veterinary Medical Center, University of Georgia, Athens, Georgia

ALONSO GUEDES, DVM, MS, PhD
Department of Veterinary Clinical Sciences, College of Veterinary Medicine, University of Minnesota, St Paul, Minnesota

HEATHER K. KNYCH, MS, DVM, PhD
Diplomate, American College of Veterinary Clinical Pharmacology; Associate Professor of Clinical Veterinary Pharmacology, K.L. Maddy Equine Analytical Chemistry Laboratory, School of Veterinary Medicine, University of California, Davis, Davis, California

MATHILDE LECLERE, DVM, PhD
Diplomate, American College of Veterinary Internal Medicine; Assistant Professor in Equine Internal Medicine, Department of Clinical Sciences, Faculty of Veterinary Medicine, Université de Montréal, Quebec, Canada

K. GARY MAGDESIAN, DVM
Diplomate, American College of Veterinary Internal Medicine; Diplomate, American College of Veterinary Emergency and Critical Care; Diplomate, American College of Veterinary Clinical Pharmacology; Henry Endowed Chair of Emergency Medicine and Critical Care, Department of Medicine and Epidemiology, School of Veterinary Medicine, University of California, Davis, Davis, California

LARA K. MAXWELL, DVM, PhD
Diplomate, American College of Veterinary Clinical Pharmacology, Professor of Pharmacology, Department of Physiological Sciences, Center for Veterinary Health Sciences, Oklahoma State University, Stillwater, Oklahoma

KRYSTA MOFFITT, PharmD
Professor of Clinical Veterinary Equine Chemistry, K.L. Maddy Equine Analytical Chemistry Laboratory, School of Veterinary Medicine, University of California, Davis, Davis, California

NICOLA PUSTERLA, DVM, PhD
Diplomate, American College of Veterinary Internal Medicine; Professor of Internal Medicine, Department of Medicine and Epidemiology, School of Veterinary Medicine, University of California, Davis, Davis, California

MEG M. SLEEPER, VMD
Diplomate, American College of Veterinary Internal Medicine (Cardiology); Clinical Professor of Cardiology, Department of Small Animal Clinical Sciences, College of Veterinary Medicine, University of Florida, Gainesville, Florida

SCOTT D. STANLEY, PhD
Professor of Clinical Veterinary Equine Chemistry, K.L. Maddy Equine Analytical Chemistry Laboratory, School of Veterinary Medicine, University of California, Davis, Davis, California

THOMAS TOBIN, MVB, MSC, PhD, MRCVS
Diplomate, American Board of Toxicology; Professor, Veterinary Science and Professor, Department of Toxicology and Cancer Research, The Maxwell H. Gluck Equine Research Center, College of Agriculture, University of Kentucky, Lexington, Kentucky

VALERIE WIEBE, PharmD, FSVHP
Diplomate, International College of Veterinary Pharmacy; Director of Pharmacy, Adjunct Professor of the Department of Medicine and Epidemiology, William R. Prichard Veterinary Medical Teaching Hospital, University of California, Davis, Davis, California

FEREYDON REZAZADEH ZAVOSHTI, DVM, DVSc
Associate Professor of Large Animal Internal Medicine, University of Tabriz, Tabriz, Iran

Contents

Nonsteroidal anti-inflammatory drugs (NSAIDs) are effective anti-inflammatory and analgesic agents and are arguably the most commonly used class of drugs in equine medicine. This article provides a brief review of the mechanism of action, therapeutic uses, pharmacokinetics, and adverse effects associated with their use in horses. The use of COX-2 selective NSAIDs in veterinary medicine has increased over the past several years and special emphasis is given to the use of these drugs in horses. A brief discussion of the use of NSAIDs in performance horses is also included.

Immune suppressive therapies target exaggerated and deleterious responses of the immune system. Triggered by exogenous or endogenous factors, these improper responses can lead to immune or inflammatory manifestations, such as urticaria, equine asthma, or autoimmune and immune-mediated diseases. Glucocorticoids are the most commonly used immune suppressive drugs and the only ones supported by robust evidence of clinical efficacy in equine medicine. In some conditions, combining glucocorticoids with other pharmacologic and nonpharmacologic treatments, such as azathioprine, antihistamine, bronchodilators, environmental management, or desensitization, can help to decrease dosages and associated side effects.

This article discusses the benefits and limitations of inhalation therapy in horses. Inhalation drug therapy delivers the drug directly to the airways, thereby achieving maximal drug concentrations at the target site. Inhalation therapy has the additional advantage of decreasing systemic side effects. Inhalation therapy in horses is delivered by the use of nebulizers or pressured metered dose inhalers. It also requires the use of a muzzle or nasal mask in horses. Drugs most commonly delivered through inhalation drug therapy in horses include bronchodilators, antiinflammatories, and antimicrobials.

Neonatal foals are at high risk of developing sepsis, which can be life-threatening. Early antimicrobial use is a critical component of the treatment of sepsis. Because the neonatal foal has unique pharmacologic physiology, antimicrobial choice and dosing are often different than in adult horses. Broad-spectrum, bactericidal, and intravenous antimicrobials should be considered first-line therapy for septic foals. A combination of aminoglycoside and beta-lactam antimicrobial or third-generation cephalosporin is an excellent empirical first choice for treating septic foals, until culture and susceptibility results are available. Renal function should be monitored carefully in foals being treated with aminoglycosides.

Pneumonia caused by *Rhodococcus equi* remains an important cause of disease and death in foals. The combination of a macrolide (erythromycin, azithromycin, or clarithromycin) with rifampin remains the recommended therapy for foals with clinical signs of infection caused by *R equi*. Most foals with small, subclinical ultrasonographic pulmonary lesions associated with *R equi* recover without therapy, and administration of antimicrobial agents to these subclinically affected foals does not hasten lesion resolution relative to administration of a placebo. Resistance to macrolides and rifampin in isolates of *R equi* is increasing.

Equine protozoal myeloencephalitis is an infectious disease of the central nervous system caused by *Sarcocystis neurona* or *Neospora hughesi*. Affected horses routinely present with progressive and asymmetrical neurologic deficits. The diagnosis relies on the presence of neurologic signs, ruling out other neurologic disorders, and the detection of intrathecally derived antibodies to either *S neurona* and/or *N hughesi*. Recommended treatment is use of an FDA-approved anticoccidial drug formulation. Medical and supportive treatment is provided based on the severity of neurologic deficits and complications. This article focuses on recent data related to diagnosis, pharmacologic treatment, and prevention.

Since vaccination may not prevent disease, antiherpetic drugs have been investigated for the therapy of several equine herpesviruses. Drug efficacy has been assessed in horses with disease, but most evidence is in vitro, in other species, or empirical. Oral valacyclovir is most often administered in the therapy of equine herpesvirus type-1 (EHV-1) to protect adult horses from equine herpesvirus myeloencephalopathy, while oral acyclovir is frequently administered for EHV-5 infection in the therapy of equine multinodular pulmonary fibrosis. Other antiherpetic drugs are promising but require further investigation. Several topical drugs are also empirically used in the therapy of equine viral keratitis.

Equine endocrine disease is commonly encountered by equine practitioners. Pituitary pars intermedia dysfunction (PPID) and equine metabolic syndrome (EMS) predominate. The most logical therapeutic approach in PPID uses dopamine agonists; pergolide mesylate is the most common. Bromocryptine and cabergoline are alternative drugs with similar actions. Drugs from other classes have a poor evidence basis, although cyproheptadine and trilostane might be considered. EMS requires management changes as the primary approach; reasonable justification for use of drugs such as levothyroxine and metformin may apply. Therapeutic options exist in rare cases of diabetes mellitus, diabetes insipidus, hyperthyroidism, and critical illness-related corticosteroid insufficiency.

Equine gastric ulcer syndrome (EGUS) is an umbrella term used to describe ulcers in the nonglandular squamous and glandular mucosa, terminal esophagus, and proximal duodenum. Gastric ulcers in the squamous and glandular regions occur more often than esophageal or duodenal ulcers and likely have a different pathogenesis. At present, omeprazole is accepted globally as the best pharmacologic therapy for both regions of the stomach; however, the addition of coating agents and synthetic prostaglandins could add to its effectiveness in treatment of EGUS. Dietary and environmental management are necessary for prevention of recurrence.

 Video content accompanies this article at http://www.vetequine. theclinics.com.

Heart disease can be defined as any abnormality of the heart whether it is a cardiac dysrhythmia or structural heart disease, either congenital or acquired. Heart failure occurs when a cardiac abnormality results in the inability of the heart to pump enough blood to meet the body's needs. Heart disease can be present without leading to heart failure. Heart failure, however, is a consequence of heart disease. There are 4 main areas where the clinician can intervene to improve cardiac output with heart failure: preload, afterload, myocardial contractility, and heart rate.

There has been great progress in the understanding of basic neurobiologic mechanisms of pain, but this body of knowledge has not yet translated into new and improved analgesics. Progress has been made regarding pain assessment in horses, but more work is needed until sensitive and accurate pain assessment tools are available for use in clinical practice. This review summarizes and updates the knowledge concerning the cornerstones of pain medicine (understand, assess, prevent, and treat). It highlights the importance of understanding pain mechanisms and expressions to enable a rational approach to pain assessment, prevention, and management in the equine patient.

Equine practitioners should follow these recommendations when using compounded medications: (1) the decision must be veterinary driven, based on a valid veterinarian-client-patient relationship and on evidence-based medicine; (2) compliance with the Animal Medicinal Drug Use Clarification Act of 1994; and (3) use limited to (a) horses for which no other method or route of drug delivery is practical; (b) those drugs for which safety, efficacy, and stability have been demonstrated; or (c) disease conditions for which a quantifiable response to therapy or drug concentration can be monitored.

Special Review by Consulting Editor Thomas J. Divers

VETERINARY CLINICS OF NORTH AMERICA: EQUINE PRACTICE

THE CLINICS ARE NOW AVAILABLE ONLINE!
Access your subscription at:
www.theclinics.com

Preface

Equine Pharmacology

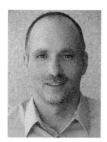

K. Gary Magdesian, DVM, DACVIM, DACVECC, DACVCP
Editor

Continued advancement of pharmacology is vital to equine practice. Medications allow clinicians to heal and improve the lives of the beloved horse. Furthering our understanding of drugs and therapeutics means better medical care for the horse. This is what I hope to accomplish with this issue.

I would like to send a heartfelt thanks to one of the finest equine veterinarians ever to practice, Dr Tom Divers, for the invitation to serve as editor for this issue. I also extend my appreciation to Donald Mumford, Patrick Manley, and the Elsevier team for their hard work and tremendous dedication. I am grateful for, and honored by, the contributions of the authors in this issue. I learned a tremendous amount from reading the manuscripts, and they have renewed my passion for pharmacology.

I dedicate this issue to all of the mentors, residents, students, clients, and especially the horses from which I learned and continue to learn pharmacology. Finally, a special thanks goes out to Dr Cynthia Cole for inspiring me to pursue training in this field.

K. Gary Magdesian, DVM, DACVIM, DACVECC, DACVCP
Professor and Henry Endowed Chair of Emergency Medicine and Critical Care
Department of Medicine and Epidemiology
School of Veterinary Medicine
University of California, Davis
1 Garrod Drive
Davis, CA 95616, USA

E-mail address:
kgmagdesian@ucdavis.edu

Vet Clin Equine 33 (2017) xi
http://dx.doi.org/10.1016/j.cveq.2017.01.001
0749-0739/17/© 2017 Published by Elsevier Inc.

vetequine.theclinics.com

Nonsteroidal Anti-inflammatory Drug Use in Horses

Heather K. Knych, MS, DVM, PhD

KEYWORDS

- Nonsteroidal anti-inflammatory drugs • Horses • Analgesia • Anti-inflammatory

KEY POINTS

- Nonsteroidal anti-inflammatory drugs (NSAIDs) are effective in the treatment of soft tissue, musculoskeletal, and abdominal inflammation and pain.
- Potential adverse effects associated with NSAIDs include gastrointestinal and renal toxicity and inhibition of bone healing.
- Over the past several decades, the focus has been on developing NSAIDs with more selectivity for cyclooxygenase-2 as a means of decreasing adverse effects while maintaining efficacy.
- As NSAIDs are commonly used in race and performance horses, it is imperative that clinicians are familiar with regulatory recommendations for the use of these drugs before performance.

THE INFLAMMATORY CASCADE

Inflammation is the body's response to tissue damage. In the acute stage, the body attempts to return normal function to the injured and inflamed tissue. However, over time, and with the development of chronic inflammation, deleterious effects can occur. The first step in the inflammatory cascade is the release of arachidonic acid, mediated by Phospholipase A2, in response to insult or injury to cellular membranes. This initiates what is termed the arachidonic acid cascade (**Fig. 1**).

Arachidonic acid serves as a substrate for the generation of a number of eicosanoids, including prostaglandins, leukotrienes, and thromboxane A_2 (TXA_2), all of which play a key role in the inflammatory cascade. Production of prostaglandins and TXA_2 is mediated by Prostaglandin H_2 synthase, otherwise known as cyclooxygenase (COX). Oxygenation of arachidonic acid by COX enzymes forms the unstable prostaglandin G_2, which is subsequently converted to prostaglandin H_2. Conversion to specific

Disclosure Statement: The authors have nothing to disclose.
K.L. Maddy Equine Analytical Chemistry Laboratory, School of Veterinary Medicine, University of California, Davis, 620 West Health Science Drive, Davis, CA 95616, USA
E-mail address: hkknych@ucdavis.edu

A

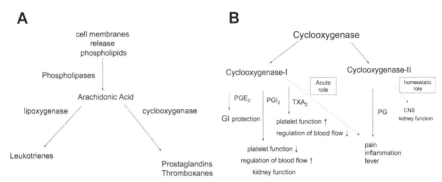

B

Fig. 1. Arachidonic acid cascade (*A*) and role of cyclooxygenase enzymes (*B*).

prostaglandins (ie, prostaglandin E_2 [PGE_2], prostaglandin $F_2\alpha$, and TXA_2) depends on the presence of specific isomerase, reductase, or synthase enzymes.[1] These inflammatory mediators are responsible for the sequelae of inflammation, including increased vascular permeability, heat, and decreased nociceptor thresholds.

CYCLOOXYGENASE ENZYMES AND NONSTEROIDAL ANTI-INFLAMMATORY DRUG INHIBITION

Nonsteroidal anti-inflammatory drugs (NSAIDs) are potent inhibitors of COX enzymes. To date, 3 COX enzymes have been identified, COX-1, COX-2, and COX-3. COX-1 and COX-2 have been well characterized (see **Fig. 1**), but less is known about COX-3. COX-1 is constitutive and present in nearly all cell types.[2] It has been deemed the "housekeeping" enzyme, as it plays a role in normal physiologic functions that help to maintain homeostasis. This includes such things as gastroprotection, gestation, and parturition. COX-2 on the other hand is constitutively expressed in most cell types with protein levels increasing in a matter of hours following stimulation.[3,4] COX-2 can be upregulated as much as 20-fold in endothelial and other cell types as part of the inflammatory process.[5–8] COX-2 induction occurs following exposure to stimuli associated with inflammation including bacterial lipopolysaccharide (LPS) and inflammatory cytokines, such as interleukins 1 and 2 and tumor necrosis factor alpha.[9] Conversely, expression of COX-2 is decreased in the presence of anti-inflammatory cytokines such as interleukins 4, 10, and 13.[3,10,11] Although in most tissues COX-2 is considered pathologic, this an oversimplification as this enzyme does contribute to homeostasis in some organs. COX-2 is constitutively expressed in certain regions of the brain[12,13] and plays a role in maintaining blood flow in the compromised kidney.[14] However, because COX-1 appears to have a greater importance in maintaining homeostasis than does COX-2, most adverse effects of NSAID administration are associated with inhibition of this enzyme (see discussion later in this article).

CYCLOOXYGENASE-1/CYCLOOXYGENASE-2 SELECTIVITY

Over the past 2 decades, the focus, both in human and veterinary medicine, has been on developing NSAIDs that are more selective for the COX-2 enzyme as compared with COX-1.[15] Depending on the relative degree of selectivity, this would ideally preserve the normal housekeeping functions of COX-1 while inhibiting the proinflammatory and potentially detrimental effects often associated with COX-2. However, as discussed previously, although minimal, the contribution of COX-2 to normal physiologic functions should be considered when selecting a COX-2 selective NSAID.

The degree to which NSAIDs inhibit the different COX isoforms and therefore their relative selectivity, is determined by in vitro COX inhibitory assays. Selectivity for the isoforms is expressed as an inhibitory ratio, usually the IC_{50} for COX-1: IC_{50} for COX-2, in which IC_{50} is the plasma concentration necessary to inhibit 50% of COX activity.[16] The higher the ratio, the more selective the NSAID is for COX-2.[16] The inhibitory ratio allows for classification of NSAIDs with specificity for COX-2 as "COX-2 preferential" or "selective," and those with no significant effect on COX-1 as "COX-1 sparing." More recently, some investigators have described selectivity using an IC_{80} or IC_{95} ratio, suggesting that this may be more clinically applicable as often times a high level of prostaglandin inhibition is necessary to achieve a therapeutically useful antipyretic, anti-inflammatory, or analgesic effect.[17,18]

It is important to note that NSAID COX-1:COX-2 selectivity varies between species[19] and therefore extrapolation of classification as a COX-2 selective or preferential inhibitor between species should be done with caution. Even within the same species, variability in inhibitory ratios between studies may be observed. Variability in the assay used, including incubation time, exogenous or endogenous substrate (arachidonic acid), use of whole cells or microsomes and presence or absence of plasma proteins in the media, can yield very different inhibitory ratios.[16] To encourage consistency, whole blood assays have been deemed the gold standard for determining COX inhibition.[16] Most inhibitory ratios reported in the literature for horses have used this assay system. Because inhibition is measured in blood samples obtained from the species of interest, the whole blood assay is considered the most physiologically relevant assay. In this assay, NSAID inhibition (IC_{50}, IC_{80}, or IC_{95}) of COX isoforms is assessed by measuring prostaglandin E_2 (PGE_2) concentrations in LPS-stimulated macrophages as a measure of COX-2 inhibition and TXB_2 concentrations in platelets as a measure of COX-1 inhibition, following incubation of different concentrations of the NSAID of interest.[20] The presence of plasma proteins in whole blood is another advantage to the whole blood assay. Most NSAIDs are highly plasma protein bound and therefore the presence of plasma proteins makes the assay more representative of the in vivo environment.[21] The whole blood assay can also be used to measure ex vivo inhibition in samples collected from animals following administration of NSAIDs in vivo. This allows for determination of COX inhibition under clinical conditions and at therapeutically achievable drug concentrations.[16]

NONSTEROIDAL ANTI-INFLAMMATORY DRUG CYCLOOXYGENASE INHIBITION IN HORSES

Inhibitory ratios (IC_{50} COX-1: IC_{50} COX-2) for selected NSAIDs used in equine medicine are listed in **Table 1**. Phenylbutazone (PBZ), flunixin meglumine (FLU), and ketoprofen (KTP) are all considered COX-1 selective NSAIDs,[18,19,22] whereas meloxicam, an NSAID approved for use only in dogs in the United States, is more selective for COX-2 than COX-1 in the horse.[22] The classification of carprofen is a little more ambiguous, with one group of investigators classifying it as nonselective[18,19] and another group as COX-2 selective.[22]

COXIBS AND CYCLOOXYGENASE INHIBITION

The coxibs are a subset of NSAIDs that were first introduced in human medicine several years ago with the promise of the same anti-inflammatory effects as other NSAIDs but with a reduction in toxicity. Coxibs are COX-2 selective and COX-1 sparing at the same time. This group of drugs is structurally different from traditional

Table 1
Inhibitory ratios (IC_{50} COX-1: IC_{50} COX-2) for nonsteroidal anti-inflammatory drugs in horses

Drug	Reference	IC_{50} COX-1: IC_{50} COX-2
Phenylbutazone	Brideau et al,[19] 2001	1.6
	Beretta et al,[22] 2005	0.30
Flunixin meglumine	Brideau et al,[19] 2001	0.3
	Beretta et al,[22] 2005	0.34
Ketoprofen	Landoni & Lees,[54] 1996	0.48
Firocoxib	Kvaternick et al,[24] 2007	268–643
Carprofen	Brideau et al,[19] 2001	1.6
	Beretta et al,[22] 2005	2.0
	Lees et al,[18] 2004	3.3
Meloxicam	Beretta et al,[22] 2005	3.8
Deracoxib	Davis et al,[29] 2010	25.7

NSAIDs in that they have a tricyclic ring and a sulfone or sulfonamide group.[23] The resultant bulky structure limits their ability to bind to the COX-1 site, thus decreasing inhibition of this enzyme. The COX-2 binding site is much larger, so coxibs are able to bind and thus "selectively" inhibit COX-2 activity.

Currently there are 4 coxibs approved for use in animals: deracoxib, firocoxib, mavacoxib, and robenacoxib. It should be noted that mavacoxib is not currently approved for use in the United States and only firocoxib is labeled for use in horses. The COX-1 sparing and COX-2 inhibitory effects of firocoxib have been demonstrated in a number of ex vivo studies.[24–27] Kvaternick and colleagues[24] reported a COX-1/COX-2 inhibitory ratio ranging from 268 to 643 (see **Table 1**). COX-2 was significantly inhibited following a single intravenous (IV) administration with PGE_2 levels decreased by 83.0% $\pm$ 22.9%.[26] Following a single oral administration, PGE_2 levels were decreased by 53.0% $\pm$ 41.1% relative to baseline.[26] Inhibition was greater following once-a-day administration for 7 days with PGE_2 levels decreased by 79% $\pm$ 8%.[25] The greater inhibition following multiple dose administration suggests a lag time until the maximal therapeutic effect is achieved and is likely attributable to the long elimination half-life for firocoxib (>24 hours).[24,26,28] A loading dose may be prudent to shorten the time to reach a therapeutic response.

Although not approved by the Food and Drug Administration (FDA) for use in horses, deracoxib (a coxib approved for use in dogs) has a COX-1/COX-2 IC_{50} ratio of 25.7 and a COX-1/COX-2 IC_{80} ratio of 22.1.[29] So, although not as COX-1 sparing/COX-2 selective as firocoxib, deracoxib appears to be much more COX-2 selective then traditional NSAIDs (PBZ, FLU, and KTP) in the horse.

THERAPEUTIC USE OF NONSTEROIDAL ANTI-INFLAMMATORY DRUGS

In horses, NSAIDs are used primarily for the treatment of soft tissue, musculoskeletal, and abdominal inflammation and pain. There are currently 6 NSAIDs approved by the FDA that are labeled for use in the horse. These include FLU, PBZ, KTP, diclofenac (DLC), meclofenamic acid, and firocoxib (**Table 2**). Other NSAIDs have been investigated in the horse and are discussed here; however, it is important to note that administration of drugs in a species other than one in which they are approved by the FDA constitutes extralabel drug use (ELDU) and therefore ELDU regulations as described in the Animal Medicinal Drug Use and Clarification Act (AMDUCA) apply.

Table 2
Nonsteroidal anti-inflammatory drugs approved by the Food and Drug Administration for use in horses

Drug	Formulation	Route	Dose, mg/kg
Phenylbutazone	Tablets, paste, powder	PO	4.4 mg/kg q24h
			2.2 mg/kg q12h
	Injectable	IV	4.4 mg/kg q24h
			2.2 mg/kg q12h
Flunixin meglumine	Injectable	IV, IM	1.1 mg/kg q24h
	Paste, granules	PO	1.1 mg/kg q24h
Ketoprofen	Injectable	IV	2.2 mg/kg q24h
Firocoxib	Injectable	IV	0.09 mg/kg q24h
	Tablets, paste	PO	0.1 mg/kg q24h
Diclofenac	Liposome cream	Topical	73 mg (5 inch strip) q12h
Meclofenamic Acid	Granules	PO	2.2 mg/kg q24h

Abbreviations: IM, intramuscular; IV, intravenous; PO, by mouth; q, every.

Musculoskeletal Pain and Inflammation

NSAIDs remain the mainstay of treatment for horses with musculoskeletal pain and inflammation, with PBZ remaining the most commonly prescribed NSAID. PBZ is an effective anti-inflammatory both in experimental models as well as naturally occurring chronic forelimb lameness.[30,31] The effects of both PBZ (4.4 mg/kg IV once per day for 4 days) and FLU (1.1 mg/kg IV once per day for 4 days) have been studied in navicular syndrome.[32] Significant improvement in force plate and clinical lameness evaluations were noted following administration of both NSAIDs compared with the saline control group.

The COX-2 selective NSAID, firocoxib, is effective in the treatment of naturally occurring osteoarthritis with improved lameness scores and mobility observed following chronic administration.[33] Improvement was most rapid within the first 7 days of treatment with continued improvement occurring at a slower rate for the next 7 days.[33] The effectiveness of firocoxib in treating osteoarthritis is comparable to that reported for PBZ.[34] In a randomized controlled clinical trial, Doucet and colleagues[34] demonstrated comparable improvement in a number of lameness parameters (lameness score, joint swelling, joint circumference, and range of motion) for PBZ paste (4.4 mg/kg by mouth every 24 hours) and firocoxib paste (0.1 mg/kg by mouth every 24 hours).

Although not approved for use in horses in the United States, meloxicam is commonly used in equine practice in other countries. Its efficacy in horses has been established for the management of orthopedic postoperative pain and inflammation.[35] Experimentally, meloxicam (0.6 mg/kg by mouth every 24 hours for 7 days) is effective in the treatment of acute synovitis,[36] producing a significant reduction in lameness and effusion and decreased synovial fluid biomarkers of inflammation, matrix metalloproteinase activity, and cartilage turnover.[36]

DLC is an NSAID used extensively in human medicine. Currently the only DLC product approved for use in veterinary medicine is a topical liposomal preparation, labeled for the control of pain and inflammation associated with osteoarthritis in horses. The purported benefit to this formulation is the lack of systemic absorption. It is applied and acts locally, and as such the potential for adverse side effects reported for systemic administration of NSAIDs is minimized. The efficacy of this preparation in the treatment of inflammatory conditions in the horse has yielded highly variable results and may be somewhat dependent on the inflammatory model used. In one study, Caldwell and colleagues[37] reported that a single topical administration of DLC resulted in DLC concentrations in transudate that significantly attenuated carrageenan-induced local production of PGE_2.[37] In a second study, DLC was used for the treatment of inflammation in a model of acute synovitis in horses.[38] The investigators of this study found no overall difference between the treatment and control groups in this model of inflammation. Also somewhat confounding was the increase in synovial PGE_2 concentrations in the DLC-treated horses as compared with the control group. This is in stark contrast to the study by Caldwell and colleagues,[37] in which PGE_2 concentrations decreased after DLC administration. Most recently, Frisbie and colleagues[39] reported on the use of DLC to treat horses with experimentally induced osteoarthritis. The results of this study led the investigators to conclude that there was a significant improvement in clinical lameness in horses treated with the DLC cream.

Colic

NSAIDs are routinely used to reduce the effects of endotoxemia and visceral pain in patients with colic and colitis.[40,41] In the case of gastrointestinal injury, endotoxin may be released, which stimulates phospholipase A2 and subsequent eicosanoid production as a result of induction of COX-2 enzymes. The most commonly used NSAID for the treatment of colic and associated endotoxemia is FLU. Experimentally, FLU has been shown to be effective in reducing the acute systemic side effects and preventing clinical signs of endotoxemia, including cardiovascular and hemodynamic alterations, hypoxemia, and lactic acidosis.[42,43] Although not used as commonly under clinical conditions, experimentally PBZ also has been shown to be effective in preventing adverse effects associated with endotoxemia.

Although FLU remains one of the mainstays for the treatment of colic, inhibition of repair mechanisms in the injured intestine and a reduction in intestinal motility following administration of nonspecific COX inhibitors has been well established.[44–46] In response to mucosal injury, intestinal villi contract, epithelial cells surrounding the denuded basement membrane migrate into the defect, and tight junctions between the apical epithelial cells are assembled to close the paracellular spaces and repair barrier integrity. Contraction of the intestinal villi and assembly of tight junctions are under the control of prostaglandins and are dependent on increases in COX enzymes. Inhibition of COX enzymes, as occurs with NSAID administration, can therefore interfere with healing of the gastrointestinal tract following injury. Although nonselective NSAIDs such as FLU slow mucosal recovery in ischemic-injured jejunum, the COX-2 selective NSAID firocoxib does not appear to affect recovery.[46] As the degree of visceral analgesia was comparable between the NSAIDs, the investigators suggested that firocoxib may be advantageous in horses recovering from ischemic intestinal injury.

Analgesia

It is well established that PGE_2 lowers nociceptor thresholds and can therefore potentiate the effects of substances that cause pain.[47–49] During inflammatory pain, prostaglandins (primarily PGE_2) are generated at peripheral terminals of sensory neurons causing hyperalgesia.[50,51] In addition to acting at peripheral sites, there is evidence that NSAIDs also act centrally to reduce hyperalgesia.[52] In addition to inhibition of PGE_2 production in the central nervous system, other central mechanisms mediated by endogenous opioid peptides as well as inhibition of serotonin or excitatory amino acids have been proposed.[53]

NONSTEROIDAL ANTI-INFLAMMATORY DRUG PHARMACOKINETICS

The pharmacokinetics of NSAIDs have been extensively reported and therefore the reader is referred to the literature for a more detailed discussion of the pharmacokinetics of these compounds. Select pharmacokinetic parameters are listed in **Table 3**. In general, NSAIDs are lipid-soluble, weak organic acids that are well absorbed following oral administration. Absorption of PBZ appears to be high regardless of the formulation. Conversely, oral absorption of KTP appears to be dependent on the specific formulation.[54,55] The bioavailability of KTP was less than 5% for an oil-based formulation, 50% when administered in a gelatin capsule[54] and 69% and 88.2% for the S (+) and R (−) enantiomers, respectively, when the FDA-approved injectable formulation (water soluble) was administered orally.[55] Food can have profound effects on the absorption of NSAIDs.[26,56] For PBZ and FLU, administration with food delays the rate of absorption but generally does not affect the extent of absorption. In vitro studies showed greater than 98% and 70% binding of drug to feed for PBZ and FLU, respectively. When administered with food, the extent of firocoxib absorption is decreased (decreased area under the curve).[26]

Most NSAIDs have relatively small volumes of distribution (0.1–0.3 L/kg) attributable to a high degree of plasma protein binding (PPB; 95%–99%). Firocoxib is an exception with a volume of distribution of 1.7 L/kg.[24,26] Although PPB limits distribution across membranes for most NSAIDs, it does allow for accumulation of NSAIDs in inflammatory exudate. Inflammatory exudate is high in plasma proteins and the high degree of affinity of NSAIDs for these proteins leads to sequestration of drug at sites of inflammation. Studies using tissue cage models have demonstrated comparable and in some cases higher concentrations of NSAIDs in inflammatory exudate in horses administered FLU, KTP, PBZ, and carprofen.[57] PPB in inflammatory exudate may also explain the prolonged duration of action of NSAIDs in spite of the short elimination half-life and only once or twice a day dosing.

The high degree of PPB limits glomerular filtration and therefore limits excretion of most NSAIDs as parent compound. Instead most NSAIDs undergo extensive hepatic metabolism to inactive metabolites. Phenylbutazone is an exception in that biotransformation produces the active metabolites, oxyphenbutazone and gamma-hydroxyphenylbutazone, which contribute to the anti-inflammatory and analgesic properties of the compound. With the exception of firocoxib, most NSAIDs have a relatively short elimination half-life. The elimination half-life for firocoxib is more than 24 hours in horses,[24,26,55] and with a once-a-day dosing interval, significant bioaccumulation occurs with concentrations at steady state being 3 to 4 times higher than after a single dose.[24,55] With a prolonged elimination half-life, time to steady state can be prolonged for firocoxib, and therefore a loading dose may be prudent to achieve maximal therapeutic effect more rapidly.

ADVERSE EFFECTS OF NONSTEROIDAL ANTI-INFLAMMATORY DRUGS
Gastrointestinal

The effects of NSAIDs on intestinal healing following an ischemic injury were discussed previously. Another commonly reported gastrointestinal adverse effect associated with NSAID use is gastric ulceration. This usually occurs following overdose (high dose administration), chronic administration, or in susceptible populations (ie, foals). These effects are attributed to both local irritation as well as decreases in cytoprotective prostaglandins. COX-1 and COX-2 are constitutively expressed in the gastrointestinal tract. COX-1 plays a major role in gastroprotection in both the healthy and diseased animal. It mediates the production of prostaglandins, such as PGE_2,

Table 3
Select pharmacokinetic parameters for commonly used nonsteroidal anti-inflammatory drugs in horses

Drug	Test Dose	Vd, L/kg	CL, mL/min/kg	T$_{1/2}$, h
Phenylbutazone				
Lees et al,[75] 1987	4.4 mg/kg IV	0.141	0.298	5.46
Flunixin meglumine				
Knych et al,[76] 2015	1.1 mg/kg IV	0.137 ± 0.012	0.767 ± 0.098	4.83 ± 1.59
Lee & Maxwell,[77] 2014	1.1 mg/kg IV	0.157 ± 0.022	1.04 ± 0.27	3.38 ± 1.14
Ketoprofen				
Knych et al,[55] 2016	2.2 mg/kg IV	0.344 ± 0.044 (R(−))	5.75 ± 0.55 (R(−))	2.49 ± 0.077 (R(−))
		0.298 ± 0.025 (S(+))	2.78 ± 0.27 (S(+))	2.86 ± 0.102 (S(+))
Landoni & Lees,[54] 1996	2.2 mg/kg IV	0.128 (R(−))	5.77 (R(−))	1.98 (R(−))
		0.117 (S(+))	6.62 (S(+))	1.09 (S(+))
Firocoxib				
Holland et al,[26] 2015	57 mg	1.81 ± 0.59	0.71 ± 0.188	31.1 ± 10.6
Knych et al,[28] 2014	1.9 mg/kg IV q 24 h 5 d	3.66 ± 1.44[a]	0.725 ± 0.180[a]	39.4 ± 17.7[a]
Kvaternick et al,[24] 2007	0.1 mg/kg IV	1.70 ± 0.53	0.611 ± 0.221	29.6 ± 7.5

Abbreviations: CL, total systemic clearance; IV, intravenous; q, every; T$_{1/2}$, terminal elimination half-life; Vd, volume of distribution.
[a] Parameters were calculated after the last dose.

which are responsible for decreasing hydrochloric acid secretion and increasing mucosal bicarbonate and mucus production, effects that protect the stomach from the erosive effects of gastric acid. Ulceration following NSAID administration is usually a result of interference with mucosal protective mechanisms. Because the gastroprotective mechanisms are associated primarily with COX-1, administration of COX-2–selective NSAIDs have been proposed as an alternative to avoid gastric ulcer formation. An alternative mechanism to gastric ulcer formation by the NSAIDs was proposed by Martinez and colleagues.[58] These investigators suggested that ulcer formation may be due to oxidative stress that resulted from PBZ overdose (4.4 mg/kg once per day by mouth for 5 days, followed by a single 13.2 mg/kg IV dose on day 6).[58]

Right dorsal colitis is another reported adverse effect associated with NSAIDs, especially PBZ administration.[59] Diarrhea, often mild (ie, cow pie consistency), and signs of colic often in conjunction with hypoalbuminemia are commonly observed. Similar to gastric ulcers, right dorsal colitis is thought to be a result of inhibition of protective prostaglandins that simulate mucous production and maintain blood flow to the colon.[60]

Renal Toxicity

PGE_2 and PGI_2 play key roles in the regulation of renal blood flow, water excretion, and electrolyte balance. Production of both are under the control of COX-1 and COX-2, both of which are constitutively expressed in the kidneys. In the hydrated animal, COX inhibition by NSAIDs likely has little effect on renal hemodynamics; however, when an animal is dehydrated, loss of prostaglandin production can result in vasoconstriction of the afferent arteriole, loss of medullary perfusion, and redistribution of blood flow to the renal cortex. The likelihood of renal toxicity does not appear to be decreased because COX-2 plays a key role in renal homeostasis.

Bone and Wound Healing

Although studies are limited in veterinary species, there is substantial evidence from human and rodent studies that NSAIDs inhibit bone healing. The exact mechanism of action is unknown, but the predominant theory is that NSAIDs inhibit prostaglandin synthesis, therefore interfering with cell signaling and leading to an uncoordinated healing process.[61] Effects on bone healing appear to be most pronounced in the early phases of bone healing[62–65] and are reversible on discontinuation of treatment.[63,66–71] Inhibition of bone healing is equally as likely with COX-2 selective as with COX-1 selective NSAIDs[62,63,66–73] because there is evidence that inflammation stimulated by the COX-2 enzyme is essential for fracture healing.

USE IN PERFORMANCE HORSES

NSAIDs are commonly used as part of treatment regimens for sports-related injuries in horses and because of their ability to affect performance, their use is tightly regulated

Table 4 Recommended thresholds and withdrawal times for nonsteroidal anti-inflammatory drugs under the model rules for horseracing				
Drug	Route	Dose, mg/kg	Plasma Threshold	Withdrawal, h
Flunixin meglumine	IV	1.1	20 ng/mL	32
Ketoprofen	IV	2.2	2.0 ng/mL	24
Phenylbutazone	IV	4.0	2.0 μg/mL	24

Abbreviation: IV, intravenous.

Table 5
Recommended thresholds and withdrawal times for nonsteroidal anti-inflammatory drugs for performance horse events

Drug	Route	Dose, mg/kg	Threshold, μg/mL	Withdrawal, h
Firocoxib	Oral	0.1	0.240	>12
Flunixin meglumine	Oral, IV	1.1	1.0	>12
Ketoprofen	IV	2.2	0.250	>12
Meclofenamic acid	Oral	2.2	2.5	>12
Naproxen	Oral	10	40.0	>12
Phenylbutazone	Oral, IV	2.2	15.0	>12

in these horses. Specific NSAIDs that are allowed, the permitted threshold concentration, and withdrawal time recommendation may vary from discipline to discipline and between regulatory groups (**Tables 4** and **5**). Although regulations for horse racing can vary between racing jurisdictions, many individual states have adopted the Racing Commissioners International's "Model Rules" (see **Table 4**). Equestrian disciplines, other than horse racing, usually follow the recommendations of the US Equestrian Federation or the Federation Equestrian International. Alternatively, individual breeds or disciplines may develop their own recommendations. Recommendations change occasionally, so it is important to visit the organization's Web sites periodically for updates (**Box 1**).

Regardless of the governing body, the intent is to establish regulatory thresholds at a concentration in which the drug has no or minimal pharmacologic activity and can be effectively regulated. In the United States, to establish appropriate regulatory recommendations, a pharmacokinetic study is conducted and a statistical approach is then used to establish a withdrawal time that is representative of the time that drug concentration will fall below the threshold value, plus a statistical margin of safety.[74] The recommended withdrawal time is based on a specific drug formulation, route of administration and dosage, and therefore if treatment deviates in any way it may be necessary to extend the withdrawal time recommendation accordingly. A published withdrawal time recommendation in the United States does not constitute a guarantee, warranty, or assurance that the use of the therapeutic medication at the dosage listed will not result in a positive post-race test. The treating veterinarian must still do his or her own risk assessment based on relevant clinical factors.

Box 1
Web sites for various equestrian disciplines

Horseracing	http://ua-rtip.org/industry_service/arci_model_rules
Model Rules	
Racing Medication and	http://rmtcnet.com
Testing Consortium (RMTC)	
US Equestrian Federation (USEF)	http://www.usef.org
Federation Equestrian International (FEI)	http://www.fei.org
American Quarter Horse Association	https://aqha.com
National Cutting Horse Association	http://www.nchacutting.com
Tennessee Walking Horse National Celebration	http://twhnc.com

REFERENCES

1. Smith WL, Marnett LJ. Prostaglandin endoperoxidase synthase: structure and catalysis. Biochim Biophys Acta 1991;1083(1):1–17.
2. Vane JR, Bakhle YS, Botting RM. Cyclooxygenases 1 and 2. Annu Rev Pharmacol Toxicol 1998;38:97–120.
3. Otto JC, Smith WL. Prostaglandin endoperoxidase synthases-1 and 2. J Lipid Mediat Cell Signal 1995;12(2–3):139–56.
4. Herschman HR. Prostaglandin synthase 1 and 2. Biochem Biophys Acta 1996; 1299(1):125–40.
5. Xie WL, Chipman JG, Robertson DL, et al. Expression of a mitogen-responsive gene encoding prostaglandin synthase is regulated by mRNA splicing. Proc Natl Acad Sci U S A 1991;88(7):2692–6.
6. Smith WL, DeWitt DL. Biochemistry of prostaglandin endoperoxidase synthase-1 and -2 and their differential susceptibility to nonsteroidal anti-inflammatory drugs. Semin Nephrol 1995;15:179–94.
7. Luong C, Miller A, Barnett J, et al. Flexibility of the NSAID binding site in the structure of human cyclooxygenase-2. Nat Struct Biol 1996;3(11):927–33.
8. O'Banion MK, Sadowski HB, Winn V, et al. A serum and glucocorticoid regulated 4-kilobase mRNA encodes a cyclooxygenase-related protein. J Biol Chem 1991; 266(34):261–7.
9. Lee SH, Soyoola E, Chanmugam P, et al. Selective expression of mitogen-inducible cyclooxygenase in macrophages stimulated with lipopolysaccharide. J Biol Chem 1992;267(36):934–8.
10. Bakhle YS, Botting RM. Cyclooxygenase-2 and its regulation in inflammation. Mediators Inflamm 1996;5(5):305–23.
11. Onoe Y, Miyaura C, Kaminakayashiki T, et al. IL-13 and IL-4 inhibit bone resorption by suppressing cyclooxygenase-2-dependent prostaglandin synthesis in osteoblasts. J Immunol 1996;156:758–64.
12. Breder CD, Dewitt D, Kraig RP. Characterization of inducible cyclooxygenase in rat brain. J Comp Neurol 1995;355(2):296–315.
13. Breder CD, Saper CB. Expression of inducible cyclooxygenase mRNA in the mouse brain after systemic administration of bacterial lipopolysaccharide. Brain Res 1996;713(1–2):64–9.
14. Vane JR, Botting RM. Biological properties of cyclooxygenase products. In: Cunningham F, editor. Lipid mediators. London: Academic; 1994. p. 61–97.
15. Mengle-Gaw LJ, Schwartz BD. Cyclooxygenase-2 inhibitors: promise or peril? Mediators Inflamm 2002;11(5):275–86.
16. Brooks P, Mery P, Evans JF, et al. Interpreting the clinical significance of the differential inhibition of cyclooxygenase-1 and cyclooxygenase-2. Rheumatology 1999;38(8):779–88.
17. Warner TD, Giuliano F, Vojnovic L, et al. Nonsteroid drug selectivities for cyclo-oxygenase-1 rather than cyclo-oxygenase-2 are associated with gastrointestinal toxicity: a full in vitro analysis. Proc Natl Acad Sci U S A 1999;96(13):7563–8.
18. Lees P, Landoni MF, Giraudel J, et al. Pharmacodynamics and pharmacokinetics of nonsteroidal anti-inflammatory drugs in species of veterinary interest. J Vet Pharmacol Ther 2004;27(6):479–90.
19. Brideau C, VanStaden C, Chan CC. In vitro effects of cyclooxygenase inhibitors in whole blood of horses, dogs and cats. Am J Vet Res 2001;62(11):1755–60.

20. Patrignani P, Panara MR, Greco A, et al. Biochemical and pharmacological characterization of the cyclooxygenase activity of human blood prostaglandin endoperoxidase synthases. J Pharmacol Exp Ther 1994;271(3):1705–12.
21. Frolich JC. A classification of NSAIDs according to the relative inhibition of cyclooxygenase isoenzymes. Trends Pharmacol Sci 1997;18(1):30–4.
22. Beretta C, Garavaglia G, Cavalli M. COX-1 and COX-2 inhibition in horse blood by phenylbutazone, flunixin, carprofen and meloxicam: an in vitro analysis. Pharmacol Res 2005;52(4):302–6.
23. Brune K, Hinz B. Selective cyclooxygenase-2 inhibitors: similarities and differences. Scand J Rheumatol 2004;33(1):1–6.
24. Kvaternick V, Pollmeier M, Fischer J, et al. Pharmacokinetics and metabolism of orally administered firocoxib, a novel second generation coxib, in horses. J Vet Pharmacol Ther 2007;30(3):208–17.
25. Barton MH, Paske E, Norton N, et al. Efficacy of cyclo-oxygenase inhibition by two commercially available firocoxib products in horses. Equine Vet J 2015; 46(1):72–5.
26. Holland B, Fogle C, Blikslager AT, et al. Pharmacokinetics and pharmacodynamics of three formulations of firocoxib in healthy horse. J Vet Pharmacol Ther 2014;38(3):249–56.
27. Duz M, Parkin TD, Cullander RM, et al. Effect of flunixin meglumine and firocoxib on ex vivo cyclooxygenase activity in horses undergoing elective surgery. Am J Vet Res 2015;76(3):208–15.
28. Knych HK, Stanley SD, Arthur RM, et al. Detection and pharmacokinetics of three formulations of firocoxib following multiple administrations to horses. Equine Vet J 2014;46(6):734–8.
29. Davis J, Marshall J, Papich M, et al. The pharmacokinetics and in vitro cyclooxygenase selectivity of deracoxib in horses. J Vet Pharmacol Ther 2010;34(1): 12–6.
30. Hu HH, MacAllister CG, Payton ME, et al. Evaluation of the analgesic effects of phenylbutazone administered at a high or low dosage in horses with chronic lameness. J Am Vet Med Assoc 2005;226(3):414–7.
31. Foreman JH, Barange A, Lawrence LM, et al. Effects of a single-dose intravenous phenylbutazone on experimentally induced, reversible lameness in the horse. J Vet Pharmacol Ther 2008;31(1):39–44.
32. Erkert RS, MacAllister CG, Payton ME, et al. Use of force plate analysis to compare the analgesic effects of intravenous administration of phenylbutazone and flunixin meglumine in horses with navicular syndrome. Am J Vet Res 2005; 66(2):284–8.
33. Orsini JA, Ryan WG, Carithers DS, et al. Evaluation of oral administration of firocoxib for the management of musculoskeletal pain and lameness associated with osteoarthritis in horses. Am J Vet Res 2012;73(5):664–71.
34. Doucet MY, Bertone AL, Hendrickson D, et al. Comparison of efficacy and safety of paste formulations of firocoxib and phenylbutazone in horses with naturally occurring osteoarthritis. J Am Vet Med Assoc 2008;232(1):91–7.
35. Walliser U, Fenner A, Mohren N, et al. Evaluation of the efficacy of meloxicam for post-operative management of pain and inflammation in horses after othopaedic surgery in a placebo controlled clinical field trial. BMC Vet Res 2015;11:113.
36. deGrauw JC, Van de Lest CHA, Brama PAJ, et al. In vivo effects of meloxicam on inflammatory mediators, MMP activity and cartilage biomarkers in equine joints with acute synovitis. Equine Vet J 2009;41(7):693–9.

37. Caldwell FJ, Mueller E, Lynn RC, et al. Effect of topical application of diclofenac liposomal suspension on experimentally induced subcutaneous inflammation in horses. Am J Vet Res 2004;65(3):271–6.
38. Schleining JA, McClure SR, Evans RB, et al. Liposome-based diclofenac for the treatment of inflammation in an acute synovitis model in horses. J Vet Pharmacol Ther 2008;31(6):554–61.
39. Frisbie DD, McIlwraith CW, Kawcak CE, et al. Evaluation of topically administered diclofenac liposomal cream for treatment of horses with experimentally induced osteoarthritis. Am J Vet Res 2009;70(2):210–5.
40. Baskett A, Barton MH, Norton N, et al. Effect of pentoxifylline, flunixin meglumine and their combination on a model of endotoxemia in horses. Am J Vet Res 1997; 58(11):1292–9.
41. Shuster R, Traub-Dargatz J, Baxter G. Survey of diplomates of the American College of Veterinary Internal Medicine and the American College of Veterinary Surgeons regarding clinical aspects and treatment of endotoxemia in horses. J Am Vet Med Assoc 1997;210(1):87–92.
42. Semrad SD, Hardee GE, Hardee MM, et al. Low dose flunixin meglumine: effects on eicosanoid production and clinical signs induced by experimental endotoxaemia in horses. Equine Vet J 1987;19(3):201–6.
43. King JN, Gerring EL. Antagonism of endotoxin-induced disruption of equine bowel motility by flunixin and phenylbutazone. Equine Vet J Suppl 1989;7:38–42.
44. Campbell NB, Blikslager AT. The role of cyclooxygenase inhibitors in repair of ischemic-injured jejunal mucosa in the horse. Equine Vet J 2000;S32:59–64.
45. Van Hoogmoed LM, Snyder JR, Harmon F. In vitro investigation of the effect of prostaglandins and nonsteroidal anti-inflammatory drugs on contractile activity of the equine smooth muscle of the dorsal colon, ventral colon and pelvic flexure. Am J Vet Res 2000;61(10):1259–66.
46. Cook VL, Meyer CT, Campbell NB, et al. Effect of firocoxib or flunixin meglumine on recovery of ischemic-injured equine jejunum. Am J Vet Res 2009;70(8): 992–1000.
47. Vane JR. Inhibition of prostaglandin synthesis as a mechanism of action for the aspirin-like drugs. Nat New Biol 1971;231(25):232–5.
48. Ferreira SH. Peripheral analgesia: mechanism of the analgesic action of aspirin like drugs and opiate antagonists. Br J Clin Pharmacol 1980;10(2):237S–45S.
49. Higgs GA. Arachidonic acid metabolism, pain and hyperalgesia: the mode of action of non-steroid analgesics. Br J Clin Pharmacol 1980;10(2):233S–5S.
50. Ferreira SH. Prostaglandins, aspirin-like drugs and hyperalgesia. Nat New Biol 1972;240(102):200–3.
51. Woolf CJ, Allchorne A, Safieh-Garabedian B, et al. Cytokines, nerve growth factor and inflammatory hyperalgesia: the contribution of tumour necrosis factor alpha. Br J Pharmacol 1997;121(3):417–24.
52. Samad TA, Moore KA, Sapirsterin A, et al. Interleukin-1beta-mediated induction of Cox-2 in the CNS contributes to inflammatory pain hypersensitivity. Nature 2001;410(6827):471–5.
53. Cashman JN. The mechanisms of action of NSAIDs in analgesia. Drugs 2012; 52(5):13–23.
54. Landoni MF, Lees P. Pharmacokinetics and pharmacodynamics of ketoprofen enantiomers in the horse. J Vet Pharmacol Ther 1996;19(6):466–74.
55. Knych HK, Arthur RM, Steinmetz S, et al. Pharmacokinetics of ketoprofen enantiomers following intravenous and oral administration to exercised Thoroughbred horses. Vet J 2016;207:196–8.

56. Lees P, Taylor JBO, Higgins AJ, et al. In vitro and in vivo studies on the binding of phenylbutazone and related drugs to equine feeds and digesta. Res Vet Sci 1988;44(1):50–6.

57. Lees P, Taylor JBO, Higgins AJ, et al. Phenylbutazone and oxyphenbutazone distribution into tissue fluids in the horse. J Vet Pharmacol Ther 1986;9(2):204–12.

58. Martinez Aranazles JR, Cnidid de Andrade BS, Silveira Alves GE. Orally administered phenylbutazone causes oxidative stress in the equine gastric mucosa. J Vet Pharmacol Ther 2014;38(3):257–64.

59. McConnico RS, Morgan TW, Williams CC, et al. Pathophysiologic effects of phenylbutazone on the right dorsal colon in horses. Am J Vet Res 2008;69(11): 1496–505.

60. Robert A. Cytoprotection by prostaglandins. Gastroenterology 1979;77(4 Pt 1): 761–7.

61. Barry S. Non-steroidal anti-inflammatory drugs inhibit bone healing: a review. Vet Comp Orthop Traumatol 2010;23(6):385–92.

62. Simon AM, O'Connor JP. Dose and time-dependent effects of cyclooxygenase-2 inhibition on fracture-healing. J Bone Joint Surg Am 2007;89(3):500–11.

63. Beck A, Krischak G, Sorg I, et al. Influence of diclofenac (group of nonsteroidal anti-inflammatory drugs) on fracture healing. Arch Orthop Trauma Surg 2003; 123(7):327–32.

64. Giordano V, Giordano M, Knackfuss IG, et al. Effect of tenoxicam on fracture healing in rat tibiae. Injury 2003;34(2):85–94.

65. Riew KD, Long J, Rhee J, et al. Time-dependent inhibitory effects of indomethacin on spinal fusion. J Bone Joint Surg Am 2003;85(4):632–4.

66. Gerstenfeld LC, Al-Ghawas M, Alkhiary YM, et al. Selective and nonselective cyclooxygenase-2 inhibitors and experimental fracture-healing. Reversibility of effects after short-term treatment. J Bone Joint Surg Am 2007;89(1):114–25.

67. Endo K, Sairyo K, Komatsubara S, et al. Cyclooxygenase-2 inhibitor delays fracture healing in rats. Acta Orthop 2005;76(4):470–4.

68. Krischak G, Augat P, Sorg T, et al. Effects of diclofenac on periosteal callus maturation in osteotomy healing in an animal model. Arch Orthop Trauma Surg 2007; 127(1):3–9.

69. Dimmen S, Nordsletten L, Engebretsen L, et al. Negative effect of parecoxib on bone mineral during fracture healing in rats. Acta Orthop 2008;79(3):438–44.

70. Goodman SB, Ma T, Mitsunaga L, et al. Temporal effects of a COX-2 selective NSAID on bone in-growth. J Biomed Mater Res 2005;72(3):279–87.

71. Dimmen S, Nordsletten L, Madsen JE. Parecoxib and indomethacin delay early fracture healing: a study in rats. Clin Orthop Relat Res 2009;467(8):1992–9.

72. Zhang X, Schwarz EM, Young DA, et al. Cyclooxygenase-2 regulates mesenchymal cell differentiation into the osteoblast lineage and is critically involved in bone repair. J Clin Invest 2002;109(11):1405–15.

73. Leonelli SM, Goldberg BA, Safanda J, et al. Effects of a cyclooxygenase-2 inhibitor (rofecoxib) on bone healing. Am J Orthop 2006;35(2):79–84.

74. The European Agency For the Evaluation of Medicinal Products. Note for guidance for the determination of withdrawal periods for milk. 2000. Available at: http://www.ema.europa.eu/docs/en_GB/document_library/Scientific_guideline/2009/10/WC500004496.pdf. Accessed May 30, 2016.

75. Lees P, Taylor JB, Maitho TE, et al. Metabolism, excretion, pharmacokinetics and tissue residues of phenylbutazone in the horse. Cornell Vet 1987;77(2):192–211.

76. Knych HK, Arthur RM, McKemie DS, et al. Pharmacokinetics and effects on thromboxane B2 production following intravenous administration of flunixin

meglumine to exercised thoroughbred horses. J Vet Pharmacol Ther 2015;38(4): 313–20.
77. Lee CD, Maxwell LK. Effect of body weight on the pharmacokinetics of flunixin meglumine in miniature horses and quarter horses. J Vet Pharmacol Ther 2014; 37(1):35–42.

Corticosteroids and Immune Suppressive Therapies in Horses

Mathilde Leclere, DVM, PhD

KEYWORDS

- Azathioprine • Equine asthma • Glucocorticoids • Glucocorticosteroids
- Immune-mediated • Immunomodulation

KEY POINTS

- Glucocorticoids are the most commonly used immune suppressive drugs and the only class supported by robust evidence of clinical efficacy in equine medicine.
- Other immune suppressive agents used in horses include azathioprine, cyclophosphamide, and cyclosporine.
- Strategies to decrease side effects of glucocorticoids include using local and combination therapy.

INTRODUCTION

Immune suppressive therapies target exaggerated and deleterious responses of the immune system. These immune responses can lead to several clinical manifestations in horses, including atopy and skin hypersensitivity reactions, equine asthma, pemphigus, vasculitis (including purpura hemorrhagica), eosinophilic granuloma, mastocytosis, inflammatory bowel syndrome, recurrent uveitis, and immune-mediated keratitis, anemia, thrombocytopenia, and myositis. Glucocorticoids are the most commonly used immune suppressive drugs and the only ones supported by robust evidence of efficacy in equine medicine. Their efficacy has been demonstrated and compared with other drugs primarily in the context of research on equine asthma. The paucity of available data on immunosuppressive therapy in horses is due in part to the complexity of the immune system as well as the chronic and recurrent manifestations of the many diseases targeted with immune suppressive therapy. Other immune suppressive agents used in horses include azathioprine, cyclophosphamide, and local cyclosporine. Alternative therapies without clearly demonstrated immunosuppressive effects (eg, acupuncture, herbal medicine) are not covered in this review.

Disclosure Statement: The author has no relevant financial or nonfinancial relationship to disclose.
Department of Clinical Sciences, Faculty of Veterinary Medicine, Université de Montréal, 3200 Sicotte, St-Hyacinthe, Quebec J2S 7C6, Canada
E-mail address: mathilde.leclere@umontreal.ca

Vet Clin Equine 33 (2017) 17–27
http://dx.doi.org/10.1016/j.cveq.2016.11.008
0749-0739/17/© 2016 Elsevier Inc. All rights reserved.
vetequine.theclinics.com

GLUCOCORTICOIDS (CORTICOSTEROIDS)

Glucocorticoids, also called corticosteroids, are the most effective anti-inflammatory and immunosuppressive drugs available for the treatment of many chronic inflammatory and immune diseases across species. The hypothalamus releases corticotropin-releasing hormone into the portal system of the pituitary gland, which in turn releases adrenocorticotropic hormone (ACTH). This ACTH induces cortisol synthesis and release by the adrenal cortex into the bloodstream. Cortisol then targets glucocorticoid receptors present in almost every cell of the body.[1,2] Synthetic corticosteroids have a similar 21-carbon steroid skeleton, with the addition of a C1-C2 double bond, and bind to the same glucocorticoid receptor as cortisol. Glucocorticoids will only be discussed in the context of immune suppressive therapy, but some glucocorticoids used in equine medicine also have an affinity for mineralocorticoid receptors (eg, prednisolone, isoflupredone).

Glucocorticoids exert most of their anti-inflammatory and immunosuppressive effects by diffusing across the cell membrane and binding the glucocorticoid receptors in the cytoplasm.[3] After releasing the receptor chaperon proteins, glucocorticoids and their receptors translocate into the cell nucleus and alter gene expression (illustrated in **Fig. 1**). Anti-inflammatory effects generally result from gene transrepression leading to transcription factor repression (such as NF-κB and AP-1) and downregulation of inflammatory chemokines and cytokines (eg, interleukin-1 [IL-1], IL-6, tumor necrosis factor) as well as adhesion molecules. Glucocorticoids also result in gene transactivation following direct DNA binding, which increases the release of anti-inflammatory mediators, but also leads to undesirable metabolic effects.

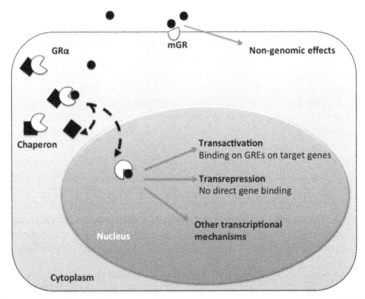

Fig. 1. Glucocorticoids (*black circles*) binding to the major receptor, the cytoplasmic glucocorticoid receptor isoform α (GRα, *white*), and displacing chaperon proteins (such as heat shock proteins; *black squares*) before entering the nucleus. mGR, membrane-associated glucocorticoid receptor. GREs, glucocorticoid response elements. (*Data from* Hall JE. Adrenocortical hormones. Guyton and Hall textbook of medical physiology. 13th edition. Philadelphia: Elsevier Health Sciences; 2015. p. 965–82; and Hapgood JP, Avenant C, Moliki JM. Glucocorticoid-independent modulation of GR activity: implications for immunotherapy. Pharmacol Ther 2016;165:93–113.)

Transrepression and transactivation are referred to as "classical genomic actions," but glucocorticoid-cell interactions are in fact much more complex. For example, glucocorticoids also have nongenomic effects mediated through membrane-associated glucocorticoid receptors and nonspecific, nonglucocorticoid receptor-dependent effects.[4,5] Some of these nongenomic effects have been observed in equine peripheral blood neutrophils exposed to dexamethasone ex vivo.[6] Because most of the positive and negative effects of glucocorticoids are mediated by their genomic effects and through the same receptor, engineering selective glucocorticoids with predominant transrepression effects has proven to be challenging.[2] These "selective" glucocorticoids have been regrouped under the term SEGRAMs for Selective Glucocorticoid Receptor Agonists and Modulators. Partial selectivity can be achieved through glucocorticoids with greater affinity for protein-protein interactions or greater nongenomic effects, but the current best practice for decreasing side effects remains through the local administration of glucocorticoids (topical, intraocular, or inhalation) whenever possible.

Glucocorticoids in Equine Asthma

The most common use of glucocorticoids in equine medicine is for the management of equine asthma (formerly known as heaves or recurrent airway obstruction, inflammatory airway disease, and summer pasture obstructive pulmonary disease). With asthma, susceptible horses develop abnormal airway inflammation and bronchoconstriction in response to inhaled antigens present in hay and barns.[7] Although there are numerous studies evaluating the effects of corticosteroids in severe equine asthma, studies assessing the effects of corticosteroids in other conditions are limited. Most studies on equine asthma are performed in controlled research settings, and although this does not perfectly reflect field conditions, it offers a unique opportunity to study and compare drug efficacy of different corticosteroids under similar environmental conditions.

Dexamethasone is the most studied corticosteroid because it is often used as a positive control for the evaluation of new anti-inflammatory drugs. Lung function improvement was observed in the vast majority of studies with intravenous, intramuscular, and oral administration of dexamethasone with dosages varying from 0.04 to 0.1 mg/kg body weight.[8–11] **Table 1** summarizes systemic and inhaled corticosteroids that have demonstrated a positive effect on lung function or clinical scores of horses with severe equine asthma. Prednisone is absent from this table because it appears to have little effect in horses because of poor bioavailability and lack of conversion to prednisolone in vivo.[12] There is also an apparent discrepancy between the reported relative potency of dexamethasone and prednisolone and the dosages used in equine practice.

Based on animal studies and in vitro experiments using transfected cells with glucocorticoid receptors, the relative potency of dexamethasone versus prednisolone is approximately 6 to 12 times greater (approximately 21–25 and 1.7–4 times the cortisol potency for dexamethasone and prednisolone, respectively).[1,13] However, in equine asthma, a prednisolone dosage 20 to 40 times that of dexamethasone does not reach a similar improvement in lung function.[11] This discrepancy could be due in part to the duration of cortisol suppression (shorter with prednisolone) or the greater stability of the dexamethasone-receptor complex,[14] but is probably not the result of differences in oral bioavailability (50%–65% for both).[12,15,16] Last, although the effect of corticosteroids on lung function can be reliably predicted, their administration does not consistently abrogate bronchoalveolar lavage neutrophilia unless environmental changes are concurrently put into place.[17–19] This apparent contradiction could be explained by a lower level of activation of the remaining neutrophils, or a better control of inflammation in the lung tissue despite persistent neutrophils in the airways.

Table 1
Glucocorticoids with demonstrated effects on lung function or clinical score in horses with equine asthma

Corticosteroid	Dosage	Route of Administration	References
Dexamethasone[a]	0.04–0.16 mg/kg every 24 h	IV, IM, PO	8–11,18–25
Dexamethasone-21-isonicotinate	0.04 mg/kg every 72 h	IM	23
Prednisolone	1–2 mg/kg every 24 h	PO	10,11
Isoflupredone[b]	0.03 mg/kg every 24 h	IM	8
Triamcinolone[a]	0.09 mg/kg	IM	26
Beclomethasone	500–3750 μg/450 kg every 12–24 h	Inhalation	25,27,28
Fluticasone	2000–6000 μg/450 kg every 12–24 h	Inhalation	17,22,29,30

Abbreviations: IM, intramuscular; IV, intravenous; PO, oral.
 [a] The dosages listed have been shown to improve lung function but are not necessarily recommended for long-term use. Dexamethasone at 0.16 mg/kg was used as a single oral administration.[24] Triamcinolone at 0.09 mg/kg was used as single IM injection.[26]
 [b] Induces hypokalemia, not recommended.

In conclusion, synthetic corticosteroids administered orally, intravenously, intramuscularly, or by inhalation are effective at improving lung function in equine asthma.[31–33] Inhaled corticosteroids should be used whenever possible because they have the advantage of reaching high concentrations in the lungs while minimizing systemic side effects due to their low bioavailability.[34]

Evidence of Corticosteroid Efficacy in Other Diseases

The list of indications for corticosteroid administration is long and includes vasculitis, numerous dermatologic conditions (atopy and hypersensitivity reactions, pemphigus, eosinophilic granuloma, mastocytosis), inflammatory bowel syndrome, recurrent uveitis, immune-mediated keratitis, anemia, thrombocytopenia, and myositis.[35,36] Cutaneous lymphoma can also regress with corticosteroids, which is often administered in combination with antineoplastic drugs.[37] Clinical efficacy of glucocorticoids in these conditions is unequivocal, but no prospective studies are available to support one treatment regimen over another.

The choice of corticosteroid, dosage, duration of administration, and combination with other immunosuppressive drugs is based on clinical experience and case reports or is extrapolated from other conditions. One of the few prospective studies on horses with a confirmed or presumptive diagnosis of inflammatory bowel disease showed a relatively good short-term response (an improvement in 15/20 cases) to a combined treatment of anthelmintic and 3-week course of prednisolone. However, the lack of a control group (untreated or anthelmintic alone) makes extrapolation to other cases difficult.[38]

Glucocorticoids and the Immune Response

Depending on the intended use of corticosteroid therapy, alteration of the immune response can be regarded as either a goal or a side effect. The effects of corticosteroids are numerous and include, but are not limited to, alteration of cytokine production, decreased adhesion molecule and immunoglobulin receptor expression, and decreased phagocytosis and cell migration.[1,39] However, these effects have not all been recognized or studied in equine cells specifically.

In horses, corticosteroids induce an increase in peripheral blood neutrophil and a decrease in lymphocyte concentrations.[40,41] With dexamethasone, this occurs within 12 hours of administration and is accompanied by a transient decrease in the CD4/CD8 lymphocyte ratio.[42] Corticosteroids can decrease phagocytosis, but administration of a short course of hydrocortisone to adult or neonatal horses did not result in decreased neutrophil phagocytic capacity.[43,44] On the other hand, horses receiving high doses of dexamethasone (0.2 mg/kg twice a week for 2 months) did not mount a normal immunoglobulin Ga (IgGa) and IgGb response to vaccination.[45] These changes are notable, but how they affect immune function in horses treated with lower doses is unknown. Dauvillier and colleagues[46] observed the effects of prolonged administration of inhaled fluticasone for almost a year in horses with asthma and could not detect significant effects on clinical and hematologic parameters, peripheral blood neutrophil gene expression, lymphocyte subpopulations, or response to vaccination.

Side Effects of Glucocorticoids

Undesirable side effects of corticosteroids can occur in several different organs. Systemic administration of corticosteroids to horses can induce hypothalamic-pituitary-adrenal axis suppression, with a resultant decrease in endogenous cortisol production.[8,12,16,47–49] Adrenocortical dysfunction, resulting in an altered response to exogenous ACTH, may also develop.[47,50] Cortisol suppression is often used as an indicator of potential adverse systemic side effects; at least in other species, however, the duration of adrenal suppression also correlates with the anti-inflammatory effects of corticosteroids.[51] This suppression lasts for approximately 24 hours after prednisolone, 48 hours after beclomethasone, and 48 to 96 hours after dexamethasone administration.[12,16,48,49] These systemic effects are reduced with inhaled corticosteroid therapy.

Cortisol suppression with inhaled fluticasone proprionate is inconsistently reported, ranging from no suppression,[30] to short-term suppression (12–24 hours),[52,53] and up to 72 hours partial suppression with high dosages.[22] Because the bioavailability of fluticasone across the nasal or gastric mucosa is low,[53] cortisol suppression is expected to be minimal and instead reflects absorption following lung deposition. Significant cortisol suppression is observed with inhaled beclomethasone, but responsiveness of the adrenal gland to ACTH administration is not altered.[47]

Hepatopathy, muscle wasting, altered bone metabolism, hyperglycemia, polyuria, polydipsia, and increased susceptibility to infection have also been described in horses on corticosteroid therapy.[54–59] Recrudescence of viral infections occurs under certain conditions,[60] and fever and suspected bacterial respiratory infections during corticosteroid treatment have also been reported anecdotally.[21,57] Potassium depletion was also demonstrated with isoflupredone administration,[8] and although it did not translate to observable clinical effects, it is not recommended for use in horses because it lacks selectivity and has mineralocorticoid effects.

Finally, laminitis has been reported in association with corticosteroid administration in horses with no prior history of laminitis, typically with high doses.[56,61,62] The occurrence of iatrogenic laminitis in healthy horses appears to be very low, however.[63] In a retrospective study involving horses with various medical conditions (including laminitis), oral prednisolone did not appear to increase the risk of laminitis.[64] Despite the lack of objective data supporting a direct causal link between laminitis and the administration of glucocorticoids at commonly used doses,[63] the prevalence of laminitis in horses with known risk factors (previous laminitis history, equine metabolic syndrome, pituitary pars intermedia dysfunction, concurrent gastrointestinal disease) is perceived to be increased. Although this requires further study, glucocorticoids should be used with caution in these cases.

OTHER IMMUNOSUPPRESSIVE DRUGS USED IN HORSES

Azathioprine interferes with DNA and RNA formation by inhibiting purine synthesis. It has been used in horses with immune-mediated conditions such as immune-mediated blood disorders (eg, immune-mediated thrombocytopenia),[65–68] skin conditions,[69] and polysynovitis.[70] Its use is supported by reports of clinical improvement after treatment failure with corticosteroids alone. A pharmacokinetic study showed apparent safety, but also low bioavailability following oral administration (1%–7%).[71] Azathioprine appears to be relatively safe in horses, because few side effects were observed after 2 months of treatment, but its efficacy remains primarily anecdotal[67–69] and inconsistent.[72]

Cyclophosphamide is cytotoxic, decreases the proliferation of rapidly dividing cells, and targets B-lymphocytes more specifically.[39] It is used in the treatment of lymphosarcoma in conjunction with other chemotherapeutic drugs. The use of cyclophosphamide and vincristine, another immunosuppressive and antineoplastic agent, in immune-mediated or inflammatory conditions is anecdotal, but has been reported in clinical equine cases.[67,73]

Cyclosporine is a potent immunosuppressive agent used to prevent graft rejection in humans through its effects on T-lymphocyte function and proliferation. Its use in horses is limited to local ocular administration for the treatment of recurrent uveitis or keratitis.[74,75] Systemic use would be cost prohibitive in most cases, and the drug is potentially nephrotoxic.

The use of sodium aurothiomalate or aurothioglucose (gold salts) has been reported as an immune suppressive therapy in horses, having been used in the treatment of pemphigus foliaceus.[69,76] However, the pharmacokinetics and efficacy have not been objectively studied.

PATIENT EVALUATION OVERVIEW

Historical and physical examinations should be aimed to determine the gravity of the condition that warrants treatment with immunomodulatory drugs. If corticosteroids are deemed to be indicated, topical or local treatment should be used whenever possible. Because of the potential side effects of corticosteroids, any history or clinical signs suggestive of previous episodes of laminitis, equine metabolic syndrome, or pituitary pars intermedia dysfunction should be investigated and taken into consideration in the treatment plan, because such horses are likely at increased risk of laminitis with corticosteroid administration.

PHARMACOLOGIC AND NONPHARMACOLOGIC TREATMENT OPTIONS

Pharmacologic and nonpharmacologic therapeutic options in horses depend on the condition being treated. The following treatments should be considered in order to decrease the dose or use entirely of immunosuppressive agents:

- Equine asthma: consider bronchodilators and antigen avoidance (environmental management including limiting access to hay).
- Urticaria: consider antihistamines, antigen avoidance, and desensitization for long-term control.

COMBINATION THERAPIES

The treatment options listed above are usually more effective when used in combination with immune suppressive therapies. However, they allow for dose or duration reductions in the immunosuppressive therapy. Furthermore, combinations of immu-nosuppressives may be used to reduce the dose of corticosteroids. For example, azathioprine is often added to corticosteroid therapy when corticosteroids alone fail to control the condition, or when dosage has to be decreased due to side effects or pre-existing conditions.

TREATMENT RESISTANCE/COMPLICATIONS

Treatment can be interrupted or tapered due to the development of side effects or the perceived risk of side effects (eg, laminitis with corticosteroids).

EVALUATION OF OUTCOMES AND LONG-TERM RECOMMENDATIONS

Medical conditions treated with glucocorticoids and immune suppressive therapies in horses are often chronic and recurrent (eg, equine asthma, urticaria, inflammatory bowel syndrome). Slow tapering of dosages and combining corticosteroids with other therapies, coupled with environmental management, can help in preventing relapses.

SUMMARY

Immunosuppressive therapies with strong evidence-based data supporting their use in horses are limited to glucocorticoids. The "ideal" glucocorticoids can be described as having the following:

- A low mineralocorticoid-to-glucocorticoid receptor affinity ratio.

  Practical consideration: aside from isoflupredone, glucocorticoids used in horses have low mineralocorticoid effects.

- Tissue specificity.

  Practical consideration: local therapy (topical, intraocular, by inhalation) should be used whenever possible.

- A low transactivation to transrepression activation ratio and increased nonge-nomic effects.

  Practical consideration: currently theoretic.

Additional strategies to decrease the risk of side effects of glucocorticoids include the following:

- Use short-acting systemic corticosteroids when local therapy is not possible.
- Use the minimum dosage and duration necessary.
- Use combinations (including pharmacologic and nonpharmacologic treatment options) whenever possible, to allow for dose and duration reductions.
- Morning administration of corticosteroids to minimize disruption of normal circadian cycles.

REFERENCES

1. Hall JE. Adrenocortical hormones. Guyton and Hall textbook of medical physiology. 13th edition. Philadelphia: Elsevier Health Sciences; 2015. p. 965–82.
2. Sundahl N, Bridelance J, Libert C, et al. Selective glucocorticoid receptor modulation: new directions with non-steroidal scaffolds. Pharmacol Ther 2015;152:28–41.

3. Nicolaides NC, Galata Z, Kino T, et al. The human glucocorticoid receptor: molecular basis of biologic function. Steroids 2010;75(1):1–12.

4. Lu NZ, Cidlowski JA. The origin and functions of multiple human glucocorticoid receptor isoforms. Ann N Y Acad Sci 2004;1024:102–23.

5. Hapgood JP, Avenant C, Moliki JM. Glucocorticoid-independent modulation of GR activity: implications for immunotherapy. Pharmacol Ther 2016;165:93–113.

6. Lecoq L, Vincent P, Lavoie-Lamoureux A, et al. Genomic and non-genomic effects of dexamethasone on equine peripheral blood neutrophils. Vet Immunol Immunopathol 2009;128(1–3):126–31.

7. Couetil LL, Cardwell JM, Gerber V, et al. Inflammatory airway disease of horses-revised consensus statement. J Vet Intern Med 2016;30(2):503–15.

8. Picandet V, Leguillette R, Lavoie JP. Comparison of efficacy and tolerability of isoflupredone and dexamethasone in the treatment of horses affected with recurrent airway obstruction ('heaves'). Equine Vet J 2003;35(4):419–24.

9. Cesarini C, Hamilton E, Picandet V, et al. Theophylline does not potentiate the effects of a low dose of dexamethasone in horses with recurrent airway obstruction. Equine Vet J 2006;38(6):570–3.

10. Courouce-Malblanc A, Fortier G, Pronost S, et al. Comparison of prednisolone and dexamethasone effects in the presence of environmental control in heaves-affected horses. Vet J 2008;175(2):227–33.

11. Leclere M, Lefebvre-Lavoie J, Beauchamp G, et al. Efficacy of oral prednisolone and dexamethasone in horses with recurrent airway obstruction in the presence of continuous antigen exposure. Equine Vet J 2010;42(4):316–21.

12. Peroni DL, Stanley S, Kollias-Baker C, et al. Prednisone per os is likely to have limited efficacy in horses. Equine Vet J 2002;34(3):283–7.

13. Grossmann C, Scholz T, Rochel M, et al. Transactivation via the human glucocorticoid and mineralocorticoid receptor by therapeutically used steroids in CV-1 cells: a comparison of their glucocorticoid and mineralocorticoid properties. Eur J Endocrinol 2004;151(3):397–406.

14. Ichii S, Satoh Y, Izawa M, et al. Stability of receptor complexes in the rat liver bound to glucocorticoids of different biopotencies. Endocrinol Jpn 1984;31(5):583–94.

15. Cunningham FE, Rogers S, Fischer JH, et al. The pharmacokinetics of dexamethasone in the thoroughbred racehorse. J Vet Pharmacol Ther 1996;19(1):68–71.

16. Grady JA, Davis EG, Kukanich B, et al. Pharmacokinetics and pharmacodynamics of dexamethasone after oral administration in apparently healthy horses. Am J Vet Res 2010;71(7):831–9.

17. Leclere M, Lavoie-Lamoureux A, Joubert P, et al. Corticosteroids and antigen avoidance decrease airway smooth muscle mass in an equine asthma model. Am J Respir Cell Mol Biol 2012;47(5):589–96.

18. Lavoie JP, Leguillette R, Pasloske K, et al. Comparison of effects of dexamethasone and the leukotriene D4 receptor antagonist L-708,738 on lung function and airway cytologic findings in horses with recurrent airway obstruction. Am J Vet Res 2002;63(4):579–85.

19. Lavoie JP, Pasloske K, Joubert P, et al. Lack of clinical efficacy of a phosphodiesterase-4 inhibitor for treatment of heaves in horses. J Vet Intern Med 2006;20(1):175–81.

20. Gerber V, Schott Ii HC, Robinson NE. Owner assessment in judging the efficacy of airway disease treatment. Equine Vet J 2011;43(2):153–8.

21. Lavoie JP, Thompson D, Hamilton E, et al. Effects of a MAPK p38 inhibitor on lung function and airway inflammation in equine recurrent airway obstruction. Equine Vet J 2008;40(6):577–83.

22. Robinson NE, Berney C, Behan A, et al. Fluticasone propionate aerosol is more effective for prevention than treatment of recurrent airway obstruction. J Vet Intern Med 2009;23(6):1247–53.
23. Robinson NE, Jackson C, Jefcoat A, et al. Efficacy of three corticosteroids for the treatment of heaves. Equine Vet J 2002;34(1):17–22.
24. Cornelisse CJ, Robinson NE, Berney CE, et al. Efficacy of oral and intravenous dexamethasone in horses with recurrent airway obstruction. Equine Vet J 2004; 36(5):426–30.
25. Rush BR, Raub ES, Rhoads WS, et al. Pulmonary function in horses with recurrent airway obstruction after aerosol and parenteral administration of beclomethasone dipropionate and dexamethasone, respectively. Am J Vet Res 1998;59(8): 1039–43.
26. Lapointe JM, Lavoie JP, Vrins AA. Effects of triamcinolone acetonide on pulmonary function and bronchoalveolar lavage cytologic features in horses with chronic obstructive pulmonary disease. Am J Vet Res 1993;54(8):1310–6.
27. Rush BR, Raub ES, Thomsen MM, et al. Pulmonary function and adrenal gland suppression with incremental doses of aerosolized beclomethasone dipropionate in horses with recurrent airway obstruction. J Am Vet Med Assoc 2000;217(3): 359–64.
28. Couetil LL, Art T, de Moffarts B, et al. Effect of beclomethasone dipropionate and dexamethasone isonicotinate on lung function, bronchoalveolar lavage fluid cytology, and transcription factor expression in airways of horses with recurrent airway obstruction. J Vet Intern Med 2006;20(2):399–406.
29. Giguere S, Viel L, Lee E, et al. Cytokine induction in pulmonary airways of horses with heaves and effect of therapy with inhaled fluticasone propionate. Vet Immunol Immunopathol 2002;85(3–4):147–58.
30. Couetil LL, Chilcoat CD, DeNicola DB, et al. Randomized, controlled study of inhaled fluticasone propionate, oral administration of prednisone, and environmental management of horses with recurrent airway obstruction. Am J Vet Res 2005;66(10):1665–74.
31. Williamson KK, Davis MS. Evidence-based respiratory medicine in horses. Vet Clin North Am Equine Pract 2007;23(2):215–27.
32. Leclere M, Lavoie-Lamoureux A, Lavoie JP. Heaves, an asthma-like disease of horses. Respirology 2011;16(7):1027–46.
33. Leguillette R. Recurrent airway obstruction–heaves. Vet Clin North Am Equine Pract 2003;19(1):63–86, vi.
34. Stoloff SW, Kelly HW. Updates on the use of inhaled corticosteroids in asthma. Curr Opin Allergy Clin Immunol 2011;11(4):337–44.
35. Lloyd DH, Littlewood JD, Craig JM, et al. Practical equine dermatology. Ames (IA): Blackwell Publishing Company; 2003.
36. Sprayberry KA, Robinson NE. Robinson's current therapy in equine medicine. St. Louis (MO): Elsevier Health Sciences; 2014.
37. Saulez MN, Schlipf JW Jr, Cebra CK, et al. Use of chemotherapy for treatment of a mixed-cell thoracic lymphoma in a horse. J Am Vet Med Assoc 2004;224(5): 733–8, 699.
38. Kaikkonen R, Niinisto K, Sykes B, et al. Diagnostic evaluation and short-term outcome as indicators of long-term prognosis in horses with findings suggestive of inflammatory bowel disease treated with corticosteroids and anthelmintics. Acta Vet Scand 2014;56:35.
39. Felippe MJ. Immunotherapy. In: Sellon DC, Long MT, editors. Equine infectious diseases. 2nd edition. St Louis (MO): Saunders/Elsevier; 2013. p. 585–97.

40. Burguez PN, Ousey J, Cash RS, et al. Changes in blood neutrophil and lympho-cyte counts following administration of cortisol to horses and foals. Equine Vet J 1983;15(1):58–60.

41. Targowski SP. Effect of prednisolone on the leukocyte counts of ponies and on the reactivity of lymphocytes in vitro and in vivo. Infect Immun 1975;11(2):252–6.

42. Flaminio MJBF, Tallmadge RL, Secor E, et al. The effect of glucocorticoid therapy in the immune system of the horse. Abstract presented at the 8th International Veterinary Immunology Symposium. Ouro Preto, Brazil, August 15–19, 2007.

43. Morris DD, Strzemienski PJ, Gaulin G, et al. The effects of corticosteroid admin-istration on the migration, phagocytosis and bactericidal capacity of equine neu-trophils. Cornell Vet 1988;78(3):243–52.

44. Hart KA, Barton MH, Vandenplas ML, et al. Effects of low-dose hydrocortisone therapy on immune function in neonatal horses. Pediatr Res 2011;70(1):72–7.

45. Slack J, Risdahl JM, Valberg SJ, et al. Effects of dexamethasone on development of immunoglobulin G subclass responses following vaccination of horses. Am J Vet Res 2000;61(12):1530–3.

46. Dauvillier J, Felippe MJ, Lunn DP, et al. Effect of long-term fluticasone treatment on immune function in horses with heaves. J Vet Intern Med 2011;25(3):549–57.

47. Rush BR, Worster AA, Flaminio MJ, et al. Alteration in adrenocortical function in horses with recurrent airway obstruction after aerosol and parenteral administra-tion of beclomethasone dipropionate and dexamethasone, respectively. Am J Vet Res 1998;59(8):1044–7.

48. Rush BR, Trevino IC, Matson CJ, et al. Serum cortisol concentrations in response to incremental doses of inhaled beclomethasone dipropionate. Equine Vet J 1999;31(3):258–61.

49. Toutain PL, Brandon RA, de Pomyers H, et al. Dexamethasone and prednisolone in the horse: pharmacokinetics and action on the adrenal gland. Am J Vet Res 1984;45(9):1750–6.

50. Dowling PM, Williams MA, Clark TP. Adrenal insufficiency associated with long-term anabolic steroid administration in a horse. J Am Vet Med Assoc 1993; 203(8):1166–9.

51. Melby JC. Clinical pharmacology of systemic corticosteroids. Annu Rev Pharma-col Toxicol 1977;17:511–27.

52. Munoz T, Leclere M, Jean D, et al. Serum cortisol concentration in horses with heaves treated with fluticasone proprionate over a 1 year period. Res Vet Sci 2015;98:112–4.

53. Laan TT, Westermann CM, Dijkstra AV, et al. Biological availability of inhaled flu-ticasone propionate in horses. Vet Rec 2004;155(12):361–4.

54. Lepage OM, Laverty S, Marcoux M, et al. Serum osteocalcin concentration in horses treated with triamcinolone acetonide. Am J Vet Res 1993;54(8):1209–12.

55. Cohen ND, Carter GK. Steroid hepatopathy in a horse with glucocorticoid-induced hyperadrenocorticism. J Am Vet Med Assoc 1992;200(11):1682–4.

56. Ryu SH, Kim BS, Lee CW, et al. Glucocorticoid-induced laminitis with hepatop-athy in a thoroughbred filly. J Vet Sci 2004;5(3):271–4.

57. Mair TS. Bacterial pneumonia associated with corticosteroid therapy in three horses. Vet Rec 1996;138(9):205–7.

58. Edington N, Bridges CG, Huckle A. Experimental reactivation of equid herpesvirus 1 (EHV 1) following the administration of corticosteroids. Equine Vet J 1985;17(5): 369–72.

59. Cutler TJ, MacKay RJ, Ginn PE, et al. Immunoconversion against Sarcocystis neurona in normal and dexamethasone-treated horses challenged with S. neurona sporocysts. Vet Parasitol 2001;95(2–4):197–210.
60. Pusterla N, Hussey SB, Mapes S, et al. Molecular investigation of the viral kinetics of equine herpesvirus-1 in blood and nasal secretions of horses after corticosteroid-induced recrudescence of latent infection. J Vet Intern Med 2010;24(5):1153–7.
61. Eustace RA, Redden RR. Iatrogenic laminitis. Vet Rec 1990;126(23):586.
62. Dutton H. The corticosteroid laminitis story: 1. Duty of care. Equine Vet J 2007; 39(1):5–6.
63. Bailey SR. Corticosteroid-associated laminitis. Vet Clin North Am Equine Pract 2010;26(2):277–85.
64. Jordan VJ, Ireland JL, Rendle DI. Does oral prednisolone treatment increase the incidence of acute laminitis? Equine Vet J 2017;49(1):19–25.
65. Winfield LS, Brooks MB. Hemorrhage and blood loss-induced anemia associated with an acquired coagulation factor VIII inhibitor in a Thoroughbred mare. J Am Vet Med Assoc 2014;244(6):719–23.
66. McGurrin MK, Arroyo LG, Bienzle D. Flow cytometric detection of platelet-bound antibody in three horses with immune-mediated thrombocytopenia. J Am Vet Med Assoc 2004;224(1):83–7, 53.
67. Messer NT, Arnold K. Immune-mediated hemolytic anemia in a horse. J Am Vet Med Assoc 1991;198(8):1415–6.
68. Humber KA, Beech J, Cudd TA, et al. Azathioprine for treatment of immune-mediated thrombocytopenia in two horses. J Am Vet Med Assoc 1991;199(5): 591–4.
69. Vandenabeele SI, White SD, Affolter VK, et al. Pemphigus foliaceus in the horse: a retrospective study of 20 cases. Vet Dermatol 2004;15(6):381–8.
70. Pusterla N, Pratt SM, Magdesian KG, et al. Idiopathic immune-mediated polysynovitis in three horses. Vet Rec 2006;159(1):13–5.
71. White SD, Maxwell LK, Szabo NJ, et al. Pharmacokinetics of azathioprine following single-dose intravenous and oral administration and effects of azathioprine following chronic oral administration in horses. Am J Vet Res 2005;66(9): 1578–83.
72. Winfield LD, White SD, Affolter VK, et al. Pemphigus vulgaris in a Welsh pony stallion: case report and demonstration of antidesmoglein autoantibodies. Vet Dermatol 2013;24(2):269-e60.
73. Schumacher J. Infiltrative bowel diseases. In: Sprayberry KA, Robinson NE, editors. Robinson's current therapy in equine medicine. St. Louis (MO): Elsevier Health Sciences; 2014. p. 439.
74. Gilger BC, Stoppini R, Wilkie DA, et al. Treatment of immune-mediated keratitis in horses with episcleral silicone matrix cyclosporine delivery devices. Vet Ophthalmol 2014;17(Suppl 1):23–30.
75. Gilger BC, Wilkie DA, Clode AB, et al. Long-term outcome after implantation of a suprachoroidal cyclosporine drug delivery device in horses with recurrent uveitis. Vet Ophthalmol 2010;13(5):294–300.
76. White SD. Pemphigus foliaceus. In: Lavoie JP, Hinchcliff KW, editors. Blackwell's five-minute veterinary consult: equine. Ames (IA): Wiley; 2008. p. 874.

Inhalation Therapy in Horses

Mandy L. Cha, BS, BVSc[a], Lais R.R. Costa, MV, MS, PhD[b],*

KEYWORDS

- Inhalation • Pharmacology • Respiratory • Equine • Nebulizer

KEY POINTS

- Inhalation therapy in horses can be accomplished with nebulizers or pressured metered dose inhalers.
- Nasal or muzzle masks can be used for delivery of inhalation therapy in horses.
- Inhalation therapy is important in the treatment of inflammatory airway disease in horses.
- Inhaled antimicrobial therapy may be adjunctive to systemic therapy for treatment of pneumonia.

INTRODUCTION

Inhalation therapy has been practiced in humans since ancient times in many cultures, including Chinese, Indian, Greek, Egyptian, Roman, and Hebrew.[1] In all of these cultures, inhalational therapy was performed using condensation of vapor by steaming liquids and combustion of plants or their derivatives, creating a smoke containing aerosolized droplets and solid particles.[1]

Inhalation therapy is the administration of aerosols into the airway and is a means of delivering topical pulmonary therapy. An aerosol is a suspension of liquid or solid particles dispersed in gas. The physical characteristics of the particles, including size, hydrophobicity, and shape, affect their ability to travel within the airways.[1,2] The size of the particles is regarded as one of the most critical physical characteristics of aerosol therapy. **Fig. 1** depicts a schematic representation of the aerosol deposition throughout the airways of the horse. Large aerosols (>10 μm) are filtered out in the upper respiratory tract (URT) or deposited in larger airways in association with turbulent airflow and do not effectively reach the lower airways. Midsized particles (10 to 6 μm) deposit in the larynx, trachea, bronchi, and large-caliber bronchioles. Particles 5 μm or

[a] Kulshan Veterinary Hospital, 8880 Benson Rd, Lynden, WA 98264, USA; [b] William R. Pritchard Veterinary Medical Teaching Hospital, University of California-Davis, One Shields Avenue, Davis, CA 95616, USA
* Corresponding author.
E-mail address: lais.costa65@gmail.com

Vet Clin Equine 33 (2017) 29–46
http://dx.doi.org/10.1016/j.cveq.2016.11.007
0749-0739/17/© 2016 Elsevier Inc. All rights reserved.

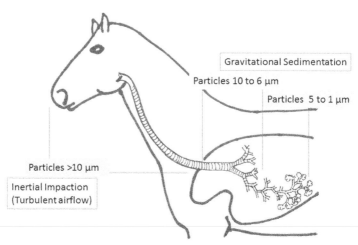

Fig. 1. Particle deposition throughout the airways of the horse. Large aerosols (>10 μm) deposit in the upper respiratory tract and larger airways; midsized aerosols (10 to 6 μm) deposit in the larynx, trachea, bronchi, and large-caliber bronchioles; aerosols less than 5 μm are deposited in smaller diameter bronchioles and in alveolar acini by gravitational sedimentation; and very small aerosols (<1 μm) remain in suspension, with part being deposited in alveoli and part exhaled.

less are deposited in smaller diameter bronchioles and in alveolar acini by gravitational sedimentation. Very small particles (<1 μm) tend to remain in suspension, and approximately 50% are deposited in alveoli and 50% are exhaled. Small particles may coalesce to make larger particles, which affects deposition. Hydrophilic particles attract water, promoting their deposition deeper in the tracheobronchial tree. More aerodynamically shaped particles are also deposited deeper within the respiratory tract. Patient factors that influence aerosol particle deposition include the depth of breathing, airway patency and reactivity, bronchospasm, and coughing.

Inhalation medications may be in the form of solutions, powders, vapors, or pressurized cartridges, when solutions or powders are administered with a propellant. The onset of action of aerosolized drugs is relatively rapid; however, the effects are usually short-lived; this is because the aerosolized drugs are partially degraded in the lung, cleared from the respiratory tract by the mucociliary escalator, and absorbed into the blood stream where they are disposed of by breakdown and excretion as are systemic drugs.

ADVANTAGES AND DISADVANTAGES OF INHALATION VERSUS SYSTEMIC ROUTE OF DRUG ADMINISTRATION

The inhalation route has long been perceived as the best route to affect the components of the airways and alveoli. The blood-bronchial barrier limits the access of systemically administered drugs to the airway lumen and to the cells lining the lower respiratory tract (LRT). In order to achieve drug penetration, high systemic doses are often required.

Some drugs, such as sympathomimetic and parasympatholytic agents used in the management of equine asthma, including recurrent airway obstruction (RAO) and inflammatory airway disease (IAD), may result in undesirable and sometimes life-threatening side effects, such as tachycardia, tremors, sweating, anxiety, decreased gastrointestinal motility, and cardiac arrhythmias, when used in large systemic doses. Administration of these drugs through the inhalational route minimizes the risks of these side effects.

In equine asthma, the potent inflammatory responses in the small airways lead to a cascade of pathophysiologic events, including the accumulation of inflammatory cells, primarily neutrophils and mucus, as well as a decrease in mucociliary clearance. Bronchoconstriction and coughing are common features of airway disease. Many of the drugs recommended for treating equine asthma are available in inhaled formulations, and current consensus indicates that inhalation is the route of choice to manage these conditions.[3,4] Directly delivering potent antiinflammatory therapy in the form of inhaled corticosteroids provides pharmacotherapy and also reduces the likelihood of adverse systemic effects. The inflammatory cascade can be modulated by the preventative use of cromones, such as cromoglycate and nedocromil sodium, medications which are only available for inhalational administration.

Drugs administered by aerosol obviate absorption, bypass degradation in the gastrointestinal tract and liver, avoid the detrimental effects on the gut flora, and allow the use of drugs that are not bioavailable when administered orally. One example is the aminoglycoside class of antimicrobials, which can be administered through the inhalational route.

Although drugs administered through the inhalational route can still cause adverse reactions, such as anaphylaxis, hypersensitivity, idiosyncratic reactions, overdose, cumulative effects, and toxicity, they are less likely to do so than the same drugs administered systemically. Tolerance, defined as resistance to standard dosages of drugs, can also occur with inhalational therapy. Tolerance of inhaled drugs may be manifested as tachyphylaxis, resistance, paradoxic effect, and rebound phenomenon.[1]

Horses with chronic pulmonary diseases, particularly severe asthma (RAO), require long-term management. Aerosol treatment is often a more acceptable means by which owners can manage their horses at home with bronchodilators and corticosteroids as opposed to injections or even oral medications.

Treatment of infections of the LRT with aerosolized antimicrobial drugs may avoid antibiotic-induced colitis associated with systemic administration. Infectious agents of bacterial pneumonia, even when secondary, are often inhaled or aspirated rather than established by a hematogenous route in adult horses. Administration of antimicrobials directly to the site where the pathogen resides potentially enhances efficacy and decreases undesirable effects.

Delivering a precise dose of a medication by inhalation therapy is challenging. Because of variable drug deposition, the determination of half-life of inhaled drugs is difficult. The efficacy of drugs administered through inhalation is best gauged by the observation of a desirable drug effect. Improvement of airflow in the case of bronchodilators is a better indicator than, for example, the measured decline in activity of the drug in bronchoalveolar lavage fluid (BALF). Knowledge of the half-life is helpful, because for an adequate response, many drugs are administered at intervals that are approximately twice that of the half-life. Drugs administered through inhalation tend to have a shorter duration of effect than when administered through the systemic route. Thus, more frequent administration may be necessary to attain a similar desired effect. Drug deposition of the inhaled drug may be even more unpredictable in diseased lung. Proper drug distribution is hampered by abnormal breathing patterns, bronchoconstriction, airway secretions, and coughing. Thus, control of bronchospasm and coughing is important to obtain an effective distribution of any drug through the inhalation route.

DELIVERY OF AEROSOLS IN INHALATION THERAPY

Particles as large as 50 μm can be suspended in gas and administered as aerosol; however, only small particles effectively reach more distal airways. Particles ranging from 1 to 5 μm suspended in gas, referred to as therapeutic aerosol, maximize deposition in lower airways deeper in the lung.[1,2,5] The relationship between particle size and deposition pattern holds true across species.

The patients' pattern of breathing impacts drug distribution with the inhalation route. Maximal distal deposition occurs when patients take slow, deep breaths, with large tidal volumes. Unlike humans, it is difficult to control the breathing pattern of animals because it is impossible to request a voluntary deep breath from equine patients.

Forms of Administration

The available forms of drug delivery by the inhalation route include nebulizers and pressurized cartridge dispensers for administration of aqueous or alcoholic solutions as well as powders in the form of aerosol. Nebulization is used for the delivery of medications formulated as a liquid, either as a solution or suspension. There are different kinds of nebulizers, including vaporizers, jet nebulizers, and ultrasonic nebulizers.

Vaporizers deliver the drug vaporized in steam and are the oldest form of inhalation therapy. With vaporizers, the particle size and drug deposition are highly variable. Vaporizers are currently used primarily for the purpose of humidification of airway secretions because they have been replaced by other devices for medication delivery. Steam vaporizers are thought to increase the fluidity of airway secretions, thereby aiding with tenacious mucus and favoring their elimination by the ciliary escalator and coughing.

Jet nebulizers draw up liquid and produce a spray, breaking up the liquid into small particles in the process. Larger droplets are returned to the reservoir and enter the next cycle, whereas smaller particles are carried in inhaled air. The primary advantage of jet nebulizers is that they are economical. The disadvantages are that they are loud, provide a slow delivery rate, particle size is highly variable, and relatively large volumes of liquid are required for a small amount of actual delivery.[6] In humans, the reported deposition of drug by jet nebulizers is approximately 7.0% to 7.5% of nebulized volume.[7] The airflow rate should be set at 6 to 8 L/min to optimize output.[6,8] If the airflow rate is too slow, there is an increase in droplet size, whereas if the flow rate is too fast, turbulent flow favors pharyngeal deposition and the droplets do not reach the lower airways.

Ultrasonic nebulizers use piezoelectric crystal vibrations to nebulize a pool of liquid into a cloud of mist. The vibration frequency is the primary determinant of particle size. Higher frequencies create smaller droplets, but droplet size and deposition are determined by several factors, including individual drug characteristics, nebulizer specifications, and tubing length and diameter. The disadvantages of ultrasonic nebulizers are that they are more expensive than jet nebulizers and they generate heat, which may degrade the medication. The primary advantage is faster delivery and creation of more specific droplet size than jet nebulizers.[9] In humans, the reported deposition of drug is around 5% of nebulized volume.[7] Both jet and ultrasonic nebulizers require good sanitation, as unhygienic use can result in deposition of bacteria into lower airways.

Pressurized cartridge dispensers or pressurized metered dose inhalers (pMDIs) are the other primary means of providing inhalation therapy. They provide a method of ensuring administration of an accurate amount of medication by delivering a set amount of drug per actuation or puff. Although this method is thought to be precise, some variability of delivery may still occur.[10] Failure to adequately shake the pMDI before use is a very common source of this variability.[10] The type of propellant and the form of delivery influence the relative deposition of the drug in the lung. Coordination of actuation of the pMDI with inhalation is important for successful delivery; failure to coordinate is the most common cause of therapeutic failure, making the use of a delivery device a requirement.[11] In humans, incorrect coordination results in oropharyngeal deposition of the drug rather than pulmonary deposition, but correct coordination results in 60% of the drug reaching the lungs.[12] Therefore, for adequate delivery by pMDI, a spacer is required in the delivery device for use in horses. Most pMDI drugs labeled for human use, including bronchodilators and corticosteroids for treatment of asthma, are designed to be inhaled through the mouth. Because horses are obligate nasal breathers, the delivery devices have been modified for nasal delivery. The type of propellant influences the relative deposition of drug in the lung. Currently, chlorofluorocarbon (CFC) propellant is no longer available, and only the hydrofluoroalkane (HFA) propellant is available in the United States.

Commercial Spacers for Use in Horses

The inability to coax a horse to breathe on command necessitates the use of spacers to deliver the pMDI-packaged therapies. These aerosol delivery devices create a reservoir of drug in a chamber that is released on subsequent inspirations. The use of a delivery device adapts the commercially available human formulations of pMDI-delivered drugs to horses. This adaptation eliminates the need to manually synchronize the actuation of the pMDI with the horse's inspirations by automatically releasing the drug from the device when there is airflow (ie, when the horse breathes in). The pMDI delivery with a spacer is thought to be a great advance as compared with the initial nebulizer systems, which deposited only small amounts into equine lungs.[13] These aerosol delivery devices are generally well tolerated and effective in horses.[14–18] If a particular horse reacts to the sound of the actuation of the pMDI, the drug may be puffed into the chamber away from horse's face. Then the spacer can be held up to the nostril until the next inhalation. Currently there are several products used as spacer devices in the horse. It is important to ensure the device is properly cleaned after each use. The devices should be cleaned with warm water and mild soap and rinsed with sterile or distilled water. The valves and crevices should be thoroughly cleaned.

There are both single nostril and entire muzzle masks available for use in horses, along with spacer devices. Single nostril masks for horses include the Equine Haler and the AeroHippus. The Equine Haler (Equine Health Care Aps Jorgensen Labs, Inc., Loveland, Colorado, USA) is a single-nostril mask connected to a handheld large ellipsoid chamber, the spacer, into which the pMDI is inserted (**Fig. 2**). On actuation of the pMDI, the aerosol particles are suspended in the chamber, which contains a one-way valve that allows flow of medication on inspiration. This device was shown to effectively provide deposition of radiolabeled fluticasone propionate with propellant CFC in lung tissue at a rate of 8.2% ± 5.2% of the administered dose (250 µg per actuation) indicating successful deposition of the drug in small airways and alveoli.[17]

The AeroHippus Equine Aerosol Chamber (Trudell Medical, London, Ontario, Canada) (https://www.trudellmed.com/animal-health/aerohippus) is also a single-nostril device (**Fig. 3**).[19] A proprietary visible valve called a Flow-Vu (Trudell Medical, London, Ontario, Canada) serves as a visual indicator of inspiration so that the operator knows when to puff the pMDI. The drug deposition of radiolabeled beclomethasone dipropionate with propellant HFA was reported to be 18.2% using 10 actuations at 80 µg per actuation with this device.[18]

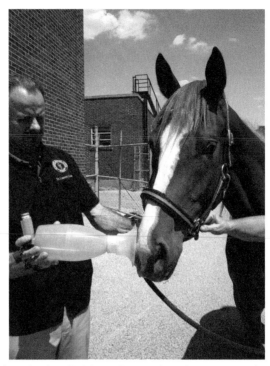

Fig. 2. Equine Haler: The handheld, single-nostril mask is connected to a large ellipsoid chamber, and the pMDI is inserted into the opposite end. On actuation of the pMDI, the suspended aerosols remain in the chamber until the horse inspires. (Jorgensen Laboratories, Loveland, CO. *Courtesy of* Dr Laurent Couetil, West Lafayette, IN.)

The studies mentioned earlier were completed using different propellants, drugs, and amounts of drug per actuation; therefore, the 2 studies cannot be directly compared. In a direct comparison between the AeroHippus and the Equine Haler as devices for the delivery of albuterol with the same propellant, at the same dose, similar improvements in clinical scores and pulmonary function were reported.[15] However, this study did not evaluate drug deposition. Nonetheless, it was concluded that both devices effectively delivered the bronchodilator albuterol and reversed the abnormalities associated with airway obstruction.[15] With either of the single-nostril devices, it is recommended to occlude the contralateral nostril temporarily in order to optimize deposition.

The AeroMask by Trudell Medical has been discontinued, but it is still in use by many veterinarians in clinical and research settings. It consists of a fitted mask placed on the horse's muzzle, thus including both nostrils (**Fig. 4**).

The Flexineb Equine Nebulizer (Flexineb Inc, Union City, TN, USA) is a fitted mask placed on the horse's muzzle (http://flexineb.us/; **Fig. 5**). The mask should be snug over the horse's face, with both nostrils exposed to the system. The mask is strapped behind the horse's ears, to ensure a tight fit around the horse's nose and minimize drug leakage. The Flexineb mask is best suited for use with nebulizers. The mask is connected to a vertical cylindrical chamber, the spacer, to which a container is attached. The solution to be nebulized is added to the container and aerosolized; the aerosols remain in the spacer until the horse inspires. The control

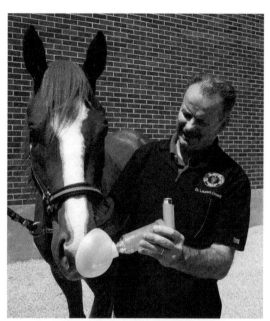

Fig. 3. Aerohippus Equine Aerosol Chamber: The handheld, single-nostril mask is connected to a small cylindrical chamber, and the pMDI is inserted into the opposite end. On actuation of the pMDI, the suspended aerosols remain in the chamber until the horse inspires. (Trudell Medical, Inc, London, ON. *Courtesy of* Dr Laurent Couetil, West Lafayette, IN.)

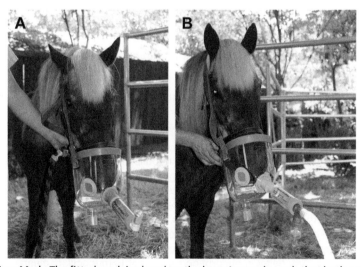

Fig. 4. AeroMask: The fitted mask is placed on the horse's muzzle, such that both nostrils are exposed to the system, and the mask is strapped behind the horse's ears. (*A*) The mask is connected to a small cylindrical chamber, and the pMDI is inserted into the opposite end. On actuation of the pMDI, the suspended aerosols remain in the chamber until the horse inspires. (*B*) The mask can be connected to a nebulization delivery system. (Trudell Medical, Inc, London, ON.)

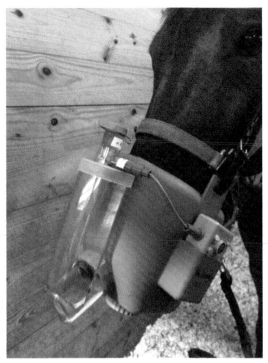

Fig. 5. Flexineb Equine Nebulizer: The fitted mask is placed on the horse's muzzle, such that both nostrils are exposed to the system, and the mask is strapped behind the horse's ears. The mask is connected to a vertical cylindrical chamber, to which the solution to be nebulized is added. (Flexineb, Inc, Union City, TN. *Courtesy of* Dr Laurent Couetil, West Lafayette, IN.)

is attached to the side of the mask. This mask can also be adapted for use with pMDIs.

PHARMACOKINETICS OF DRUGS ADMINISTERED THROUGH THE INHALATION ROUTE TO HORSES
Dead Space, Drug Absorption, and Drug Clearance

Inhaled drug administration systems contain dead space. This dead space occurs in the reservoir chamber or in the tubing of the nebulizer. Dead space in nebulizers and spacers serves to create a reservoir of drug available to patients on a subsequent inspiration. Reducing dead space volume and using a reservoir with a round or conical shape is best for recuperating any lost droplets.[9]

The airway epithelial lining readily absorbs drugs in aqueous form.[20,21] Most drugs administered through the inhalation route into the lung are relatively bioavailable.[21] In contrast to aqueous solutions, a suspension of drug still in particulate form may not be readily absorbed. Any delay in absorption may result in mucociliary clearance of the drug before it has a chance to achieve full effect.[20] The more soluble the drug, the faster it is absorbed. The lungs, although possessing some ability of drug clearance, do not do so as efficiently or as rapidly as the liver.

Drugs administered into the airway can be systemically absorbed through alveolar capillaries into the bloodstream. The absorption of the drug into the systemic circulation is of concern with drugs that have undesirable side effects, such as immunosuppression from corticosteroids or the anticholinergic effects of atropinelike drugs (ie, ipratropium). However, the zona occludens that limits entry of systemically administered drugs into the airways generally allows little of the inhaled drug to reach the circulation. Indeed, several studies have shown only small increases in plasma concentrations of inhaled drugs.[22–24]

Physiologic changes in the lungs, such as age-related changes or pathologic conditions as a result of the disease process, may decrease the effectiveness of inhalation therapy and, thus, the amount of drug that can be deposited in the lung. Although this is outside the control of the operator, it should be considered when designing therapy. For example, a 25-year-old horse with severe equine asthma (RAO) may require more drug than a 7-year-old horse with mild asthma (IAD).

Therapy Design and Drugs Used for Inhalation

In order to maximize efficacy, the therapeutic plan must be designed with appropriate duration of treatment and frequency of administration in mind. This point is especially important for inhalation treatments. Patient compliance and tolerance are maximized when nebulization time is short.[10] There is an inverse correlation between droplet size and time to aerosolize the drug; thus, larger droplets get aerosolized faster. Viscous substances take longer to nebulize and have larger droplet sizes.[25] Frequency of administration must be feasible for the client to comply with.

Reported values of effective doses of inhaled drugs serve as general guidelines, because each drug will interact with the delivery system and create a particle size distribution unique to that combination. **Tables 1** and **2** depict recommended doses for commonly used drugs administered by inhalation to horses. Some drugs used in humans and small animals, such as xanthine derivatives (eg, theophylline), are not currently used in horses.

Mucolytic drugs

Mucus is held together by covalent, ionic, and hydrogen bonds, van der Waals forces and parallel DNA network formation. Mucus binds bacteria and other debris and is then cleared through the ciliary escalator. Excessive mucus, resulting from increased production due to inflammation or decreased clearance, can be detrimental by

Table 1
Bronchodilators used as inhalation therapy in horses

Type of Bronchodilator	Drug	Formulations Brand Names (in the United States)	Dosage
Short-acting beta2 adrenergic agonists	Albuterol (Salbutamol)	Proventil-HFA Ventolin-HFA ProAir-HFA	1–2 µg/kg, q 1–4 h
	Levalbuterol	Xopenex-HFA	0.5 µg/kg, q 4 h
Long-acting beta2 adrenergic agonists	Salmeterol	Serevent-CFC free	0.25–1.0 µg/kg, q 6–8 h
Muscarinic cholinergic antagonist	Ipratropium	Atrovent-HFA	1–3 µg/kg, q 6–8 h

These inhalers are formulated as pMDIs and should be used with a delivery device, such as Equine Haler, AeroHippus, AeroMask, or Flexineb.

Table 2
Antiinflammatories used as inhalation therapy in horses

Type of Antiinflammatory	Drug Formulations	Brand Names (in the United States)	Dosage
Corticosteroid	Beclomethasone: HFA	QVAR Beclazone	2–8 µg/kg q 12 h
	Fluticasone: HFA	Flovent Flixotide	2–4 µg/kg q 12 h
	Flunisolide: HFA	Aerospan	1–4 µg/kg q 8 h (anecdotal)
Mast cell stabilizer	Nedocromil: CFC free	Tilade (2 mg per actuation)	8–14 mg per 500 kg q 4–8 h
	Cromoglycate: CFC free	Intal (5 mg per actuation)	10–15 mg per 500 kg q 4–8 h

These inhalers are formulated as pMDIs and should be used with a delivery device, such as Equine Haler, AeroHippus, AeroMask, or Flexineb.

altering gas exchange properties and retaining harmful substances or bacteria within the respiratory tract.

The amount and viscosity of mucus, along with ciliary activity, determine mucus clearance. Mucus production and viscosity are increased during pulmonary diseases, such as severe equine asthma. Mucokinetic agents that reduce mucus in airways are candidates for inhalation therapy in the management of diseases like severe asthma.

Physiologic saline exerts mucolytic activity when applied topically to respiratory mucus. Inhalation of droplets of isotonic fluid can help to breakdown the oligosaccharide cross-linking and disrupt van der Waals forces, thus, reducing the viscosity of mucus and making it easier to clear.[26] Diseases such as pneumonia and moderate to severe equine asthma result in increased mucus secretion. The inhalation of vaporized or nebulized isotonic fluid in such cases can have a therapeutic effect by facilitating clearance of these secretions.[27] Although isotonic solutions are beneficial, the use of vaporized or nebulized sterile water or hypertonic saline is controversial because of possible bronchoconstriction in response to the altered osmolariy.[28]

Other mucokinetic agents that have been administered by inhalation include hygroscopic agents, such as propylene glycol, as well as true mucolytics, such as acetylcysteine.[1,8]

Bronchodilators

The 2 major classes of inhaled bronchodilators are the beta-2-adrenergic agonists and the muscarinic antagonists. Beta-2 agonists include albuterol (salbutamol), levalbuterol, salmeterol, and fenoterol. The muscarinic antagonists include ipratropium, oxitropium, and tiotropium. Inhaled nitric oxide (NO) also promotes bronchodilation.

Beta-2 adrenergic agonists The beta-2 adrenergic agonists are sympathomimetic drugs that inhibit smooth muscle contraction by decreasing intracellular calcium stores and the activity of smooth muscle cell protein kinase. This inhibition of smooth muscle contraction is done through activation of adenyl cyclase, which in turn stimulates cyclic adenosine monophosphate and protein kinase A. Beta-2 agonists enhance mucociliary clearance by stimulating ciliary activity and increasing the fluidity of the mucus secretion. In addition, these drugs may also decrease proinflammatory cytokine release from mononuclear cells and neutrophils.[29]

Beta-2 agonists mediate smooth muscle relaxation leading to bronchodilation.[30] Short-acting beta-2 agonists have a quick onset of action and are the most effective drug class for relieving acute bronchoconstriction in patients with asthma.[31] Diseases associated with smooth muscle hypertrophy, hyperplasia, or metaplasia are particularly prone to the occurrence of life-threatening bronchoconstriction, making short-acting beta-2 agonists critical for the management of these diseases in several animal species.[18]

Short-acting beta-2 adrenergic agonists have a rapid onset of action within 5 to 15 minutes, and duration as short as 2 to 4 hours. Long-acting beta-2 agonists have a slower onset time of 30 minutes, with peak activity 3 hours after administration, and duration of 8 hours.[32] Available formulations are listed in **Table 1**.

Reversing bronchoconstriction is symptomatic therapy only, and it does not treat the underlying disease. Nonetheless, it helps to reestablish normal gas exchange and comfort. In addition, provision of bronchodilation first will aid in improved delivery of inhalational corticosteroids or other therapies.

The systemic side effects of beta-2 adrenergic agonists include trembling, sweating, anxiousness, tachycardia, and cardiac arrhythmias. These side effects are very uncommon when the drugs are administered through the inhalation route as compared with systemic routes.

Muscarinic cholinergic antagonists Muscarinic cholinergic antagonists are parasympatholytic drugs. They block muscarinic receptors in a fashion similar to atropine, resulting in inhibition of calcium release from myocytes, and thus preventing contraction of airway smooth muscles. They are therefore very potent inhibitors of bronchoconstriction. Side effects include decreased salivation, tachycardia, mydriasis, and decreased gastrointestinal motility; however, they are significantly less common after inhalation as compared with systemic administration. The onset of action is slow, 30 to 60 minutes, making these drugs less suitable as rescue remedies for acute respiratory distress associated with bronchospasm as compared with short-acting beta-2 agonists.

Formulations of muscarinic cholinergic antagonists for inhalation therapy include ipratropium, oxitropium and tiotropium. Currently only ipratropium is recommended for use in the horse. **Table 1** depicts details in the formulation and dosage of inhalational ipratropium in horses. Muscarinic cholinergic antagonists can be given in combination with beta-2 adrenergic agonists; a combination of ipratropium and albuterol inhalation aerosol (Combivent Respimat) is commercially available in the United States.

Nitric oxide NO is a gaseous, highly reactive molecule with a free radical electron, produced in neuronal and non-neuronal tissues from the conversion of L-arginine to L-citrulline. In lungs its exact source is uncertain, but it may be produced by pneumocytes, pulmonary macrophages, or from the respiratory epithelium. At the cellular level, NO binds to guanylyl cyclase, changing its shape and increasing its activity to increase production of cyclic guanosine 3'5'-monophosphate (cGMP). cGMP then acts on smooth muscle, causing vasodilation and bronchodilation. The pulmonary effects of inhaled NO are pulmonary vasodilation, with an accompanying decrease in pulmonary blood pressures. Therefore, NO can reverse pulmonary vasoconstriction and may be used as a therapy in acute respiratory distress syndrome and pulmonary hypertension.[33] It also serves as a bronchodilator by acting directly on airway smooth muscles and may even play a role in mast cell stabilization, which would assist in controlling exacerbation of asthma and other obstructive airway diseases.[34] It must be remembered that NO in large amounts can be toxic because of the formation of nitrite and peroxynitrite radicals, particularly in the presence of oxygen. These toxic byproducts may cause increased airway responsiveness.[35]

Mast cell stabilizers
The cromone drugs inhibit mast cell degranulation, thus preventing the release of several mediators of inflammation, including prostaglandins, leukotrienes and histamine by blocking calcium channels. The overall effect is to inhibit bronchoconstriction by means of decreasing the inflammatory cascade. These drugs are considered prophylactic or preventative. For optimal results, they require a period of 1 to 2 weeks of steady use before the onset of signs in order to provide any notable benefit. Therefore, they are particularly indicated in horses with seasonally recurrent asthma, particularly when an increased percentage of mast cells is present on BALF cytology. Available inhalational formulations of cromones include nedocromil (Tilade) and cromoglycate (Intal) (see **Table 2**).

Corticosteroids
Corticosteroids bind to intracellular glucocorticoid receptors leading to inhibition of nuclear factor–kβ and ultimate downregulation of the gene expression of inflammatory cytokines. The side effects of glucocorticoids include hyperglycemia, sodium and water retention, hypokalemia, suppression of the hypothalamic pituitary axis, impaired healing, immunosuppression, gastrointestinal ulceration and laminitis. Because of the concerns about the use of systemic corticosteroids, inhaled corticosteroids have become quintessential to the treatment of inflammatory bronchoconstrictive diseases, such as RAO and IAD in horses, especially for long-term management. One limiting factor for the use of inhaled corticosteroids is that they are more expensive than the formulations available for systemic use. The adverse effects are significantly less likely with the inhaled versus systemic formulations.[36] Inhaled corticosteroids can be delivered through various spacers. Formulations of pMDI currently available include beclomethasone, fluticasone and flunisolide (see **Table 2**).

Beclomethasone dipropionate Beclomethasone dipropionate is currently available in various formulations with an HFA propellant. The receptor binding half-life of beclomethasone administered through this route is 7.5 hours. Very fine particle size can be achieved with the propellant, which increases lower airway and lung deposition.[37,38] Beclomethasone dipropionate is transformed to the more active 17-beclamethasone dipropionate on absorption.[39] It reverses airway obstruction and improves pulmonary function in horses affected with severe equine asthma.[40,41] Inhaled beclomethasone at doses greater than 1500 µg per 500 kg of body weight in horses has been shown to cause adrenal suppression.[42] Because of this, the dose must be tapered at cessation of treatment.[41,42] In humans, the most common side effect of inhalational beclomethasone is oral candidiasis, possibly associated with local immunosuppression.[43] In horses, mild respiratory infections have been reported after inhaled beclomethasone therapy.[40]

Fluticasone Fluticasone is currently formulated with HPA propellants, such as Flovent or Flixotide. The receptor binding half-life in humans is 10.5 hours.[38] In humans, fluticasone is detectable in the lungs for up to 20 hours after inhalation.[23] In comparing the two inhalational corticosteroids, fluticasone has better potency, less systemic absorption, and a longer half-life than beclomethasone. The primary disadvantage of fluticasone is the increased cost. The recommended dosage is similar to beclomethasone for resolution of airway obstruction during severe equine asthma attacks.[4,36,44,45] No evidence of immunosuppression was noted in horses treated for as long as 11 months based on markers of immune function.[36] Administration of 2000 µg per 500 kg of body weight through inhalation does not result in adrenal suppression, whereas higher doses, including 3000 µg per 500 kg of body weight, may do so.[25]

Flunisolide Flunisolide is also formulated with an HPA propellant. It has a receptor-binding half-life of 3.5 hours and is less potent than fluticasone.[38] There are no published recommended doses for flunisolide in horses.

Antimicrobials

There is great interest in inhaled antimicrobials for use in lower airway infections in human medicine, especially in patients affected with cystic fibrosis and non–cystic fibrosis bronchiectasis. Several classes of antibiotics are reported to be administered through the inhalation route in humans with these infections. These classes include tobramycin, amikacin, and gentamicin (aminoglycoside antibiotics); aztreonam (monobactam antibiotic); colistin (polymyxin antibiotic); ciprofloxacin (fluoroquinolone antibiotic); and ceftazidime (third-generation cephalosporin).[46,47] Only tobramycin, colistin, and aztreonam are specifically formulated for aerosol delivery.

Selection of an antibiotic for use as inhalation therapy should be made with care, as some drug formulations contain preservatives or stabilizers that could be harmful if inhaled.[48] Among these are phenols, thioglycerol, cresol, and disodium edetate, which can cause bronchial irritation, coughing, and bronchospasm.[47,48] Use of sterile water as a diluent should be avoided because hypotonicity of the solution can cause bronchoconstriction. Drugs may be reconstituted in saline (either 0.23% or 0.45%) instead of water to avoid the ill effects of hypotonicity.[24] Hyperosmolarity can also induce bronchial irritation.

Inhalation allows delivery of antibiotics that are not well absorbed orally without having to perform an injection. In addition, it reduces systemic side effects of antimicrobials. None of the antibiotics discussed are labeled for aerosol use (**Table 3**).

Gentamicin Gentamicin is an aminoglycoside antibiotic with primarily aerobic gram-negative coverage.[49] It may also affect some aerobic gram-positive bacteria, such as *Staphylococcus* species and *Rhodococcus equi*.[49,50] Resistance to gentamicin is developing in many genera of bacteria.[51]

The bactericidal activity of gentamicin is concentration dependent. When administered systemically, gentamicin is primarily distributed in extracellular fluid. As such, it easily reaches therapeutic levels in fluids associated with the respiratory tract, like pleural fluid, sputum, and bronchial secretions.[49] It also reaches therapeutic concentrations in lung tissue.[49] The most significant side effect of gentamicin administered systemically is nephrotoxicity. Administration of gentamicin in an aerosol can lower

Table 3
Antimicrobials studied for inhalation administration in horses

Antimicrobial	Delivery Method	Volume of Injectable and Diluent	Dosage
Gentamicin	Ultrasonic nebulizer[22,24]	Gentamicin diluted to 50 mg/mL (from 100 mg/mL) using sterile water[22] or sterile saline[24]	20 mL total volume of diluted solution per adult horse q 24 h (approximately 2 mg/kg daily)
Ceftiofur (Naxcel)	Nebulized with Flexineb[53]	Diluted with sterile water to a concentration of 50 mg/mL[53]	2.2 mg/kg q 24 h[53] (or 1.1 mg/kg q 12 h)
Cefquinome	Jet nebulizer[57]	5 mL injectable cefquinome + 2.5 mL saline[57]	0.5 mg/kg q 24 h

the total-body dose while providing a high concentration of drug within the respiratory system, an important consideration for a concentration-dependent drug.[22]

The recommended concentration for nebulization of gentamicin is 50 mg/mL.[22] When gentamicin was administered to adult horses through inhalation of 20 ml of 50 mg/ml or intravenous injection at 6.6 mg/kg, the concentration of gentamicin in BALF was higher after inhalation than after systemic administration.[22] Seven days of once-a-day administration of gentamicin through inhalation at 1000 mg (20 ml of 50 mg/ml) per day per horse did not result in side effects. There was also no evidence of inflammation in BALF.[24] The primary disadvantage of gentamicin and other aminoglycosides is that they poorly penetrate abscessed pulmonary tissue.[32]

Ceftiofur Ceftiofur has the spectrum of a third-generation cephalosporin, which provides broad-spectrum antimicrobial coverage against gram-positive and gram-negative bacteria, including *Streptococcus equi ss zooepidemicus*. Ceftiofur is effective in the treatment of respiratory infections in adult horses when given systemically and is labeled for treatment of *Streptococcus equi ss zooepidemicus*.[52] The recommended concentration for nebulization is 25 mg/mL, but the concentration of 50 mg/mL did not result in any adverse effects in one study.[53] In a comparison of ceftiofur administered to foals through inhalation using a Flexineb (Flexineb North America, Jiffy Steamer Equine Division, Union City, Tennessee) mask and systemic administration, the inhalation route was found to be adequate. Ceftiofur was administered with the nebulization system or through intramuscular injection at a dosage of 2.2 mg/kg once daily for 5 days; the concentration in BALF was higher, and the BALF concentrations lasted longer after inhalation than after the intramuscular injection.[52] No adverse effects were reported following the use of ceftiofur given through inhalation.[53]

Cefquinome Cefquinome is a fourth-generation cephalosporin that provides broad-spectrum coverage, particularly against gram-negative aerobes and cephalosporinase-producing bacteria.[54] When given systemically, it has efficacy against common equine respiratory pathogens.[55] It is also used to treat septicemia in neonatal foals.[56] In a comparison study, cefquinome was given to adult horses through inhalation at 225 mg (0.5 mg/kg) or systemically at 1 mg/kg (intramuscularly or intravenously).[57] The inhalation route resulted in BAL concentrations that were much higher than after systemic administration. For aerosol administration, the total dose of 225 mg resulted in BALF concentrations that were greater than the reported minimal inhibitory concentrations (MICs) for respiratory pathogens within 30 minutes after nebulization. After 5 days of treatment, the horses showed no adverse effects.[57] In pulmonary epithelial lining, high concentrations were detected immediately after nebulization, but they were rapidly cleared (less than 4 hours after administration).[58] As cephalosporins are time-dependent antimicrobials, this may affect their ability to control infections in the lower airways unless given at frequent intervals.[55]

Marbofloxacin Marbofloxacin is a fluoroquinolone antimicrobial that exhibits broad-spectrum bactericidal activity, although it does not have anaerobic or adequate anti-streptococcal activity.[49] It frequently has activity against multidrug-resistant bacteria, such as *Pseudomonas aeruginosa*, *Klebsiella spp*, and methicillin-resistant *Staphylococcus aureus*.[49] When administered at a dose of 300 mg with nebulization, using a concentration of 25 mg/mL, the concentrations of marbofloxacin in BALF were higher compared with those after systemic administration.[59] However, concentrations did not reach published MIC values for most bacterial pathogens.[39,60] Therefore, studies regarding dose and safety are required before it can be recommended for administration. No adverse pulmonary effects have been noted after a single administration, as determined by pulmonary function testing.[59]

ADJUNCTIVE MEASURES
Environmental and Feed Management

In airway disease, such as mild, moderate, and severe equine asthma syndromes, identifying and controlling environmental breathable particulates, including organic and inorganic dust, mold, and pollen, are critical in reducing the exacerbation of disease. Factors such as seasonality (summer, winter), indoor and outdoor management, and dusty or moldy hay are important triggers of clinical signs of RAO and IAD. Soaking hay, using low-dust bedding (such as shredded cardboard), and providing misters and adequate ventilation to decrease particulate matter in the affected horse's breathing zone are some of the important environmental management measures. In fact, environmental and feeding management are even more important than medical therapy in the treatment of horses with airway disease.[45]

Key Points

Inhaled therapy provides 2 particular benefits: (a) the ability to deliver a drug directly to the airways for immediate or relatively rapid effects and (b) decreased systemic absorption of medication, which helps to avoid unwanted drug side effects. In addition, inhaled drugs can be delivered at a maximal concentration to the target site, as compared with systemic administration of the drug.

Inhalational drug therapy depends on a complex combination of drug characteristics (such as size, solubility, and hydrophilicity), the method of delivery, and patient breathing pattern. There are numerous potential combinations of drugs and delivery forms.

Some general rules to use during inhalational therapy include the following:

- Use equipment known to have optimal droplet size and flow rate.
- Ensure drug formulation is of optimal viscosity, dilution, and tonicity for aerosolization.
- Minimize dead space volume in the nebulization delivery system.
- Optimize actuation of pMDIs with inhalation, by using a delivery device appropriate for horses.
- Ensure delivery apparatus is clean before use.

REFERENCES

1. Ziment I. Respiratory pharmacology and therapeutics. Philadelphia (PA): Saunders; 1978.
2. Derksen F. Applied respiratory physiology. Beech J, editor. Equine respiratory disorders. Philadelphia (PA): Lea & Febiger; 1991. p. 1–26.
3. Couëtil LL, Hoffman AM, Hodgson J, et al. ACVIM consensus statement inflammatory airway disease of horses. J Vet Intern Med 2007;21:356–61.
4. Couëtil L, Cardwell J, Gerber V, et al. Inflammatory airway disease of horses—revised consensus statement. J Vet Intern Med 2016;30(2):503–15.
5. Clay MM, Clarke SW. Effect of nebulised aerosol size on lung deposition in patients with mild asthma. Thorax 1987;42(3):190–4.
6. Clay MM, Newman SP, Pavia D, et al. Assessment of jet nebulisers for lung aerosol therapy. Lancet 1983;2(8350):592–4.

7. Votion D, Ghafir Y, Munsters K, et al. Aerosol deposition in equine lungs following ultrasonic nebulisation versus jet aerosol delivery system. Equine Vet J 1997; 29(5):388–93.

8. Duvivier DH, Votion D, Roberts C, et al. Inhalation therapy of equine respiratory disorders. Equine Veterinary Education 1999;11(3):124–31.

9. Flament M-P, Leterme P, Gayot A. Factors influencing nebulizing efficiency. Drug Dev Ind Pharm 1995;21(20):2263–85.

10. Durham A. Inhalation therapy for LRT disease. Paper presented at: Proceedings of the 50th British Equine Veterinary Association Congress. Liverpool, United Kingdom, September 7–10, 2011.

11. Lenney J, Innes J, Crompton G. Inappropriate inhaler use: assessment of use and patient preference of seven inhalation devices. Respir Med 2000;94(5): 496–500.

12. Leach CL, Davidson PJ, Hasselquist BE, et al. Influence of particle size and patient dosing technique on lung deposition of HFA-beclomethasone from a metered dose inhaler. J Aerosol Med 2005;18(4):379–85.

13. Viel L, Tesarowski D. Radioaerosol deposition in equids. Paper presented at: 40th Annual American Association Equine Practitioners Convention. Vancouver, December 4–7, 1994.

14. Tesarowski DB, Viel L, McDonell WN, et al. The rapid and effective administration of a beta 2-agonist to horses with heaves using a compact inhalation device and metered-dose inhalers. Can Vet J 1994;35(3):170.

15. Bertin F, Ivester K, Couetil L. Comparative efficacy of inhaled albuterol between two hand-held delivery devices in horses with recurrent airway obstruction. Equine Vet J 2011;43(4):393–8.

16. Derksen F, Olszewski M, Robinson N, et al. Use of a hand-held, metered-dose aerosol delivery device to administer pirbuterol acetate to horses with 'heaves'. Equine Vet J 1996;28(4):306–10.

17. Funch-Nielsen H, Roberts C, Weekes J, et al. Evaluation of a new spacer device for delivery of drugs into the equine respiratory tract. Paper presented at: Proceedings of the World Equine Airways Society Symposium. Edinburgh, Scotland, July 19–23, 2001.

18. Hoffman A, Foley M, Spendlove P. Respiratory medicine: new advances in interspecies aerosol delivery. Paper presented at: Proceedings of the Australasian Equine Science Symposium. Queensland, Australia, June 4–6, 2008.

19. Anonymous. AeroHippus equine aerosol chamber. 2016. Available at: https://www.trudellmed.com/animal-health/aerohippus. Accessed May 5, 2016.

20. Olsson B, Bondesson E, Borgström L, et al. Pulmonary drug metabolism, clearance, and absorption. Controlled pulmonary drug delivery. New York: Springer; 2011. p. 21–50.

21. Brown R, Schanker L. Absorption of aerosolized drugs from the rat lung. Drug Metab Dispos 1983;11(4):355–60.

22. McKenzie HC III, Murray MJ. Concentrations of gentamicin in serum and bronchial lavage fluid after intravenous and aerosol administration of gentamicin to horses. Am J Vet Res 2000;61(10):1185–90.

23. Esmailpour N, Hogger P, Rabe K, et al. Distribution of inhaled fluticasone propionate between human lung tissue and serum in vivo. Eur Respir J 1997;10(7): 1496–9.

24. McKenzie HC III, Murray MJ. Concentrations of gentamicin in serum and bronchial lavage fluid after once-daily aerosol administration to horses for seven days. Am J Vet Res 2004;65(2):173–8.

25. Munoz T, Leclere M, Jean D, et al. Serum cortisol concentration in horses with heaves treated with fluticasone propionate over a 1 year period. Res Vet Sci 2015;98:112–4.

26. King M. Relationship between mucus viscoelasticity and ciliary transport in guaran gel/frog palate model system. Biorheology 1979;17(3):249–54.

27. King M, Rubin BK. Pharmacological approaches to discovery and development of new mucolytic agents. Adv Drug Deliv Rev 2002;54(11):1475–90.

28. Mann J, Howarth P, Holgate S. Bronchoconstriction induced by ipratropium bromide in asthma: relation to hypotonicity. Br Med J (Clinical Res Ed) 1984; 289(6443):469.

29. Robinson NE. Clenbuterol and the horse. Paper presented at: Proceedings of the American Association of Equine Practitioners Annual Convention. San Antonio, Texas, November 26–29, 2000.

30. Olson L, Perkowski S, Mason D, et al. Isoproterenol-and salbutamol-induced relaxation of acetylcholine-and histamine-induced contraction of equine trachealis muscle in vitro. Am J Vet Res 1989;50(10):1715–9.

31. US Department of Health and Human Services, Public Health Service, National Institutes of Health, National Heart, Lung, and Blood Institute. National Asthma Education and Prevention Program: Expert panel report: guidelines for the diagnosis and management of asthma: update on selected topics, 2002. Washington D.C.

32. Mazan MR, Ceresia ML, Cole C, et al. Clinical pharmacology of the respiratory system. Equine Pharmacology: John Wiley & Sons, Inc; 2014. p. 137–82.

33. Rossaint R, Falke KJ, Lopez F, et al. Inhaled nitric oxide for the adult respiratory distress syndrome. N Engl J Med 1993;328(6):399–405.

34. Valentovic M, Ball J, Morenas M, et al. Influence of nitrovasodilators on bovine pulmonary histamine release. Pulm Pharmacol 1992;5(2):97–102.

35. Barnes PJ, Belvisi M. Nitric oxide and lung disease. Thorax 1993;48(10):1034.

36. Dauvillier J, Felippe M, Lunn DP, et al. Effect of long-term fluticasone treatment on immune function in horses with heaves. J Vet Intern Med 2011;25(3):549–57.

37. Kelly HW. Comparison of inhaled corticosteroids: an update. Ann Pharmacother 2009;43(3):519–27.

38. Dubois EF. Clinical potencies of glucocorticoids: what do we really measure? Curr Respir Med Rev 2005;1(1):103–8.

39. Würthwein G, Rohdewald P. Activation of beclomethasone dipropionate by hydrolysis to beclomethasone-17-monopropionate. Biopharm Drug Dispos 1990;11(5): 381–94.

40. Ammann V, Vrins A, Lavoie JP. Effects of inhaled beclomethasone dipropionate on respiratory function in horses with chronic obstructive pulmonary disease (COPD). Equine Vet J 1998;30(2):152–7.

41. Rush BR, Raub ES, Thomsen MM, et al. Pulmonary function and adrenal gland suppression with incremental doses of aerosolized beclomethasone dipropionate in horses with recurrent airway obstruction. J Am Vet Med Assoc 2000;217(3): 359–64.

42. Rush BR, Trevino I, Matson C, et al. Serum cortisol concentrations in response to incremental doses of inhaled beclomethasone dipropionate. Equine Vet J 1999; 31(3):258–61.

43. Pedersen S, O'Byrne P. A comparison of the efficacy and safety of inhaled corticosteroids in asthma. Allergy 1997;52(s39):1–34.

44. Giguère S, Viel L, Lee E, et al. Cytokine induction in pulmonary airways of horses with heaves and effect of therapy with inhaled fluticasone propionate. Vet Immunol Immunopathol 2002;85(3):147–58.

45. Couëtil LL, Chilcoat CD, DeNicola DB, et al. Randomized, controlled study of inhaled fluticasone propionate, oral administration of prednisone, and environmental management of horses with recurrent airway obstruction. Am J Vet Res 2005;66(10):1665–74.

46. Brodt AM, Stovold E, Zhang L. Inhaled antibiotics for stable non-cystic fibrosis bronchiectasis: a systematic review. Eur Respir J 2014;44:382–93.

47. Quon BS, Goss CH, Ramsey BW. Inhaled antibiotics for lower airway infections. Ann Am Thorac Soc 2014;11(3):425–34.

48. Kuhn RJ. Formulation of aerosolized therapeutics. Chest 2001;120(supplement 3):94S–8S.

49. Plumb DC. Plumb's veterinary drug handbook. Stockholm (WI); Ames (IA): PharmaVet; Distributed by Wiley; 2011.

50. McNeil M, Brown J. Distribution and antimicrobial susceptibility of Rhodococcus equi from clinical specimens. Eur J Epidemiol 1992;8(3):437–43.

51. Erol E, Locke SJ, Donahoe JK, et al. Beta-hemolytic Streptococcus spp. from horses a retrospective study (2000–2010). J Vet Diagn Invest 2012;24(1):142–7.

52. Folz S, Hanson B, Griffin A, et al. Treatment of respiratory infections in horses with ceftiofur sodium. Equine Vet J 1992;24(4):300–4.

53. Fultz L, Giguère S, Berghaus LJ, et al. Pulmonary pharmacokinetics of desfuroyl-ceftiofur acetamide after nebulisation or intramuscular administration of ceftiofur sodium to weanling foals. Equine Vet J 2015;47(4):473–7.

54. Rose M, Thomas V, Nordmann P. In vitro activity of third and fourth generation cephalosporins against E. coli strains expressing plasmid-encoded AmpC cephalosporinases. Risk management for the limitation of antibiotic resistance. Berlin, Germany: Federal Office of Consumer Protection and Food Safety (BVL); 2004.

55. Thomas E, Thomas V, Wilhelm C. Antibacterial activity of cefquinome against equine bacterial pathogens. Vet Microbiol 2006;115(1):140–7.

56. Rohdich N, Zschiesche E, Heckeroth A, et al. Treatment of septicaemia and severe bacterial infections in foals with a new cefquinome formulation: a field study. Dtsch Tierarztl Wochenschr 2009;116(9):316–20.

57. Art T, Ramery E, Fraipont A, et al. Pulmonary function, airway cytology and bronchoalveolar lavage fluid drug concentration after aerosol administration of cefquinome to horses. Equine Vet Education 2010;22(9):473–9.

58. Winther L, Baptiste KE, Friis C. Antimicrobial disposition in pulmonary epithelial lining fluid of horses, part III. cefquinome. J Vet Pharmacol Ther 2011;34(5):482–6.

59. Art T, De Moffarts B, Bedoret D, et al. Pulmonary function and antimicrobial concentration after marbofloxacin inhalation in horses. Vet Rec 2007;161(10):348.

60. Carretero M, Rodriguez C, Andrés MS, et al. Pharmacokinetics of marbofloxacin in mature horses after single intravenous and intramuscular administration. Equine Vet J 2002;34(4):360–5.

Antimicrobial Pharmacology for the Neonatal Foal

K. Gary Magdesian, DVM

KEYWORDS

- Neonatal foal • Equine • Antibiotics • Antimicrobials • Pharmacology
- Pharmacokinetics • Sepsis

KEY POINTS

- Sepsis is one of the leading causes of death in neonatal foals and requires early antimicrobial intervention.
- Neonatal foals have unique pharmacology that makes antimicrobial choice and dosage different than in adult horses.
- Front-line antimicrobial use should consist of bactericidal, broad-spectrum, and intravenously administered drugs.
- A combination of aminoglycoside–beta-lactam antimicrobial or third-generation cephalosporin is an excellent choice for antimicrobial therapy in septic foals.
- Renal function must be monitored carefully in foals on aminoglycosides.

INTRODUCTION

Sepsis is the leading cause of death in the neonatal foal during the first week of life. Sepsis results from a dysregulated immune response to infection, often leading to organ dysfunction and hypotension.[1] It can lead to localized infections in foals, with life-threatening consequences, including osteomyelitis, physitis, septic arthritis, meningitis, and umbilical infections. The treatment of sepsis consists of antimicrobial therapy, hemodynamic support, and supportive care.[1] Because failure of passive transfer of colostral antibodies is a marker of or risk factor for sepsis, serum immunoglobulin concentrations should be measured to ensure they are greater than 800 mg/dL; if failure of passive transfer is present, a plasma transfusion should be administered if the foal is older than 12 hours of age and beyond the time point of absorbing colostral immunoglobulin G (IgG). Septic foals may benefit from plasma regardless of IgG status.

The initial antimicrobial choice for the treatment of sepsis should include bactericidal, intravenous (IV), and broad-spectrum drugs. They should be cidal, because

The author has nothing to disclose.
Department of Medicine and Epidemiology, School of Veterinary Medicine, University of California, 1 Shields Avenue, Davis, Davis, CA 95616, USA
E-mail address: kgmagdesian@ucdavis.edu

Vet Clin Equine 33 (2017) 47–65
http://dx.doi.org/10.1016/j.cveq.2016.12.004

septic foals are often neutropenic, and the immune system of foals is less robust than that of adult horses. The antimicrobials should be administered IV, because gut and muscle perfusion may be reduced, thereby decreasing bioavailability of the drugs administered through those routes. Although blood culture results can aid in directing antimicrobial therapy, particularly for longer-term administered drugs, they cannot be relied on for the initial selection because of the time delay in obtaining results. In addition, false negative results occur frequently.[2] Antimicrobial administration to foals should not be delayed for the sake of obtaining blood cultures, because delays allow for continued bacterial growth and cytokine production and increase the risks of developing localized infections such as septic arthritis. In human medicine, early antimicrobial administration, before septic shock ensues, has been associated with improved outcome.[3]

Broad-spectrum antimicrobials are required because both gram-negative and -positive bacteria are commonly found in foal sepsis. The most common isolate cultured from blood cultures obtained from septic foals worldwide is *Escherichia coli*, and other enteric gram-negative bacteria are frequently isolated, including *Enterobacter* and *Klebsiella*.[2,4–8] Gram-negative nonenteric bacteria are also commonly isolated from septic foals, especially *Actinobacillus* and *Pasteurella* isolates. Mixed infections with both gram-positive and -negative bacteria are also common. Gram-positive bacteria associated with foal sepsis include *Streptococcus*, *Enterococcus*, and *Staphylococcus*. Anaerobes are uncommon, but possible, so some degree of anaerobic coverage is also indicated. In a study evaluating the prevalence of bacteria causing sepsis in foals admitted to UC Davis demonstrated that *E coli* was the most common isolate at 29%, with *Actinobacillus* being second at 14%, and beta-hemolytic *Streptococcus* comprising 9%. *Klebsiella* (7.3%) and *Enterococcus* (7.2%) rounded out the top 5 isolates.[8] These data demonstrate the importance of *E coli* in foals sepsis, but also of the need for covering for a wide spectrum of bacteria, including gram-negative enteric, gram-negative nonenteric, and gram-positive bacteria.[8] A review compiling data from 3 additional studies had very similar results, with the top 5 most prevalent isolates from blood cultures of neonatal foal, in descending order, consisting of *E coli*, *Actinobacillus*, *Enterobacter*, *Enterococcus*, and *Streptococcus*. *Klebsiella* came in at number 6. Anaerobes comprised 4% of isolates.[9]

Antimicrobial Classes Available for Use in Foals

Beta-lactam antimicrobials: penicillin, ampicillin, amoxicillin

Beta-lactam antimicrobials are bactericidal drugs that inhibit cell wall synthesis and are synergistic with aminoglycosides. They bind to penicillin-binding proteins, especially transpeptidase, thereby inhibiting the crosslinking of peptidoglycan strands of the bacterial cell wall. They are time-dependent drugs, so that the duration of time that plasma concentrations are above the minimum inhibitory concentration (MIC) of the isolate is important (T>MIC). Plasma concentrations of beta-lactams should remain above the MIC for at least 50% of the dosing interval for gram-positive infections, and at least 80% of the interval for gram-negative infections. For example, if the dosing interval is every 6 hours for ampicillin, the plasma concentrations should remain above the MIC of the microbes for at least 3 and 5 hours for susceptible gram-positive and -negative bacteria, respectively.

The classic beta-lactam drugs are penicillin, ampicillin, and amoxicillin. In general, these have primarily a gram-positive spectrum; however, many staphylococci are now resistant to these beta-lactams. Penicillin G has high efficacy against many gram-positive bacteria, especially beta-hemolytic streptococci, as well as most gram-positive and gram-negative anaerobic bacteria, except for *Bacteroides fragilis*.

Variably, some gram-negative nonenteric microbes, including some *Pasteurella* and *Actinobacillus* isolates, are also susceptible to penicillin. Penicillin should be administered slowly IV, whether as potassium or sodium salt, because horses can react to rapid administration.[9] The potassium form can induce myoelectrical activity of the equine gastrointestinal tract, causing cramping and loose stool, whereas some have anecdotally observed hypotension with rapid administration of the sodium salt.[9]

The semisynthetic penicillins (aminopenicillins), ampicillin and amoxicillin, are similar in spectrum to penicillin G, with increasing activity against gram-negative bacteria. Ampicillin is available as sodium and trihydrate forms; amoxicillin trihydrate can be administered orally (PO) to foals, as can ampicillin trihydrate (**Table 1**). This is a feature unique to the young foal, whereas in the older foal and adult horse, beta-lactam antimicrobials have very low bioavailability, and oral administration risks induction of enterocolitis.

Amoxicillin has a very similar spectrum of activity as ampicillin, primarily gram-positive, with some gram-negative coverage. Some gram-negative nonenteric microbes, as well as some *E coli*, *Klebsiella*, and *Proteus* isolates, historically have been susceptible to ampicillin, whereas they were not susceptible to penicillin. However, after decades of use, ampicillin has lost some of its efficacy against these enteric microbes. *Pseudomonas* and many *Enterobacter* isolates are resistant to both penicillin and ampicillin.[10] A somewhat unique advantage of ampicillin is that it is one of the few antimicrobials with efficacy against some of the multidrug-resistant *Enterococcus faecalis* and *Enterococcus faecium* isolates. Of the commonly used antimicrobials prescribed in equine practice, ampicillin and chloramphenicol are often the most consistently effective against these enterococci.

The combination of ampicillin with amikacin yields the highest percentage of susceptible isolates among those cultured from blood of foals with sepsis.[11] A recent study of 306 bacterial isolates demonstrated that 91.5% were susceptible to this combination. Penicillin can also be administered in combination with aminoglycosides in place of ampicillin; however, a lower percentage of enterococcal isolates is susceptible to penicillin than to ampicillin.[11]

Beta-lactam antimicrobials: extended-spectrum penicillins

These formulations of beta-lactam antimicrobials are considered "antipseudomonal" antimicrobials. They include carbenicillin, piperacillin, and ticarcillin, and their clinical use is primarily targeting *Pseudomonas aeruginosa* infections in foals, because *Pseudomonas* tends to be multidrug resistant and difficult to treat. They also have activity against *Proteus* isolates that are often resistant to other penicillins.[10] However, most *Klebsiella*, *Citrobacter*, *Serratia*, and *Enterobacter* isolates are resistant to even these extended-spectrum penicillins, so they are not a complete replacement for gram-negative coverage, except for the case with *Pseudomonas* and *Proteus* (*Klebsiella* may be susceptible to piperacillin specifically).[10] These antibiotics also have similar activity against gram-positive aerobic bacteria and anaerobes as do the other penicillins. In addition, they are more likely to be effective against *B fragilis*, which tends to be resistant to penicillin and ampicillin.[10] As might be expected from their specific and extended antimicrobial spectrum, this subclass of beta-lactam drugs is not routinely used in horses, unless dictated by culture and susceptibility testing results, or when *Pseudomonas* is cultured.

Beta-lactam antimicrobials: cephalosporins

Cephalosporins are also beta-lactam antimicrobials based on chemical structure. They penetrate well into most body fluids and the extracellular fluids of most tissues, better

Table 1
Suggested dosages for beta lactam antimicrobials in foals

Drug	Dosage	Comment
Penicillins		
Ampicillin	22–30 mg/kg IV or PO, every 6–8 h	Oral pivampicillin 19.9 mg/kg
Amoxicillin	13–30 mg/kg PO, every 8 h	—
Penicillin, potassium, or sodium	22,000–44,000 IU/kg IV, every 6 h	Always infuse slowly
Ticarcillin-clavulanic acid	50 mg/kg IV, every 6 h	Slow and dilute infusion (dose based on ticarcillin)
Imipenem	15 mg/kg IV, every 6–8 h	Use only when culture dictated
Meropenem	15 mg/kg IV, every 6 h	Use only when culture dictated
First-generation cephalosporins		
Cefazolin	15–22 mg/kg IV, every 6–8 h	—
Cephalothin	10–20 mg/kg IV, every 6 h	—
Cefadroxil	20–40 mg/kg PO, every 8–12 h	—
Cefalexin	25 mg/kg PO, every 6, or 30 mg/kg PO, every 8 h	—
Second-generation cephalosporins		
Cefuroxime Na	16–33 mg/kg IV, every 8 h	—
Cefoxitin	20 mg/kg IV, every 6 h	—
Third-generation cephalosporins		
Ceftazidime	20–50 mg/kg IV, every 6 h, slow infusion	Crosses the BBB
Cefoperazone	30 mg/kg IV, every 8 h, slow infusion	—
Cefotaxime	40–50 mg/kg IV, every 6 h, slow infusion	Crosses the BBB
Cefotaxime continuous infusion	40 mg/kg loading dose, then 6.7 mg/kg/h IV	Can go up to 8.3 mg/kg/h
Ceftizoxime	20–50 mg/kg IV, every 6 h, slow infusion	—
Cefpodoxime proxetil	10 mg/kg PO, every 6–8–12 h	q 6 h dosing for E coli
Ceftriaxone	25–50 mg/kg IV, every 12 h	Crosses the BBB
Ceftiofur	5–10 mg/kg IV, SC, IM, every 6–12 h	Author most often uses 5–10 mg/kg IV, every 12 h; high doses should be given slowly
Ceftiofur continuous infusion	5 mg/kg loading dose, then 0.42 mg/kg/h	Can double the dose depending on MIC
Fourth-generation cephalosporins		
Cefepime	11 mg/kg IV, every 8 h	Crosses the BBB
Cefquinome	1 mg/kg IM or IV, every 12 h	Has been used up to 2.5 mg/kg, every 6–8 h

than penicillin and ampicillin, and this penetration is enhanced by inflammation. Cephalosporins penetrate poorly into the intracellular space, however. They are bactericidal and time dependent as are other beta-lactam drugs. In general, they are very safe drugs, with rare hypersensitivity reactions and antimicrobial-associated diarrhea as possible adverse reactions in foals, as for penicillin or ampicillin. In foals with reduced glomerular filtration rate, the dosage interval may need to be increased due to reduced clearance. Cephalosporins should be administered slowly, as per label instructions.

Cephalosporins are similar to penicillins, with some important differences. Penicillins are primarily excreted into the urine; although cephalosporins are also primarily excreted into urine, a portion of the administered drug is eliminated into bile. This property may make the cephalosporins more likely than penicillins to induce antimicrobial-associated diarrhea. Cefoperazone and ceftriaxone, both third-generation cephalosporins, have significant biliary excretion.

Cephalosporins are categorized into 5 "generations" based on their activity, with first-generation cephalosporins having primarily gram-positive activity, while third-, fourth- and fifth-generation drugs include potent gram-negative coverage as well. Fifth-generation cephalosporins have not been studied in horses to date.

First-generation cephalosporins In general, first-generation cephalosporins are similar to aminopenicillins in that they have excellent streptococcal coverage, some gram-negative nonenteric spectrum, and minimal anaerobic activity. Cephalothin, cephapirin, cephalexin, and cefadroxil are examples of first-generation cephalosporins. As for amoxicillin, first-generation cephalosporins can be administered orally to young foals because they absorb them well, whereas older animals have poor absorption and are at risk for dysbiosis from PO administered beta-lactam drugs. Cephalexin can be administered to neonatal foals PO (see **Table 1**). Cefadroxil has also been studied in foals. In 2-week-old foals, a dose of 10 mg/kg PO showed almost 100% bioavailability.[12] Based on the studies, cefadroxil can be administered at a dose of 20 to 40 mg/kg PO, every 8 to 12 hours.[12]

Second-generation cephalosporins Second-generation cephalosporins are similar in gram-positive spectrum to the first-generation cephalosporins, but they have increased activity against gram-negative bacteria. Examples include cefoxitin and cefuroxime. Cefoxitin in particular has anaerobe activity, whereas many cephalosporins do not, including efficacy against *B fragilis*.

Third-generation cephalosporins As discussed above, the first- and second-generation cephalosporins can be used to treat sepsis in foals, but they must be combined with aminoglycosides because of their limited activity against gram-negative organisms. Because of their broader spectrum, particularly their activity against gram-negative enteric microbes, the third- and fourth-generation cephalosporins are more conducive to treating sepsis as monotherapy in foals. A third-generation cephalosporin, ceftiofur, is labeled for use in horses in both sodium salt and crystalline free acid forms.

The third-generation cephalosporins are bactericidal with a relatively broad spectrum of activity that includes many gram-positive and gram-negative aerobic and anaerobic organisms. They represent an excellent alternative to aminoglycoside–beta-lactam combinations in foals with renal azotemia (see **Table 1**). The anaerobic spectrum of ceftiofur is limited, however. In a study of equine anaerobe isolates, the MIC of 90% of isolates, or MIC_{90}, of *Fusobacterium necrophorum* and *Peptostreptococcus anaerobius* to ceftiofur was conducive with efficacy (≤ 0.0625 and 0.125 µg/mL, respectively). However, *B fragilis*, other species of *Bacteroides*, and *Prevotella* species had high MIC_{90} values for ceftiofur, consistent with resistance.[13]

Resistance to ceftiofur among bacteria isolated from septic foals is slightly more common than resistance to aminoglycoside–beta-lactam combinations. Publications report that as many as 30% of the isolates obtained from septic foals may be resistant to ceftiofur.[2,6,14–16] Therefore, the decision to use ceftiofur should be made based on culture and susceptibility testing results, or at least from historical, regional antimicrobial susceptibility data. In addition, because the labeled dose of ceftiofur (2.2–4.4 mg/kg every 24 hours) is for treatment of respiratory infections associated with *Streptococcus zooepidemicus*, which is considered particularly sensitive to ceftiofur (MIC of $\leq$0.25 μg/mL), ceftiofur should be administered to septic foals at higher than labeled doses in order to target gram-negative enteric microbes like *E coli*. Ceftiofur's high safety profile in newborn foals also allows this. At the Veterinary Medical Teaching Hospital, University of California, Davis, only approximately 60% to 89% of *E coli* isolates are susceptible to ceftiofur with an MIC value of 2 μg/mL. That percentage is even lower when considering *Klebsiella* or *Enterobacter* isolates. In fact, doses as high as 10 mg/kg every 6 to 12 hours have been administered to foals in order to achieve plasma concentrations likely to be effective against gram-negative enteric microbes often associated with sepsis in foals, which tend to have much higher MIC values than *S zooepidemicus*.[17,18] *Actinobacillus* and *Pasteurella* isolates, both gram-negative nonenteric microbes, tend to be very susceptible to ceftiofur, similar to *Streptococcus*.

There are geographic and publication differences among reported MIC values for ceftiofur among bacteria isolated from foals. One published study showed that ceftiofur administered at a dose of 5 mg/kg every 12 hours would be predicted to have efficacy against 90% of the *E coli*, *Pasteurella*, *Klebsiella*, and *Streptococcus* organisms isolated from blood cultures in that study, based on their MIC ($MIC_{90} \leq$0.5 μg/mL).[19] However, even at that dose, which is greater than 2 times the labeled dose, 27% of *Salmonella* isolates and most *Enterococcus* isolates in that study were considered resistant to ceftiofur ($MIC_{90} >$4 μg/mL). Another study of blood culture isolates from septic foals found that 23% of all bacterial isolates were resistant to ceftiofur.[16] It should be pointed out that ceftiofur sodium can be administered IV to septic foals, and that is the optimal dosing route early on when foals have hypoperfusion. Later, it can be changed to intramuscular (IM) or subcutaneous (SC) route of delivery. Despite the label recommendations for IM administration, the IV and SC routes are also acceptable.[20]

A crystalline-free acid formulation of ceftiofur has been studied in neonatal foals.[21] In order to target the MIC of common enteric microorganism (2 μg/mL), although the product is labeled for treating infections with *Streptococcus* (MIC typically $\leq$0.25 μg/mL), the conclusion was that the dose needed to be doubled. A dose of 13.2 mg/kg SC administered every 48 to 72 hours of crystalline-free acid ceftiofur maintains therapeutic concentrations for enteric microorganisms.[21] The second dose should be administered at 48 hours, but after that it can be administered every 72 hours. Although the drug was well tolerated in that study, the author has seen occasional firm swellings at injection sites in foals. In addition, it should be highlighted that it takes approximately 6 hours for ceftiofur free acid equivalents to reach 2 μg/mL in plasma, which is a long delay in septic foals. In addition, the pharmacokinetics will likely be altered in sick foals, particularly because perfusion to the SC tissues will likely be reduced. In such foals, IV administration of ceftiofur sodium is far preferable.

Aside from ceftiofur, there are several other third-generation cephalosporins used in human medicine, which can also be used in foals. These third-generation cephalosporins are structurally slightly different than ceftiofur, allowing them even greater gram-negative potency and the ability for some of them to penetrate into the central nervous system (CNS). These other third-generation cephalosporins can be used in foals with sepsis that is associated with bacteria that are not susceptible to ceftiofur or amino-glycoside–beta-lactam combinations. These drugs include cefotaxime, ceftizoxime, cefpodoxime, and ceftizoxime, among others. Because these antimicrobials are used to treat serious human infections, and there is concern for the development of antimicrobial resistance against cephalosporins, these antimicrobials should be used judiciously and only when antimicrobial susceptibility data indicate no other viable options; the other time they are indicated is when meningitis is present in foals, because they penetrate the blood-brain barrier (BBB) well, whereas ceftiofur and ami-noglycosides do not under normal circumstances.[19] Those third-generation cephalo-sporins that penetrate the BBB well include ceftriaxone, cefotaxime, and ceftazidime; among these, ceftriaxone achieves the highest concentration within the cerebral spi-nal fluid. One of these 3 should be used for empirical treatment of meningitis, and their highest recommended doses should be used. Cefpodoxime does not cross into the CNS well and is therefore not a good choice for treatment of meningitis.

These third-generation cephalosporins have very broad-spectrum efficacy against a wide range of bacteria, including both gram-positive and -negative bacteria, with some individual variation among the specific drugs. For example, cefotaxime is the third-generation cephalosporin with the highest degree of anaerobe coverage. Cefta-zidime and cefoperazone have the most potent activity of all of the third-generation cephalosporins against *Pseudomonas* isolates, but ceftazidime has poor anaerobic coverage. Cefpodoxime is formulated for oral administration and has been studied in foals.[22]

Fourth-generation cephalosporins Fourth-generation cephalosporins have the broad-est spectrum of activity, with similar gram-positive activity as the first-generation cephalosporins, although they may be slightly less potent than first- and second-generation agents against methicillin-susceptible *Staphylococcus aureus*. They do not have activity against methicillin-resistant *S aureus* (MRSA). They have even greater gram-negative activity than the third-generation cephalosporins because they have greater resistance to beta-lactamase enzymes. Because of this spectrum, they should be reserved for culture-directed or nonresponsive sepsis.

A limited number of fourth-generation cephalosporins, including cefquinome and cefepime, have been studied in horses (see **Table 1**).[23,24] Others used in human med-icine include cefluprenam, cefozopran, and cefpirome. Cefquinome is labeled to treat foal septicemia in Europe. It has a very broad spectrum of activity, including good ac-tivity against *Actinobacillus equuli*, streptococci, enteric bacteria such as *E coli*, *Clos-tridium perfringens*, and staphylococci.[24,25] It is labeled to treat foals with septicemia at a dose of 1 mg/kg IV or IM every 12 hours, but it has been used at extralabel doses up to 2.5 mg/kg IV every 6 to 8 hours.[9] The pharmacokinetics of cefepime, another fourth-generation cephalosporin, has been studied in foals.[23] It requires further study, but may be potentially useful for treatment of gram-negative sepsis in foals. The MIC values of cefepime for equine isolates have not been reported; however, *E coli*, *Kleb-siella pneumonia*, and *C perfringens* isolated from human patients are generally considered susceptible to cefepime (MIC ≤ 8 μg/mL). *E faecalis* and methicillin-resistant staphylococci are considered resistant to cefepime, as they are to many other cephalosporins. Cefepime, like some of the third-generation agents, penetrates the CNS well and can be used to treat meningitis.

Fifth-generation cephalosporins Relatively new, this subclass has not been studied in horses. Ceftaroline is an example of a fifth-generation cephalosporin. Importantly, it is active against MRSA and other gram-positive bacteria, but also retains the activity of third- and fourth-generation cephalosporins against gram-negative bacteria. The use of ceftaroline should be restricted.

Beta-lactam antimicrobials: carbapenems

Carbapenems are modified beta-lactams that are considered to have among the broadest spectrum of activity of any of the commercially available antimicrobials. Examples include imipenem, meropenem, and doripenem. Imipenem, which is the only carbapenem that has been studied in horses, has activity against many bacteria that are resistant to first-line antimicrobials, including many *Enterococcus* and *Pseudomonas* isolates. It also has excellent anaerobic activity.[25] The primary limitation of the carbapenems is MRSA as well as some *Enterobacter*, *Pseudomonas*, and *E faecium* isolates.

Imipenem is formulated with cilastatin, a compound that inhibits the imipenem-degrading renal enzyme dehydropeptidase, in order to prolong its elimination half-life. In adult horses, imipenem-cilastatin was well tolerated in an experimental model, and there were no significant adverse events reported.[25] Because it is time dependent and has a short half-life like most beta-lactam drugs, it should be dosed frequently, up to every 6 to 8 hours.[25] Potential uncommon to rare adverse effects of imipenem in foals include seizures, antimicrobial-induced diarrhea, and thrombophlebitis if not diluted as per label instructions.

Meropenem has not been studied in horses. The author has used meropenem in foals with culture-directed therapy or those with severe sepsis that were nonresponsive to other antimicrobials. Meropenem has a similar spectrum as imipenem; however, it has advantages of bolus administration options with less thrombophlebitis potential as well as greater in vitro activity against gram-negative bacteria. It may be safer in terms of seizure induction than imipenem. Finally, it does not require coadministration with cilastatin.

Because of concerns over the increasing development of antimicrobial resistance in both human and veterinary medicine, carbapenems should be used sparingly and only when indicated by culture and susceptibility testing, or when severe infections in foals are clinically nonresponsive to beta-lactam–aminoglycoside or third-generation cephalosporins.

Continuous Infusions of Beta-Lactam Antimicrobials

A relatively novel mode of antimicrobial administration, currently being evaluated in human medicine, is that of continuous rate infusion (CRI) for beta-lactam antimicrobials. Beta-lactam antimicrobials are particularly suited to this mode of administration because they are time dependent and have little postantibiotic effect (PAE). PAE is a persistent inhibition of bacterial growth after the plasma concentrations drop below the MIC of the microbe and is exerted by concentration-dependent and some time-dependent antimicrobials. Because beta-lactam drugs have little to no PAE, their plasma concentration time above MIC (T>MIC) of the offending microbe should be at least 50% of the dosing interval, and ideally longer. With CRI administration, the plasma concentrations can be maintained above the MIC of the microbe at all times. Although intuitively it seems that this dosing protocol should be more effective than intermittent bolus dosing, it requires further study. Early clinical trials have shown survival benefits of CRI administration as compared with bolus administration of beta-lactam antimicrobials in humans; however, there are also studies that have not demonstrated clear benefits.[26]

The pharmacokinetics of CRI administration of ceftiofur to neonatal foals has been studied.[27] From the pharmacokinetic values obtained in that study, the investigators predicted that a bolus loading dose of 1.26 mg/kg, followed by a CRI of 2.86 μg/kg/min, would maintain plasma concentrations of desfuroylceftiofur, the active metabolite of ceftiofur, greater than 2 μg/mL at all times.[27] This would serve to keep the time greater than MIC at 100% for microbes with an MIC ≤2 μg/mL. The cumulative daily dose of ceftiofur with this CRI rate is 5.4 mg/kg/d. Higher doses would be required for bacteria with MICs greater than 2 μg/mL. If the plan is to change the foal from CRI dosing to standard every 12-hour bolus dosing, for example, after an initial few day period of CRI dosing when the sepsis appears to be controlled, the first bolus dose should be administered 12 hours after the end of the CRI.

Cefotaxime has also been studied as a CRI administration in 1-day-old pony foals.[28] The standard bolus dosing of 40 mg/kg IV every 6 hours was compared with CRI administration at 160 mg/kg/d (6.7 mg/kg/h, after an initial loading bolus dose of 40 mg/kg), so that the total daily dose of cefotaxime was the same in the 2 groups. With CRI dosing, plasma concentrations of cefotaxime were constantly maintained at approximately 16.10 μg/mL, which is greater than the MIC of susceptible pathogens. In contrast, standard intermittent dosing allowed for plasma concentrations to decrease to 0.78 μg/mL 6 hours after dosing, just before the next dose. Importantly, synovial fluid cefotaxime concentrations were higher with CRI dosing (5.02 μg/mL) than with intermittent dosing (0.78 μg/mL).[28] Thus, CRI dosing represents a potentially significant advantage for foals with septic arthritis. Continuous rate infusion is well suited to cefotaxime, because the diluted formulation is stable for at least 24 hours at room temperature, as long as it is protected from light.

Continuous infusions can be used for other beta-lactam antimicrobials intended for IV use. The goal is to administer the same total daily dose during continuous infusion as would be administered during standard intermittent bolus administration. For example, if a drug is usually administered at a dose of 30 mg/kg every 6 hours, the CRI dosing rate would be 5 mg/kg/h to keep the same total daily dose the same. Automated fluid or syringe pumps should be used to deliver the infusion accurately. The stability of the reconstituted and diluted antimicrobial should be considered. Ceftazidime, cefotaxime, cefepime, ticarcillin/clavulanic acid, sodium or potassium penicillin, and cefazolin are stable for 24 hours at room temperature. The duration of stability of ampicillin depends on the concentration of the reconstituted solution and should be verified with the product label. Ceftiofur is stable for 12 hours at room temperature after reconstitution, but it should be protected from light.

Aminoglycosides

The aminoglycoside class of antimicrobials includes amikacin, gentamicin, and netilmicin, each of which has been studied pharmacokinetically in horses. Amikacin and gentamicin are the 2 that have been evaluated in foals.[29,30] These drugs are bactericidal drugs, which bind to the 30S ribosome, thereby inhibiting bacterial protein synthesis. They are concentration dependent and polar, so that they distribute primarily to the extracellular fluids. Amikacin is the aminoglycoside of choice for foals with sepsis. This is because it has the broadest spectrum and most potent activity against gramnegative enteric bacteria. It also has the best activity and highest predicted efficacy against *Staphylococcus*, including MRSA in many cases.

The most common and significant potential adverse effect of aminoglycosides is renal injury. Foals with sepsis, hypoxic-ischemic injury, or prematurity are at highest risk of kidney injury from aminoglycosides because of concurrent hypoperfusion or reduced oxygen delivery already placing kidneys at risk for injury during sepsis.[31,32] Ototoxicity is also possible, although it is much less recognized in veterinary medicine as compared with human medicine. Neuromuscular blockage is another potential, although it is rarely clinically significant except perhaps during anesthesia or in foals with neuromuscular diseases such as botulism.

The pharmacokinetics of aminoglycosides can be altered by changes in renal blood flow, age, or renal function. They have been shown to be altered with hypoxic injury, prematurity, and sepsis.[32] The concurrent presence of hypoxic injury and prematurity caused an increased elimination half-life of amikacin in foals of one study.[32] Another study showed different results, whereby sepsis, prematurity, and hypoxemia did not alter the serum amikacin concentrations.[33] These contrasting results likely reflect case differences, with differences in foal populations and renal function.

Precaution should be used with aminoglycosides in foals with azotemia. The author prefers to use other options, such as third- or fourth-generation cephalosporins, when azotemia is present, because foals with renal injury have reduced clearance and are at risk for aminoglycoside toxicity. Foals with concurrent azotemia and hypoxia had reduced clearance of amikacin and resultant increases in peak and trough serum amikacin concentrations.[31] Despite this reduction in clearance and higher trough serum concentrations, amikacin-induced nephrotoxicity was not evident by laboratory testing or postmortem examination.[31] These alterations in amikacin pharmacokinetics during illness highlight the importance of therapeutic drug monitoring (TDM) of amikacin in foals with critical illness (**Table 2**).[34]

In addition to TDM, monitoring of foals on aminoglycosides should include frequent measurement of plasma creatinine concentration. Because critically ill foals are at risk of hypotension or perfusion-related disorders, creatinine should be monitored daily in such foals. Premature foals should also have daily creatinine measurement, because of reduced clearance. Frequent creatinine monitoring should not stop at evaluating for abnormal values. Rather, increasing trends, even when still within the normal range, should be concerning and warrant re-evaluation of the dosing protocol. Other tools to minimize nephrotoxicity in foals on amikacin therapy include evaluation of urine output and urinalyses. The author cautions against use of aminoglycosides in foals with decreased urine output. Hematuria and glucosuria can indicate tubular damage, provided it is present after the first 24 hours of life, because mild hematuria may be present on the first day of life.

TDM is a means of ensuring appropriate dosing protocol to maximize efficacy and minimize nephrotoxicity. Because aminoglycosides are concentration dependent, their efficacy is associated with high peak concentrations. Peaks that are 8- to 10-fold the MIC of the offending bacterial isolate are considered optimal for rate and extent of bacterial killing. If the MIC is known from blood culture and susceptibility testing, it can be used to determine the target peak. For example, if the MIC for a cultured *E coli* isolate for amikacin is 2 μg/mL, the desired peak would be 16 to 20 μg/mL. Because cultures are often negative in many cases of sepsis, then an empirical target should be used. A target of 40 μg/mL is used by the author for a 1-hour peak, because it is readily achievable in horses and foals at recommended

Table 2			
Therapeutic drug monitoring of aminoglycosides			
Drug	Peak (μg/mL)	8-h Level (μg/mL)	Trough (μg/mL)
Amikacin	30 min: ≥53–60 60 min: ≥40	15–20	20 h: <2 24 h: <1
Gentamicin	30 min: ≥30–40 60 min: ≥20	3–5	20 h: <1

doses, while still being safe. In addition, many gram-negative bacteria affecting septic foals have MIC values ≤ 4 μg/mL. Some clinicians use a 30-minute peak instead (see **Table 2**); for the 30-minute sample, the concentration should be ≥53 to 60 μg/mL, in order to approximate 40 μg/mL at 1 hour. With a 1-hour peak of 40 μg/mL, bacteria with an MIC of ≤4 to 5 μg/mL will be considered highly susceptible with optimal bactericidal effect. Even those up to 8 μg/mL might also be considered susceptible, if the 30-minute peak concentration is at least 60 to 64 μg/mL.

The second necessary sample to complete TDM is termed the "trough" concentration. This "trough" concentration is taken shortly before the subsequent daily dose and ensures that the drug has been cleared enough to minimize the potential for toxicity, because the uptake of aminoglycosides by the renal tubular epithelium is saturable. Allowing plasma amikacin concentrations to "trough" provides the renal tubular epithelium with the opportunity to evacuate any accumulated aminoglycosides before lysosomal rupture and cell damage can occur. With amikacin, the desired trough concentration should be drawn 20 to 24 hours after the dose is administered; in other words, it should be drawn just before or up to 4 hours before the subsequent dose. Recommended trough targets have varied considerably in the literature and textbooks over the years. The author seeks amikacin trough concentrations to be less than 2 μg/mL for the 20-hour sample, and less than 1 μg/mL for the 24-hour sample. The 20-hour sample is preferred whenever possible, because it would ensure that the tubules have a 4-hour window in which to evacuate intracellular accumulations of aminoglycoside. Recommended peak and trough concentrations for amikacin and gentamicin are listed in **Table 2**. If calculation of elimination half-life is desired, a third concentration should be measured at approximately 8 hours, because the 20- to 24-hour sample is often at or below the limit of detection of the assays (see **Table 2**).

The Clinical Laboratory Standards Institute (CLSI) provides guidelines for susceptibility and resistance breakpoints for human and veterinary infections. For amikacin, the CLSI susceptibility breakpoint is ≤16 μg/mL. However, with current recommended dosing protocols for foals, it would be difficult to obtain peak plasma concentrations of 128 to 160 μg/mL (ie, 8–10 times MIC). Several equine studies, including those done in foals, have found that most gram-negative bacterial isolates have an MIC ≤4 μg/mL, so the current dosing protocols are acceptable in the absence of positive cultures (**Table 3**).[33,35–37]

Potentiated sulfonamides

Potentiated sulfonamides consist of trimethoprim and sulfonamides, most commonly either sulfamethoxazole or sulfadiazine. Although sulfonamides and trimethoprim alone are bacteriostatic, the combination is synergistically bactericidal for many

Table 3
Aminoglycoside dosing for foals

Drug	Dosage	Comment
Antimicrobial agents		
Aminoglycosides		
Amikacin	25 mg/kg IV, every 24 h	TDM recommended Monitor creatinine + UA
Gentamicin	8–16 mg/kg IV, every 24 h	TDM recommended Monitor creatinine + UA

Abbreviation: UA, Urinalysis.

bacteria. They are time-dependent antimicrobials and work through inhibition of folate synthesis. Sulfonamides are para-aminobenzoic acid (PABA) analogues, and trimethoprim acts as an inhibitor of dihydrofolate reductase, the enzyme necessary to produce tetrahydrofolic acid in the pathway toward folate synthesis. It should be noted that the activity of potentiated sulfonamides is reduced in the presence of purulent exudates, because of excessive amounts of free PABA or thymidine. Because procaine is metabolized to PABA, procaine penicillin G and potentiated sulfonamides should not be used together.[10]

Potentiated sulfonamides, including trimethoprim-sulfamethoxazole or trimethoprim-sulfadiazine (TMS), have a moderate spectrum of activity, meaning they are relatively broad spectrum; however, they do not target all enteric gram-negative microbes and enterococci and have relatively poor anaerobe coverage. Because gram-negative bacteria are the most common isolates from septic foals, TMS is generally not considered a first-line antimicrobial combination for the treatment of sepsis in foals. Instead, they are sometimes used to prolong the course of antimicrobial treatment after foals have been initially treated with beta-lactam–aminoglycoside or cephalosporins and once the foal is stabilized.[38] Potentiated sulfonamides have activity against *Pneumocystis carinii*, a yeastlike fungal infection that has been associated with pneumonia in immunocompromised foals.

Because they can be PO administered, TMS formulations are convenient for continued antimicrobial therapy after the initial period of treatment; for example, they are often administered upon discharge from the hospital, depending on susceptibility results on the cultured isolate. They can also be used for less serious infections, including umbilical infections that are not extensive or rapidly progressive in foals. The pharmacokinetics of IV trimethoprim-sulfamethoxazole has been studied in neonatal foals, but additional studies evaluating the oral pharmacology are warranted.[39] Foals on trimethoprim sulfonamides should be monitored for diarrhea, liver enzyme increases, as well as bone marrow suppression with long-term use. IV formulations of TMS are available for horses, but they should not be used in any foal sedated with alpha-2 agonists (eg, xylazine, romifidine, detomidine), because of concerns over cardiovascular collapse.[9]

Chloramphenicol

Chloramphenicol is a relatively broad-spectrum, bacteriostatic, and time-dependent antimicrobial. It acts by binding the 50S ribosomal unit and inhibiting protein synthesis. It penetrates tissues well and enters the intracellular fluids, bone, and CNS because of its lipophilicity. Because it is bacteriostatic, and does not have a high percentage susceptibility among enteric microbes, its use in foal sepsis is limited. It may be used when oral antimicrobials are necessary for longer term therapy after initial therapy with IV and bactericidal antimicrobials, based on culture and susceptibility results.

If chloramphenicol is used in foals, the elimination half-life is age-dependent due to hepatic metabolism through glucuronyl transferase activity. After an IV dose of 25 mg/kg, for example, the mean elimination half-life for chloramphenicol was 5.29 hours in 1-day-old foals, 1.35 hours in 3-day-old foals, 0.61 hours in 7-day-old foals, and 0.51 hours in 14-day-old foals.[40] It is absorbed well in foals, in contrast to adults, with a high oral bioavailability (83%) in foals 1 to 9 days of age.[41] Chloramphenicol dosing should be based on age (**Table 4**).

Two advantages of chloramphenicol include its excellent anaerobic spectrum as well as reasonably high activity against *Enterococcus* isolates, which tend to be multidrug resistant. Ampicillin and chloramphenicol are the most consistent first-line antimicrobials effective against enterococci.

Table 4
Other antimicrobials available for use in foals

Drug	Dosage	Comment
Azithromycin	10 mg/kg PO, every 24 h; every 48 h after 5 d	Keep foal out of sunlight/heat
Clarithromycin	7.5 mg/kg PO, every 12 h	Keep foal out of sunlight/heat
Chloramphenicol[+]	40–50 mg/kg PO, every 12 h days 1–2 of age; every 8 h days of age 3–5	Handlers should wear gloves Should be used with caution in first few days of life; although not reported in foals, gray baby syndrome is a risk in human infants
Doxycycline	10 mg/kg PO, every 12 h	May cause tendon laxity
Minocycline	4 mg/kg PO, every 12 h	—
Rifampin	5 mg/kg PO, every 12 h	Stains urine and mucous membranes pink
Metronidazole for enteric clostridiosis	10 mg/kg PO, IV every 8–12 h for 1st 2 wk	—
Trimethoprim-sulfonamide	25–30 mg/kg PO, every 12 h	—

Other limitations of chloramphenicol, aside from its limited gram-negative enteric spectrum and bacteriostatic nature, include a potential for human toxicity in susceptible individuals. Humans are susceptible to bone marrow toxicity, which can occur in both reversible and, rarely, irreversible forms. Even contact exposure can rarely lead to toxicity. Therefore, clients should be warned of this risk, and gloves should be worn when handling chloramphenicol; the medication should not be aerosolized (ie, it should not be crushed). In addition, chloramphenicol is an inhibitor of hepatic microsomal metabolic activity, which can delay the clearance of other hepatic-metabolized drugs, including phenobarbital, which is a consideration in seizuring foals. This may warrant dose reductions in phenobarbital.

In human neonates, chloramphenicol poses a risk of "gray baby syndrome." Gray baby syndrome is a syndrome of hypotension, cyanosis, and often death. It results from lack of the hepatic enzymes necessary for metabolism, leading to chloramphenicol accumulation. Premature babies are at particular risk, and because of this syndrome, chloramphenicol is generally not administered to newborn or premature babies. Although this syndrome has not yet been described in foals, it should be used with caution in premature foals and with increased dosing intervals (eg, every 12 hours initially, then every 8 hours). Even in term foals, the drug should be administered twice daily for the first 1 to 2 days of life, then every 8 hours after that (**Table 4**). If it is used in newborn foals, they should be monitored for hypotension and hypoxemia. In addition, damage to the small intestinal mucosa was noted in young calves that were administered chloramphenicol powder for 5 days, resulting in reduced glucose absorption.[42] These actual and theoretic drawbacks of chloramphenicol significantly limit its use in the newborn foal with sepsis. It may have a place in older foals with umbilical and other localized infections, owing to its penetrability.

Tetracycline, doxycycline, and minocycline
The tetracycline group of antimicrobials is widely used in equine practice, but only occasionally used for the treatment of foals with infections, largely because of spectrum. They have excellent gram-positive aerobic coverage, with efficacy against

gram-negative nonenteric microbes as well. They have some activity against specific anaerobic bacteria. The primary deficit of this class of antimicrobials is in the gram-negative enteric microbial spectrum, which limits their usefulness as primary treatments for sepsis in foals. The fact that they are static is another limiting factor.

The tetracycline class includes tetracycline, oxytetracycline, doxycycline, and minocycline. These drugs are primarily bacteriostatic and lipophilic and have characteristics of both time and concentration dependency as far as efficacy. They penetrate intracellularly and into the CNS to varying degrees, with minocycline having the greatest degree of penetration, followed by doxycycline. Their mechanism of action is by binding the 30S ribosomal subunit, thereby inhibiting protein synthesis. Oxytetracycline and tetracycline are excreted primarily through renal elimination. Doxycycline and minocycline are also eliminated through the biliary route in addition to the renal route. Doxycycline also has some gastrointestinal elimination.

Potential adverse side effects of these antimicrobials include enamel discoloration in young animals, and potential effects on bone formation because they are incorporated into developing bone. Enamel and bone effects have not been reported in foals to date, despite both clinical and experimental use in foals.[43,44] Although doxycycline can cause staining of the teeth in children, it is less common than with other tetracyclines. Diarrhea and antimicrobial-associated colitis can also result. Oxytetracycline and tetracycline can cause nephrotoxicity, especially at high doses, whereas doxycycline and minocycline are generally considered safe for renal failure patients.

Oxytetracycline and tetracycline have very similar spectrums. The differences in coverage among tetracycline, doxycycline, and minocycline are primarily that doxycycline and minocycline have slightly expanded spectrums of coverage as compared with tetracycline. They have improved activity against gram-positive microbes as compared with oxytetracycline and tetracycline. Whereas in adult horses, doxycycline is recommended for the treatment of highly susceptible pathogens (MIC $\leq 0.25\ \mu g/mL$) because of very poor bioavailability, the absorption in foals (4–8 weeks of age) is such that microbes with an MIC $\leq 3\ \mu g/mL$ can be targeted.[43] This includes most *Pasteurella*, *Actinobacillus*, *Staphylococcus* (non-MRSA), *Streptococcus*, and *Rhodococcus equi* equine isolates.[43] Some *E coli* and *Klebsiella* isolates would also be expected to be susceptible at this concentration. Similarly, minocycline has significantly higher oral bioavailability in 6- to 9-week-old foals (57.8% $\pm$ 19.3%) than in adult horses (32.0% $\pm$ 18.0%).[44] Based on the pharmacokinetics of minocycline in adult horses, it has been recommended that minocycline be used to treat only those infections caused by bacteria with MIC values less than 0.25 $\mu g/mL$.[44] With the increased bioavailability in foals, bacteria with MIC values $\leq 1.0\ \mu g/mL$ can be targeted. This MIC target would include *Actinobacillus*, *Staphylococcus*, *R equi*, and *Streptococcus*. Some isolates of *E coli* would also be susceptible to this concentration.[44]

Oxytetracycline is administered at supra-antimicrobial doses to treat foal flexural limb contracture along with bandages and/or splints. When it is used for this purpose, it should be administered slowly and diluted in fluids. The formulations of oxytetracycline designed for IV use should be used, because the intramuscular formulations may contain propylene glycol. Serum creatinine concentration and urine output should be monitored in treated foals, because this high dose of oxytetracycline can result in acute kidney injury.[45] Doxycycline should not be administered IV, due to potential for fatal hemodynamic effects.

Macrolides

Macrolides used in foals include erythromycin and clarithromycin. Azithromycin is a closely related azalide. These antimicrobials have primarily gram-positive aerobic activity, with some gram-negative nonenteric efficacy (eg, *Pasteurella*, *Actinobacillus*), which severely limits their use in neonatal foals with sepsis. They can be used when foals have gram-positive or susceptible infections. They are primarily used for *R equi* infections in older foals, along with rifampin. Macrolides may be useful for foals with umbilical or other localized infections based on culture and susceptibility results, because of their limited spectrum. The reader is referred to the article (see Steeve Giguère's article, "Update on the Treatment of Infections Caused by *Rhodococcus equi*," in this issue) for further information on macrolide use in foals. It should be noted that the dams of foals being treated with macrolides should be monitored closely for acute diarrhea or colitis. In addition, foals on macrolides or azalides should be kept cool, because they result in thermoregulatory problems that may be associated with hypohidrosis or anhidrosis and can lead to hyperthermia.[46]

Rifampin

The pharmacokinetics of rifampin has been studied in 6- to 8-week-old foals.[47] Rifampin is in the rifamycin class of antimicrobials and has an excellent gram-positive spectrum, including many *Staphylococcus* isolates.[10] It also has efficacy against a few gram-negative nonenteric microbes, such as *Actinobacillus*, and some anaerobic coverage. The drug acts by inhibiting DNA-dependent RNA polymerase, is very lipophilic, penetrates into the CNS well, and concentrates inside white blood cells. It is time dependent and is either cidal or static depending on the specific isolate. Rifampin is primarily metabolized by the liver and eliminated in bile.[48]

The primary potential adverse effects of rifampin include antimicrobial-associated diarrhea, and it innocuously colors the urine and other body fluids red. It should not be administered IV, because that has been associated with weakness, hyperhidrosis, defecation, and distress during injection, even when performed slowly over 10 minutes.[48] It should be noted that rifampin is an inducer of hepatic microsomal enzymes, opposite to that of chloramphenicol. Therefore, it may increase the elimination of other liver-metabolized drugs such as phenobarbital. Another important note is that the elimination half-life of rifampin is longer in foals than adults, and it has greater oral bioavailability in young foals as compared with 6- to 10-week-old foals and adults.[48]

Its use is primarily in combination with macrolides or azalides for the treatment of *R equi* infection in foals ≥3 weeks of age. It is also occasionally used in combination with other antimicrobials for susceptible infections in younger foals that require good penetration for gram-positive or susceptible infections, such as umbilical abscesses. Unfortunately, bacteria can develop rapid resistance to rifampin when used as monotherapy; to avoid resistance, it should be used with other antimicrobials such as potentiated sulfonamides, macrolides, or aminoglycosides depending on the cultured isolate and corresponding susceptibility.

Fluoroquinolones

Fluoroquinolones, such as enrofloxacin and marbofloxacin, have excellent spectrum of activity against gram-negative bacteria and many *Staphylococcus* isolates. They lack in vivo activity against *Streptococcus* isolates and have poor anaerobic coverage. They are bactericidal, penetrate intracellularly well, and are concentration-dependent antimicrobials. They act through inhibition of DNA gyrase activity, inhibiting DNA replication and transcription. A topoisomerase IV enzyme, mediating unlinking and relaxation of DNA after replication, is another target of fluoroquinolone activity.

Despite their potent gram-negative activity, fluoroquinolones should not be used routinely in foals, especially in neonatal foals, because they can be associated with cartilage toxicity and subsequent arthropathy and lameness.[38] This has been demonstrated in neonatal foals administered enrofloxacin (10 mg/kg daily) for 8 days, starting at 14 days of age.[49,50] With IV administration, neurologic signs are also possible. One author has anecdotally used marbofloxacin in foals without obvious joint complications, but the risks are still a potential.[9]

Metronidazole

Metronidazole is a nitro-imidazole antimicrobial. It is bactericidal and lipid soluble and has excellent anaerobic activity. It has both concentration and time-dependent features in terms of antimicrobial efficacy. Metronidazole has no aerobic spectrum, but has antiprotozoal effects against *Giardia*. It has a high degree of efficacy against gram-negative anaerobes, whereas its activity against gram-positive anaerobes is slightly less. Notably, it is highly effective against *B fragilis* isolates that are resistant to beta-lactams, as well as clostridial agents. Its mechanism of action is through metabolism to free radicals by anaerobic bacteria, which damage their DNA. Potential side effects of metronidazole include diarrhea, anorexia, neurotoxicity, and hepatopathy. Metronidazole undergoes hepatic metabolism and excretion, with some additional excretion of metabolites into urine.

Metronidazole can be used IV, PO, or rectally. It has very high (>90%) oral bioavailability and has a longer elimination half-life in foals than in adults.[51] Because of this high bioavailability and longer half-life, it should be administered at a lower dose and less frequently to foals less than 14 days of age.[51] The author uses metronidazole at a dosage regimen of 10 mg/kg PO or IV, every 12 hours during the first 2 weeks of life in foals (**Table 4**).[51]

Metronidazole is used clinically when anaerobic infections are suspected, especially for walled off or abscessed infections that require penetration. In addition, it is a highly effective therapeutic for clostridial enteritis in foals, both *C perfringens* and *Clostridium difficile* enteritis.

SUMMARY

The combination of aminoglycosides and beta-lactam/cephalosporin has one of the broadest spectrums available for use in septic foals. Amikacin has the broadest gram-negative coverage of the available aminoglycosides and also has high activity against *Staphylococcus*. Amikacin can be paired with penicillin, ampicillin, first-generation cephalosporins, or ceftiofur. However, the most active of these beta-lactam drugs against *Enterococcus* isolates is ampicillin. When enterococci are cultured, or suspected as with urinary or umbilical infections, then ampicillin should be administered. Otherwise, the combination of ceftiofur and amikacin is nearly as effective in terms of percentage of susceptible isolates.[11]

Specifically, the combination of amikacin and ampicillin is a leading pairing of antimicrobials that is effective against 91.5% of isolates cultured from septic foals in a recent study.[11] Others with a close spectrum were ceftizoxime with 89.7% of isolates being susceptible, a combination of ceftiofur and amikacin with 89.6%, and a combination of amikacin and penicillin with 88.6% of isolates considered susceptible. Ceftiofur alone was effective against 86.3% of isolates in vitro, a combination of gentamicin and ampicillin with 83.6% efficacy, and a combination of gentamicin and penicillin with 82%.[11] Imipenem actually had the highest percentage in vitro efficacy with 92.6%[11]; however, carbapenems should be reserved for culture-directed therapy or for those foals where other antimicrobials have failed to provide clinical improvement in order to limit their use.

Once clinical improvement has occurred, and the foals are stabilized after 7 to 10 days of IV antimicrobial therapy, then they can be maintained on SC, IM, or PO medication to lengthen the duration of antimicrobial therapy. Ideally the choice of oral antimicrobial would be based on culture and susceptibility data, but if unavailable, there are several choices listed in **Tables 1** and **4**. These choices include oral cephalosporins, such as cefpodoxime. Ceftiofur can be administered SC or IM. Other oral choices, with narrower spectrums, include chloramphenicol, TMS, minocycline/doxycycline, and azithromycin. These latter drugs have better gram-positive than gram-negative spectrum. In the study by Theelen and colleagues,[11] chloramphenicol was effective, based on susceptibility data, against 81.6% of cultured isolates from septic foals, and TMS was effective against 59.6%.

REFERENCES

1. Fielding CL, Magdesian KG. Sepsis and septic shock in the equine neonate. Vet Clin Equine 2015;31:483–96.
2. Wilson WD, Madigan JE. Comparison of bacteriologic culture of blood and necropsy specimens for determining the cause of foal septicemia: 47 cases (1978-1987). J Am Vet Med Assoc 1989;195:1759–63.
3. Puskarich MA, Trzeciak S, Shapiro NI, et al. Association between timing of antibiotic administration and mortality from septic shock in patients treated with a quantitative resuscitation protocol. Crit Care Med 2011;39:2066–71.
4. Koterba AM, Brewer BD, Tarplee FA. Clinical and clinicopathological characteristics of the septicaemic neonatal foal: review of 38 cases. Equine Vet J 1984;16:376–82.
5. Raisis AL, Hogdson JL, Hodgson DR. Equine neonatal septicaemia: 24 cases. Aust Vet J 1996;73:137–40.
6. Marsh PS, Palmer JE. Bacterial isolates from blood and their susceptibility patterns in critically ill foals: 543 cases (1991-1998). J Am Vet Med Assoc 2001;218:1608–10.
7. Stewart AJ, Hinchcliff KW, Saville WJ, et al. Actinobacillus sp bacteremia in foals: clinical signs and prognosis. J Vet Intern Med 2002;16:464–71.
8. Theelen MJP, Wilson WD, Edman JM, et al. Temporal trends in prevalence of bacteria isolated from foals with sepsis: 1979-2010. Equine Vet J 2014;46:169–73.
9. Corley KTT, Hollis AR. Antimicrobial therapy in neonatal foals. Equine Vet Educ 2009;21:436–48.
10. Cole C. Basics of antimicrobial therapy for the horse. In: Cole C, Bentz B, Maxwell L, editors. Equine pharmacology. Amers (IA): Wiley Blackwell; 2015. p. 16–43.
11. Theelen MJP, Wilson WD, Byrne BA, et al. Cumulative antimicrobial susceptibility of bacteria isolated from foals with sepsis: 1990-2015. In: Proceedings of the 62nd Annual Convention of the American Association of Equine Practitioners. Orlando (FL); 2016. p. 497–8.
12. Duffee NE, Stang BE, Schaeffer DJ. The pharmacokinetics of cefadroxil over a range of oral doses and animal ages in the foal. J Vet Pharmacol Ther 1997;20:427–33.
13. Samitz EM, Jang SS, Hirsh DC. In vitro susceptibilities of selected obligate anaerobic bacteria obtained from bovine and equine sources. J Vet Diagn Invest 1996;8:121–3.
14. Brewer B, Koterba A. Bacterial isolates and susceptibility patterns in foals in a neonatal intensive care unit. Compend Contin Educ Pract Vet 1990;12:1773–81.

15. Henson S, Barton M. Bacterial isolates and antibiotic susceptibility patterns from septicemic neonatal foals: one 15 year retrospective study (1986–2000). The Dorothy Havemeyer Foundation. 2001. p. 50–2.
16. Sanchez LC, Giguere S, Lester GD. Factors associated with survival of neonatal foals with bacteremia and racing performance of surviving thoroughbreds: 423 cases (1982-2007). J Am Vet Med Assoc 2008;233:1446–52.
17. Wilkins PA. Disorders of foals. In: Reed SM, Bayly WM, Sellon DC, editors. Equine internal medicine. St Louis: Saunders; 2004. p. 1381–440.
18. Wilson WD. Rational selection of antimicrobials for use in horses. Proceedings of the American Association of Equine Practitioners, 47. 2001. p. 75–93.
19. Meyer S, Giguere S, Rodriquez R, et al. Pharmacokinetics of intravenous ceftiofur sodium and concentration in body fluids of foals. J Vet Pharmacol Ther 2009;32: 309–16.
20. Slovis NM, Wilson WD, Stanley SD, et al. Comparative pharmacokinetics and bioavailability of ceftiofur in horses after intravenous, intramuscular, and subcutaneous administration. Proc Am Assoc Equine Pract 2006;52:329–30.
21. Pusterla N, Hall TL, Wetzlich SE, et al. Pharmacokinetic parameters for single- and multi-dose regiments for subcutaneous administration of a high-dose ceftiofur crystalline-free acid to neonatal foals. J Vet Pharmacol Ther 2017;40:88–91.
22. Carrillo NA, Giguere S, Gronwall RR, et al. Disposition of orally administered cefpodoxime proxetil in foals and adult horses and minimum inhibitory concentration of the drug against common bacterial pathogens of horses. Am J Vet Res 2005; 66:30–5.
23. Gardner SY, Papich MG. Comparison of cefepime pharmacokinetics in neonatal foals and adult dogs. J Vet Pharmacol Ther 2001;24:187–92.
24. Rohdich N, Zschiesche E, Heckeroth A, et al. Treatment of septicaemia and severe bacterial infections in foals with a new Cefquinome formulation: a field study. Dtsch Tierarztl Wochenschr 2009;116:316–20.
25. Thomas E, Thomas V, Wilhelm C. Antibacterial activity of Cefquinome against equine bacterial pathogens. Vet Microbiol 2006;115:140–7.
26. Osthoff M, Siegemund M, Gianmarco B, et al. Prolonged administration of β-lactam antibiotics—a comprehensive review and critical appraisal. Swiss Med Wkly 2016;146:w14368.
27. Wearn JMG, Davis JL, Hodgson DR, et al. Pharmacokinetics of a continuous rate infusion of ceftiofur sodium in normal foals. J Vet Pharmacol Ther 2013;36(1): 99–101.
28. Hewson J, Johnson R, Arroyo LG, et al. Comparison of continuous infusion with intermittent bolus administration of cefotaxime on blood and cavity fluid drug concentrations in neonatal foals. J Vet Pharmacol Ther 2013;36:68–77.
29. Magdesian KG, Wilson WD, Mihalyi J. Pharmacokinetics of a high dose of amikacin administered at extended intervals to neonatal foals. Am J Vet Res 2004;65: 473–9.
30. Burton JA, Giguere S, Arnold RD. Pharmacokinetics, pulmonary disposition and tolerability of liposomal gentamicin and free gentamicin in foals. Equine Vet J 2015;47:467–72.
31. Green SL, Conlon PD, Mama K, et al. Effects of hypoxia and azotaemia on the pharmacokinetics of amikacin in neonatal foals. Equine Vet J 1992;24:475–9.
32. Green SL, Conlon PD. Clinical pharmacokinetics of amikacin in hypoxic premature foals. Equine Vet J 1993;25:276–80.

33. Bucki EP, Giguere S, Macpherson M, et al. Pharmacokinetics of once-daily amikacin in healthy foals and therapeutic drug monitoring in hospitalized equine neonates. J Vet Intern Med 2004;18:728–33.
34. Adland-Davenport P, Brown MP, Robinson JD, et al. Pharmacokinetics of amikacin in critically ill neonatal foals treated for presumed or confirmed sepsis. Equine Vet J 1990;22:18–22.
35. Adamson PJ, Wilson WD, Hirsh DC, et al. Susceptibility of equine bacterial isolates to antimicrobial agents. Am J Vet Res 1985;46:447–50.
36. Orsini JA, Soma LR, Rourke JE, et al. Pharmacokinetics of amikacin in the horse following intravenous and intramuscular administration. J Vet Pharmacol Ther 1985;8:194–201.
37. Jacks SS, Giguere S, Nguyen A. In vitro susceptibilities of Rhodococcus equi and other common equine pathogens to azithromycin, clarithromycin, and 20 other antimicrobials. Antimicrob Agents Chemother 2003;47:1742–5.
38. Magdesian KG. Foals are not just mini horses. In: Cole C, Bentz B, Maxwell L, editors. Equine pharmacology. Ames (IA): Wiley Blackwell; 2015. p. 99–117.
39. Brown MP, McCartney JH, Gronwall R, et al. Pharmacokinetics of trimethoprim-sulphamethoxazole in two-day-old foals after a single intravenous injection. Equine Vet J 1990;22:51–3.
40. Adamson PJ, Wilson WD, Baggot JD, et al. Influence of age on the disposition kinetics of chloramphenicol in equine neonates. Am J Vet Res 1991;52:426–31.
41. Brumbaugh GW, Martens RJ, Knight HD, et al. Pharmacokinetics of chloramphenicol in the neonatal horse. J Vet Pharmacol Ther 1983;6:219–27.
42. Rollin RE, Mero KN, Kozisek PB, et al. Diarrhea and malabsorption changes in calves associated with therapeutic doses of antibiotics: absorptive and clinical changes. Am J Vet Res 1986;47:987–91.
43. Womble A, Giguere S, Lee EA. Pharmacokinetics of oral doxycycline and concentrations in body fluids and bronchoalveolar cells of foals. J Vet Pharmacol Ther 2007;30:187–93.
44. Giguere S, Burton AJ, Berghaus LJ, et al. Comparative pharmacokinetics of minocycline in foals and adult horses. J Vet Pharmacol Ther 2016. [Epub ahead of print].
45. Vivrette S, Cowgill LD, Pascoe J, et al. Hemodialysis for treatment of oxtetracycline-induced acute renal failure in a neonatal foal. J Am Vet Med Assoc 1993;203:105–7.
46. Stieler AL, Sanchez LC, Mallicote MF, et al. Macrolide-induced hyperthermia in foals: role of impaired sweat responses. Equine Vet J 2016;48:590–4.
47. Castro LA, Brown MP, Gronwall R, et al. Pharmacokinetics of rifampin given as a single oral dose in foals. Am J Vet Res 1986;47:2584–6.
48. Burrows GE, Macallister CG, Ewing P, et al. Rifampin disposition in the horse: effects of age and method of oral administration. J Vet Pharmacol Ther 1992;15:124–32.
49. Davenport CL, Boston RC, Richardson DW. Effects of enrofloxacin and magnesium deficiency on matrix metabolism in equine articular cartilage. Am J Vet Res 2001;62:160–6.
50. Vivrette SL, Bostian A, Bermingham E, et al. Quinolone-induced arthropathy in neonatal foals. In: Proceedings of the 47th Annual Convention of the American Association of Equine Practitioners. Denver (CO); 2001. p. 376–7.
51. Swain EA, Magdesian KG, Kass PH, et al. Pharmacokinetics of metronidazole in foals: influence of age within the neonatal period. J Vet Pharmacol Ther 2014;38:227–34.

Treatment of Infections Caused by *Rhodococcus equi*

Steeve Giguère, DVM, PhD

KEYWORDS

- *Rhodococcus equi* • Pneumonia • Macrolide • Rifampin

KEY POINTS

- The combination of a macrolide (erythromycin, azithromycin, or clarithromycin) with rifampin remains the recommended therapy for foals with clinical signs of infection caused by *Rhodococcus equi*.
- Most foals with mild subclinical ultrasonographic pulmonary lesions associated with *R equi* recover without therapy, and administration of antimicrobial agents to these subclinically affected foals does not hasten lesion resolution relative to administration of a placebo.
- Emergence of widespread resistance to macrolides and rifampin in isolates of *R equi* at some farms complicates selection of antimicrobial agents. There are no data to indicate the preferred antimicrobial agent or agents for the treatment of foals infected with isolates resistant to macrolides and rifampin.

INTRODUCTION

Pneumonia is the leading cause of disease and death in foals in some states[1] and ranks third as a cause of morbidity and second (after a combined category of trauma, injury, and wounds) as a cause of mortality in the United States.[2] Although many microorganisms cause respiratory disease in foals, *Rhodococcus equi* is considered the most common cause of severe pneumonia.[3] The most common clinical manifestation of disease caused by *R equi* is pyogranulomatous bronchopneumonia with abscessation. *R equi* can also be cultured from a large variety of extrapulmonary sites of infection. Extrapulmonary disorders might occur concurrent with or independent of pneumonia, and some foals have multiple extrapulmonary disorders concurrently.[4,5] Because ultrasonographic screening for early detection has become routine practice at many farms endemic for pneumonia caused by *R equi*, the most frequently recognized form of *R equi* infection on those farms is a subclinical form in which foals

Department of Large Animal Medicine, Veterinary Medical Center, University of Georgia, Athens GA 30605
E-mail address: gigueres@uga.edu

Vet Clin Equine 33 (2017) 67–85
http://dx.doi.org/10.1016/j.cveq.2016.11.002
0749-0739/17/© 2016 Elsevier Inc. All rights reserved.

develop sonographic evidence of peripheral pulmonary consolidation or abscessation without manifesting clinical signs.[6,7]

Because *R equi* is a facultative intracellular pathogen that can survive and replicate in macrophages, there is an apparent disconnect between in vitro activity of antimicrobial agents and their in vivo efficacy. Since the 1980s, the standard treatment recommendation for foals infected with *R equi* has been the combination of a macrolide (erythromycin initially and more recently clarithromycin or azithromycin) with rifampin. Based on the information currently available, this recommendation still stands. However, 3 very important discoveries have recently muddled what we thought we knew regarding antimicrobial therapy of infections caused by *R equi* in foals. First, most foals with subclinical pulmonary lesions associated with *R equi* recover without therapy, and administration of antimicrobial agents to many subclinically affected foals does not necessarily hasten lesion resolution relative to administration of a placebo.[8,9] These findings underscore the importance of inclusion of a placebo control group in studies designed to evaluate therapy and cast doubt on prior uncontrolled studies commonly cited in the literature. Second, recent studies demonstrate that concurrent therapy with rifampin considerably decreases concentrations of clarithromycin and potentially other macrolides, which has led some to question the use of the combination.[10,11] Finally, emergence of widespread resistance to macrolides and rifampin in isolates of *R equi* at some farms further complicates selection of antimicrobial agents.

This text reviews available data regarding treatment of infections caused by *R equi*. Because of the high rate of spontaneous resolution in foals with subclinical ultrasonographic lesions, treatment trials performed in this population cannot be directly applied to the treatment of foals with severe clinical disease. Therefore, treatment recommendations for these 2 clinical manifestations are addressed.

EXPERIMENTAL EVIDENCE
Activity of Antimicrobial Agents Against Rhodococcus equi

In vitro activity of antimicrobial agents against Rhodococcus equi
Drugs with the highest in vitro activity against *R equi* based on minimal inhibitory concentrations (MIC) are clarithromycin, rifampin, imipenem, telithromycin, erythromycin, gentamicin, vancomycin, azithromycin, gamithromycin, doxycycline, enrofloxacin, and linezolid (**Table 1**). Timethoprim-sulfonamide combinations are also active in vitro against most isolates. Not all macrolides are equally active, with tildipirosin, tilmicosin, tulathromycin, and tylosin being poorly active against *R equi* in vitro. Most drugs including macrolides and rifampin exert only bacteriostatic activity against *R equi* with only amikacin, gentamicin, enrofloxacin, and vancomycin being bactericidal.[12] It is important to emphasize that the Clinical and Laboratory Standards Institute has not established interpretive criteria for the classification of isolates of *R equi* as susceptible, intermediate, or resistant. Therefore, interpretive criteria reported by diagnostic laboratories are extrapolated from criteria established for other bacterial agents and, for most drugs, based on therapeutic concentrations achievable in humans or other animal species.

Combinations including a macrolide (erythromycin, clarithromycin, or azithromycin) and either rifampin or doxycycline, and the combination doxycycline-rifampin, are highly synergistic against *R equi* in vitro.[12–14] In contrast, combinations containing amikacin and erythromycin, clarithromycin, azithromycin, or rifampin and the combination gentamicin-rifampin are antagonistic.[12–14] However, the clinical significance of these in vitro findings has not been established.

Given the recent emergence of resistance to macrolides and rifampin among isolates of *R equi* (see later discussion), the relative propensity of currently available

Table 1
Minimal inhibitory concentrations data for *Rhodococcus equi* isolates susceptible to macrolides and rifampin

Antimicrobial Classes/Agents	n	MIC (μg/mL)		
		MIC_{90}[c]	MIC_{50}[d]	Range
Macrolides/azalides/ketolides				
Azithromycin	264	1	1	0.06–4
Clarithromycin	264	0.06	0.06	0.008–0.5
Erythromycin	263	0.5	0.5	0.06–1
Gamithromycin	30	1	1	0.5–1
Telithromycin	25	0.25	0.25	0.25–0.5
Tildipirosin	40	32	16	8–32
Tilmicosin	278	64	32	0.5– >64
Tulathromycin	278	>64	64	8– >64
Tylosin	200	32	32	1–64
Rifamycins				
Rifampin	194	0.12	0.06	0.008–0.25
Beta-lactams				
Ampicillin	264	8	4	0.06–8
Amoxicillin-clavulanic acid[a]	264	8	4	0.06–16
Penicillin G	200	4	4	0.03–8
Cefazolin	64	16	≤2	≤2– >16
Cefotaxime	200	8	8	0.12–16
Ceftiofur	278	16	8	0.25–16
Cefquinome	200	4	2	0.12–8
Imipenem	200	0.12	0.12	0.015–0.25
Aminoglycosides				
Amikacin	64	4	≤2	≤2–8
Gentamicin	264	0.5	0.5	0.12–1
Tetracycline				
Tetracycline	264	8	4	0.5–16
Doxycycline	278	1	1	0.25–2
Other classes				
Chloramphenicol	342	16	8	≤4–32
Clindamycin	264	8	2	0.8–8
Enrofloxacin	264	1	1	0.25–4
Florfenicol	200	16	16	4–32
Linezolid	78	1	1	0.5–2
Trimethoprim/sulfamethoxazole[b]	342	1	0.5	0.06– >4
Vancomycin	278	0.5	0.5	0.12–1

[a] Expressed as MIC of ampicillin.
[b] Expressed as MIC of trimethoprim.
[c] MIC that inhibits at least 90% of the isolates tested.
[d] MIC that inhibits at least 50% of the isolates tested.
Adapted from Refs.[18,57,60,83]

antimicrobial agents to selectively enrich for resistant mutant subpopulations among *R equi* isolates has been studied. A common way to compare drugs for selective enrichment of resistant mutants is based on measurement of the mutant prevention concentration (MPC). The MPC is defined as the drug concentration that prevents selective enrichment of first-step resistant mutants within a large susceptible bacterial population. The range of concentrations between the MIC and the MPC is known as the mutant selection window (MSW), which represents the danger zone for emergence of resistant mutants.[15] Minimizing the length of time that the drug concentrations remain in the MSW may reduce the likelihood for development of resistance during therapy. Of 10 antimicrobial agents studied, rifampin had the highest MPC, indicating that rifampin monotherapy is likely to select for resistance.[16] However, combining rifampin with erythromycin, clarithromycin, or azithromycin resulted in a profound and significant decrease in MPC, indicating that the combination of a macrolide with rifampin considerably decreases the in vitro emergence of resistant mutants of *R equi* relative to monotherapy.[16]

Activity of antimicrobial agents against intracellular Rhodococcus equi
The ability of *R equi* to survive and replicate in macrophages is at the basis of its pathogenicity, and strains unable to replicate intracellularly are avirulent for foals.[17] Many drugs active against *R equi* in vitro have been hypothesized to be ineffective in vivo because of poor cellular uptake and resultant low intracellular concentrations. Studies with facultative intracellular bacterial pathogens have shown that evaluation of the bactericidal activity of antimicrobial agents against intracellular bacteria is more closely associated with in vivo efficacy than traditional in vitro susceptibility testing. In one study, clarithromycin was more active than azithromycin, erythromycin, and gamithromycin against intracellular *R equi*.[18] More recently, equine monocyte-derived macrophages were infected with virulent *R equi* and exposed to erythromycin, clarithromycin, azithromycin, rifampin, ceftiofur, gentamicin, enrofloxacin, vancomycin, imipenem, or doxycycline at concentrations achievable in plasma at clinically recommended dosages in foals. Enrofloxacin, gentamicin, and vancomycin were significantly more active than other drugs against intracellular *R equi*, whereas doxycycline was the least active drug.[12] Despite having the highest activity against intracellular *R equi*, the clinical applications of enrofloxacin are limited due to the risk of arthropathy in treated foals.[19]

Pharmacodynamics
The pharmacokinetics of most antimicrobial agents active against *R equi* has been studied in foals. However, determination of the appropriate dose and dosing interval of antimicrobial agents requires knowledge and integration of their pharmacokinetics and pharmacodynamic properties. Pharmacodynamic properties address the relationship between drug concentration and antimicrobial activity. Although the pharmacodynamic parameters best predicting the efficacy of a given drug are often similar across bacterial species, this is not always the case. In time-kill curve experiments, gentamicin, amikacin, enrofloxacin, and doxycycline exhibit concentration-dependent activity against virulent *R equi*, whereas erythromycin, clarithromycin, azithromycin, rifampin, ceftiofur, imipenem, and vancomycin exhibit time-dependent activity.[12]

The postantibiotic effect (PAE) is defined as persistent suppression of bacterial growth after a brief exposure of bacteria to an antibiotic. The presence and length of the PAE vary considerably for different antibiotics and microorganisms. The PAEs of rifampin, erythromycin, clarithromycin, vancomycin, and doxycycline against

R equi are relatively long with median values ranging between 4.5 and 6.5 hours. Azithromycin, gentamicin, and imipenem have intermediate PAEs ranging between 3.3 and 3.5 hours. Amikacin, enrofloxacin, and ceftiofur have shorter PAEs ranging between 1.3 and 2.1 hours.

In general, plasma concentrations of macrolides in humans and cattle are considerably lower than the MIC of the pathogens against which these drugs have been proven to be effective. Thus, plasma concentrations of macrolides are considered poor predictors of in vivo efficacy against respiratory pathogens, whereas concentrations at the site of infection provide more clinically relevant information.[20] Measurement of drug concentration in pulmonary epithelial lining fluid (PELF) and cells collected by bronchoalveolar lavage (BAL) is a widely used method to estimate antimicrobial concentrations at the site of infection for antimicrobials intended to treat lower respiratory tract infections in humans.[20,21]

Pulmonary Pharmacokinetics of Antimicrobial Drugs Used to Treat Infections Caused by Rhodococcus equi in Foals

Macrolides

The pharmacokinetics of azithromycin, clarithromycin, and azithromycin has been studied in foals. Several formulations of erythromycin are commercially available. Although they all show slight differences in bioavailability and elimination, they all result in therapeutic plasma concentrations at recommended dosages. However, the bioavailability of erythromycin in foals is considerably lower when foals are not fasted (mean $\pm$ SD: 26 $\pm$ 15% when fasted and 8 $\pm$ 7% when fed).[22] Advantages of azithromycin and clarithromycin over erythromycin in foals include enhanced oral bioavailabilities especially in the absence of fasting, prolonged half-lives, and much higher concentrations in BAL cells and PELF.[23–26] These properties of the newer generation macrolides contribute to their lower dosages and longer dosing intervals. After equivalent doses, concentrations of clarithromycin in PELF and BAL cells of foals are considerably higher than concentrations reported after administration of azithromycin or erythromycin to foals (**Table 2**).[24–26] However, clarithromycin concentrations at

Table 2
Plasma and pulmonary concentrations (mean ± SD) of macrolides commonly used for the treatment of *Rhodococcus equi* infections in foals

	Erythromycin	Azithromycin	Clarithromycin
Oral bioavailability (%)	25 ± 15^{a}; 8 ± 7^{b}	54 ± 23^{b}	57 ± 12^{b}
Single oral dose (10 mg/kg; fasted)			
C_{max} plasma (μg/mL)	0.80 ± 0.74	0.83 ± 0.19	0.94 ± 0.31
C_{max} PELF (μg/mL)	ND	10.0 ± 7.5	49.0 ± 13.3
C_{max} BAL cells (μg/mL)	1.02 ± 1.11	49.9 ± 26.9	74.2 ± 45.8
$t_{1/2}$ plasma (h)	2.2 ± 2.6	25.7 ± 15.4	4.0 ± 2.1
$t_{1/2}$ PELF (h)	ND	34.8 ± 30.9	8.6 ± 4.2
$t_{1/2}$ BAL cells (h)	ND	54.4 ± 17.5	10.7 ± 7.1

Abbreviations: C_{max}, maximum concentration; ND, not determined because quantifiable erythromycin activity was not detected in a sufficient number of animals or time points; $t_{1/2}$, terminal half-life.
[a] Mean ($\pm$SD) oral bioavailability after fasting.
[b] Mean ($\pm$SD) bioavailability with ad libitum access to milk, water, and hay.
Adapted from Refs.[22–24,26,84]

these sites decrease rapidly, whereas the release of azithromycin from cells is much slower, resulting in sustained concentrations of azithromycin in the lungs for days following discontinuation of therapy.[23-26]

Availability of a long-acting macrolide antimicrobial agent providing sustained therapeutic concentrations at the site of infection would result in less frequent administration, which in turn might improve compliance. Tulathromycin and tilmicosin, 2 semisynthetic macrolides approved for use in cattle, have been shown to concentrate and persist in BAL cells of foals after intramuscular administration.[25,27] However, clinically achievable concentrations in BAL cells after intramuscular administration at recommended dosages are much lower than the MIC of these drugs against R equi. In contrast, gamithromycin, another long-acting macrolide approved for the treatment and control of respiratory disease in cattle, is active against R equi in vitro and intramuscular administration of gamithromycin at a dosage of 6 mg/kg maintains BAL cell concentrations above the MIC against R equi for approximately 7 days.[18]

Rifampin
The pharmacokinetics of rifampin has been studied in foals and adult horses. The oral bioavailability of rifampin is approximately 49% (range 26%–61%) in adult horses.[28] Although absolute bioavailability has not been determined in foals, relative bioavailability is significantly higher in foals up to 10 weeks of age than in adult horses.[29] Although rifampin concentrations in PELF and BAL cells are lower than concurrent plasma concentrations, they are well above the MIC_{90} of susceptible isolates of R equi (**Table 3**).

Table 3
Pulmonary disposition of rifampin (10 mg/kg orally every 12 h) in foals and effect of coadministration of rifampin on the disposition of clarithromycin (7.5 mg/kg orally every 12 h) concentrations in plasma, pulmonary epithelial lining fluid, and bronchoalveolar lavage cells

Study/Variable	Rifampin	Clarithromycin	
		Without Rifampin	With Rifampin
Administration for 5 d			
AUC_{0-12h} (µg · h/mL)	160 ± 48.8	4.76 ± 3.50	1.17 ± 0.93
C_{max} plasma (µg/mL)	18.1 ± 5.59	0.61 ± 0.37	0.18 ± 0.14
C_{12h} plasma (µg/mL)	10.8 ± 3.66	0.21 ± 0.23	0.05 ± 0.06
$t_{1/2}$ plasma	14.7 ± 3.18	7.17 ± 1.92	7.25 ± 2.11
C_{12h} PELF (µg/mL)	8.49 ± 4.10	9.95 ± 19.9	3.34 ± 5.54
C_{12h} BAL cells (µg/mL)	4.01 ± 1.04	116 ± 137	24.8 ± 29.0
Administration for 10 d			
AUC_{0-12h} (µg · h/mL)	ND	5.54 ± 4.42	0.35 ± 0.31
C_{max} plasma (µg/mL)	ND	0.61 ± 0.37	0.07 ± 0.01
C_{12h} plasma (µg/mL)	ND	0.30 ± 0.27	0.01 ± 0.01
$t_{1/2}$ plasma	ND	6.11 ± 0.83	6.88 ± 3.44
C_{12h} PELF (µg/mL)	ND	9.49 ± 6.12	0.69 ± 0.66
C_{12h} BAL cells (µg/mL)	ND	264 ± 375	10.2 ± 10.2

Abbreviations: AUC_{0-12h}, area under the plasma concentration versus time curve from time 0 to 12 h; C_{12h} BAL cells, concentration in BAL cells 12 h after administration; C_{12h} PELF, concentration in PELF 12 h after administration; C_{12h}, plasma concentration 12 h after administration; C_{max}, peak plasma concentration; ND, not determined.
Adapted from Refs.[10,30]

Interactions between macrolides and rifampin

Recent studies demonstrate that concurrent therapy with rifampin considerably decreases plasma, PELF, and BAL cell concentrations of clarithromycin most likely through inhibition of intestinal uptake transporters.[10,30] In contrast, the disposition of rifampin is not affected by concurrent administration of clarithromycin.[30] Despite the profound decrease in clarithromycin bioavailability caused by concurrent administration with rifampin, concentrations of clarithromycin in PELF and BAL cells are well in excess of the MIC_{90} (0.06 µg/mL) and even the MPC (0.24 µg/mL when combined with rifampin) of clarithromycin against *R equi* (see **Table 3**),[10,30] which likely explains the apparent clinical efficacy of the combination (see later discussion) despite the decrease in bioavailability. Administration of rifampin 4 hours after administration of clarithromycin results in a statistically significant improvement in the bioavailability of clarithromycin, although the modest improvement is unlikely to be of clinical relevance.[31]

In rats, concurrent administration of rifampin inhibits absorption of clarithromycin and azithromycin by 45% and 65%, respectively.[32] Although not studied in foals, it is likely that absorption of other oral macrolides is also impaired by coadministration of rifampin. Interactions between macrolides and rifampin might not be only limited to orally administered drugs because concentrations of tulathromycin in the lung of foals after intramuscular administration are significantly lowered by co-medication with rifampin.[11]

Other drugs

The pulmonary pharmacokinetics of doxycycline, gentamicin, and telithromycin has also been studied in foals. A dosage of doxycycline of 10 mg/kg every 12 hours orally results in plasma, PELF, and bronchoalveolar doxycycline activity above the MIC_{90} of *R equi* isolates (1.0 µg/mL) for the entire dosing interval.[33] Gentamicin sulfate administered intravenously or by nebulization at a dose of 6.6 mg/kg every 24 hours also results in potentially therapeutic concentrations in PELF and BAL cells.[34] In the same study, encapsulation of gentamicin into liposomes was found to result in significantly higher concentrations of the drug in BAL cells relative to free gentamicin when administered intravenously or by nebulization at the aforementioned dose.[34] Telithromycin is a semisynthetic ketolide antibiotic chemically derived from the 14-membered lactone ring structure of the macrolides. The structural modifications allow dual binding to bacterial ribosomal RNA, conferring the advantage of overcoming some of the current mechanisms of resistance to macrolides. Although telithromycin results in therapeutic concentrations in PELF and BAL cells of foals, it is unlikely to offer a considerable advantage over macrolides because isolates of *R equi* resistant to macrolides are also resistant, albeit to a slightly lower degree, to telithromycin.[35]

Comparisons of Treatments Based on Experimental Infection with Rhodococcus equi

Mice

Although immunocompetent mice clear a large inoculum of *R equi* that would be sufficient to cause severe pneumonia in foals, immunodeficient mice lacking functional T lymphocytes develop chronic infection after intravenous or intranasal challenge with *R equi*. Immunodeficient mice have been used to assess the virulence of *R equi* and to compare in vivo efficacy of antimicrobial drugs. In an experimental model of *R equi* infection in athymic nude mice, the most effective drugs in monotherapy were vancomycin, imipenem, and rifampin.[36] Amikacin, erythromycin, ciprofloxacin, or minocycline in monotherapy did not lead to a significant decrease in bacterial counts. The combination of erythromycin with rifampin was significantly more effective than either drug alone.[36]

Given that concurrent administration of rifampin considerably decreases bioavailability of clarithromycin in foals (see above), a similar mouse infection model was used to compare the in vivo activity of clarithromycin and rifampin alone or in combination. Despite significantly lower clarithromycin concentrations in mice treated with the combination, treatment with clarithromycin and rifampin in combination significantly decreased the number of R equi in the organs of nude mice compared with treatment with either drug alone.[37] The numbers of R equi in the organs of mice treated with clarithromycin or rifampin alone were not significantly different from that of saline controls.[37] Again using a similar model, treatment with liposomal gentamicin resulted in a significantly greater reduction in the number of R equi in the spleen compared with treatment with free gentamicin and in the liver compared with treatment with clarithromycin in combination with rifampin.[38] Liposomal gentamicin has also been shown to colocalize with R equi in equine alveolar macrophages, indicating that the drug reaches the intracellular vacuole where R equi replicates.[38]

Foals

Few studies have compared the efficacy of various therapies using experimental infection of foals. In addition to the obvious ethical concerns and cost associated with such studies, there are also technical difficulties with model refinement. The success and outcome of experimental infection of foals with R equi depend on the virulence of the isolate, size of the inoculum, age at time of infection, and prior exposure of the foal to R equi with resulting immunity.[17,39–42] Administration of a large inoculum to a very young foal will likely prove fatal regardless of treatment.[43] In contrast, a lower inoculum or infection of an older foal previously exposed to R equi might result in spontaneous resolution even without therapy. It is difficult to find the perfect combination of inoculum size and age that produces consistent lesions in all foals without the possibility of spontaneous resolution. In one study using a high inoculum in 4-day-old foals, streptolysin O used as an adjunct to clarithromycin and rifampin resulted in significantly lower bacterial counts in the lungs and longer survival times relative to foals receiving either antibiotics or streptolysin O alone.[43] In a small pilot study, liposomal gentamicin was of similar efficacy as the combination of clarithromycin with rifampin.[44] However, the study was underpowered and lacked an untreated control group, and evidence of nephrotoxicity in 2 foals indicated that a longer dosing interval or alternative route (such as nebulization) would be needed before liposomal gentamicin can be considered adequately safe for clinical use. Liposomal gentamicin is not commercially available currently.

RECOMMENDATIONS FOR THE TREATMENT OF FOALS WITH CLINICAL PNEUMONIA OR EXTRAPULMONARY INFECTIONS
Antimicrobial Therapy

There are no randomized controlled studies comparing various treatments in foals with clinical signs of pneumonia caused by R equi. The only data available come from retrospective cohorts and comparisons to historical controls. In a retrospective cohort of 48 foals referred to a veterinary teaching hospital between 1978 and 1985, all 10 foals treated with erythromycin-rifampin survived compared with 2 of 4 with trimethoprim-sulfa, 2 of 6 with chloramphenicol, 0 of 4 treated with oxytetracycline, and 0 of 17 with penicillin-gentamicin.[45] In the aforementioned study, the combination of erythromycin-rifampin was introduced in 1981, and it is unknown if disease severity influenced treatment allocation. In another report published in the same issue of

Veterinary Microbiology, 50 of 57 (88%) foals with culture-confirmed pneumonia caused by *R equi* survived between 1981 and 1986. These reports, in association with the previously reported in vitro activity and synergism of erythromycin and rifampin,[14] became the basis of recommended therapy with erythromycin and rifampin. Since the early 2000s, azithromycin and clarithromycin have replaced erythromycin in the combination with rifampin for the pharmacologic reasons described above. Several retrospective cohorts of foals with severe culture-confirmed *R equi* pneumonia referred to veterinary teaching hospitals have reported survival proportions ranging between 69% and 82% in foals treated with a macrolide in combination with rifampin.[4,46,47] The survival proportion in presumptively less severe clinical cases treated at the farm is likely higher, ranging between 87% and 97%.[3,48,49] The survival proportion of foals with extrapulmonary infections such as osteomyelitis or abdominal abscesses is much lower.[4]

There are no data from randomized prospective studies comparing the relative efficacy of erythromycin, clarithromycin, and azithromycin in pneumonic foals. In a retrospective study, the combination clarithromycin-rifampin was significantly more effective than erythromycin-rifampin or azithromycin-rifampin, especially in foals with severe radiographic lesions.[47] Although data analysis was adjusted for disease severity, these results must be interpreted with caution because foals were not randomly assigned to treatment groups and because of potential biases inherent to retrospective data. Nevertheless, these data are the best available evidence to guide macrolide selection in foals with *R equi* pneumonia.

The recent discovery of the pharmacologic interactions between rifampin and macrolides (see above) has led some to question the value of the combination. A well-designed, large-scale blinded clinical trial is needed to determine the benefit (or detriment) of combining a macrolide with rifampin for treating foals with severe *R equi* pneumonia. However, such study is unlikely to be performed owing to the very large sample size that would be required, clinician preferences, and logistical and financial requirements for its conduct. In the meantime, 30 years of clinical experience and retrospective data document the efficacy of the combination in foals and animal models indicate the superiority of the combination relative to macrolide monotherapy. Conversely, there is a complete lack of evidence that macrolide monotherapy is effective in foals with severe clinical pneumonia. Until it is documented that a macrolide alone is as effective as the combination with rifampin, the combination of a macrolide (erythromycin, azithromycin, or clarithromycin) with rifampin remains the recommended treatment (**Table 4**).[50,51] Recommended dosages are presented in **Table 5**.

Table 4
Antimicrobial treatment recommendations for foals with clinical infections caused by *Rhodococcus equi* or with subclinical pulmonary lesions detected by ultrasonography

Clinical Scenario	Recommended Therapy
Clinical pulmonary or extrapulmonary infection	Macrolide (erythromycin, clarithromycin, or azithromycin) in combination with rifampin
Small subclinical pulmonary lesions detected by ultrasonography	Daily clinical monitoring and weekly thoracic ultrasonography. Antimicrobial therapy not indicated unless the foal develops clinical signs or the lesions become progressively more severe over time
Large or numerous subclinical pulmonary lesions	Macrolide (erythromycin, clarithromycin, or azithromycin) in combination with rifampin; alternatively, macrolide monotherapy with erythromycin, clarithromycin, azithromycin, or gamithromycin may be used

Table 5
Recommended dosages for antimicrobial drugs used for the treatment of infections caused by *Rhodococcus equi*

Drug	Dose (mg/kg)	Route	Dosing Interval
Azithromycin	10	PO	Every 24–48 h[a]
Clarithromycin	7.5	PO	Every 12 h
Erythromycin	25	PO	Every 6–8 h
Gamithromycin	6	IM	Every 7 d
Rifampin	5	PO	Every 12 h

Abbreviations: IM, intramuscularly; PO, orally.
[a] Every 24 h for 5 d and every 48 h thereafter.

Resolution of clinical signs, normalization of plasma fibrinogen concentrations, and radiographic or ultrasonographic resolution of lung lesions are commonly used to guide the duration of therapy, which generally ranges between 3 and 12 weeks, depending on the severity of the initial lesions and response to therapy. Foals treated based on subclinical lesions identified during ultrasonographic screening typically do not require as long a treatment period as foals in respiratory distress with severe pulmonary lesions (see later discussion).

Mixed bacterial infections
A variety of bacteria and fungi are often isolated from tracheobronchial aspirates along with *R equi*. The most common concurrent bacterial isolates are beta-hemolytic streptococci and *Escherichia coli*.[52] However, isolation of multiple types of bacteria or fungi from a tracheobronchial aspirate does not negatively impact survival, and mixed infections are significantly more likely to be encountered in tracheobronchial aspirates than in lung tissue, suggesting that many bacteria isolated from a tracheobronchial aspirate colonize the trachea without necessarily contributing to pulmonary abnormality.[52] It is common practice to add a third antimicrobial agent if heavy growth of a gram-negative pathogen resistant to macrolides and rifampin is isolated along with *R equi*. However, recent retrospective data indicate that this practice may not be beneficial.[52]

Treatment of foals infected with isolates of Rhodococcus equi resistant to macrolides and/or rifampin
Although the vast majority of *R equi* isolates from foals are highly susceptible to macrolides and rifampin, strains resistant to either drug class have been encountered. In a recent study, the overall prevalence of macrolide and rifampin–resistant isolates in Texas and Florida over a 10-year-period was 4%.[53] In the same study, the odds of death were 7 times higher in foals infected with resistant isolates.[53] In addition, the study demonstrated that isolates of *R equi* susceptible to macrolides were sometimes misclassified as resistant; therefore, it is reasonable to request retesting/revalidation of resistance by the testing laboratory. More recently, it has been documented that mass antimicrobial treatment of subclinically affected foals has selected for antimicrobial resistance over time with isolates of *R equi* resistant to all macrolides and rifampin now being cultured from up to 40% of the foals at some farms.[54] Macrolide resistance in *R equi* is conferred by acquisition of a new ribosomal RNA methylase gene designated *erm*(46).[55] This gene confers resistance to all macrolides, lincosamides, and streptogramins type B but not to other classes of antimicrobial agents.[55] The gene can be transferred from resistant to susceptible isolates of *R equi* by conjugation.[55] Most macrolide-resistant isolates of *R equi* that have been identified so far are also

resistant to rifampin. Rifampin resistance in *R equi* is the result of mutations in the *rpoB* gene.[56–59]

Treatment of foals that develop severe diarrhea during macrolide therapy or of foals infected with resistant isolates is problematic because of the limited range of effective alternatives. Macrolide- and rifampin-resistant isolates of *R equi* are susceptible in vitro to fluoroquinolones, gentamicin, linezolid, and vancomycin.[53,60,61] In one study, 18 of 24 isolates were also susceptible to chloramphenicol, tetracycline, and trimethoprim-sulfamethoxazole.[53] Currently, there are no data to indicate the preferred antimicrobial agent or agents for the treatment of foals infected with isolates resistant to macrolides and rifampin. Vancomycin, imipenem, or linezolid in foals should only be used for the treatment of life-threatening *R equi* infections caused by isolates confirmed to be resistant to all other possible alternatives. The use of gentamicin might not be unreasonable in foals infected with macrolide- and rifampin-resistant isolates. Although gentamicin is highly active against intracellular *R equi*, its efficacy in foals infected with *R equi* has been widely reported as being poor. This belief is mainly based on the results of a retrospective case series of foals with pneumonia caused by *R equi* in which all 17 foals treated with gentamicin died, whereas all 10 foals treated with erythromycin in combination with rifampin survived.[45] In contrast, in another retrospective case series of 39 foals with pneumonia caused by *R equi*, all 19 survivors were treated with gentamicin, whereas nonsurvivors were treated with a variety of other antimicrobial agents, including erythromycin, kanamycin, or chloramphenicol.[62] These studies were not controlled and did not account for lesion severity at the time of initiation of therapy. In addition, the dosages of gentamicin used in those studies were lower than dosages currently recommended based on the fact that gentamicin is now known to be concentration dependent. Additional studies will be necessary to assess the clinical efficacy of intravenous or nebulized gentamicin in foals infected with *R equi*.

Ancillary therapies

Nursing care, provision of adequate nutrition and hydration, and maintaining the foal in a cool and well-ventilated environment are important. Humidified oxygen delivered by pharyngeal insufflation in moderately hypoxemic foals, or by percutaneous transtracheal oxygenation in severely hypoxemic patients, is indicated.[63] Judicious use of nonsteroidal anti-inflammatory drugs might reduce fever and improve attitude and appetite in febrile, lethargic, anorectic foals. Nebulization with saline, antimicrobial agents, or bronchodilators has been advocated, but there are no data to either support or refute these therapeutic practices. Immune-mediated extrapulmonary disorders, such as polysynovitis, generally resolve with successful treatment of the accompanying pneumonia. In addition to appropriate systemic antimicrobial therapy, foals with *R equi* septic arthritis or osteomyelitis often require aggressive local therapy such as joint lavage, surgical debridement, and intravenous or intraosseous regional limb perfusion with antimicrobial agents. The prognosis for foals with abdominal abscesses is poor, although rare cases will respond to long-term antimicrobial therapy.[4,64] Surgical removal or marsupialization have been attempted in some foals, but abdominal adhesions usually result in inability to resect the abscess.

RECOMMENDATIONS FOR THE TREATMENT OF FOALS WITH SUBCLINICAL PULMONARY LESIONS

R.equi pneumonia is often not recognized until it is well advanced and, therefore, difficult to treat. Even severely affected foals may appear to suckle and behave normally to a casual observer. In an attempt to decrease mortality, control of *R equi* infections at many farms where the disease is endemic over the past 15 years has relied on early detection of subclinical pulmonary disease using thoracic ultrasonography and initiation of treatment with antimicrobial agents before development of clinical signs.[6,7,65] Periodic ultrasonography of the chest appears to have decreased mortality due to *R equi* pneumonia at some farms compared with historical controls, but controlled studies are lacking.[6,7,65] Historically, the recommendation was to treat all foals with pulmonary lesions diameter/depth 1 cm or greater.[6,7,65] This approach has resulted in a considerable increase in the number of foals treated for presumptive *R equi* pneumonia. The temporal association between this widespread use of macrolides and rifampin as a result of ultrasonographic screening and a perceived increase in the frequency of detection of resistant isolates in the last decade suggests that this practice may not be innocuous. Emergence of widespread macrolide and rifampin resistance at a farm after widespread use of these drugs was instituted as part of an ultrasonographic screening program has been documented.[54] On that particular farm, 20% to 40% of *R equi* isolates from pneumonic foals were resistant to macrolides and rifampin.[54]

Several uncontrolled studies have reported the apparent efficacy of various antimicrobial agents in foals with mild subclinical lesions. However, recent blinded randomized placebo controlled studies have documented that approximately 88% of foals with lesion scores (defined as the sum of the largest diameter of all pulmonary lesions $\geq$ 1 cm) between 1 and 10 cm recover without antimicrobial therapy.[9] Furthermore, antimicrobial treatment of foals with such ultrasonographic lesions does not significantly hasten lesion resolution compared with administration of a placebo.[8,9] These results underscore the importance of including a placebo control group in the design of studies assessing the relative efficacy of various antimicrobial agents in foals with subclinical pneumonia at farms endemic for *R equi*.

Only studies enrolling foals with lesions scores 10 cm or greater have been able to document a significant difference in recovery between foals treated with the positive control (azithromycin with rifampin) and the placebo groups.[66,67] In 2 separate blinded placebo-controlled studies, azithromycin alone (10 mg/kg orally every 24 hours) or gamithromycin alone (6 mg/kg intramuscularly every 7 days) were found to be noninferior to the combination azithromycin-rifampin.[66,67] In contrast, the proportion of foals treated with tulathromycin that recovered was not significantly different from that of foals treated with a placebo.[67] However, despite a statistically significant difference between groups for some drugs, it is important to note that up to 78% of the foals receiving the placebo recovered without the need for antimicrobial therapy. Therefore, the apparent efficacy of macrolide monotherapy in foals with subclinical ultrasonographic lesions should not be interpreted as evidence of similar efficacy in foals with severe pneumonia. It is also unknown if macrolide monotherapy is more likely to induce and select for resistance than combination therapy in vivo. In vitro evidence suggests that resistance is less likely to occur with the combination.

In a recent study, 270 foals at a different endemic farm were subjected to thoracic ultrasonography every 2 weeks for the entire season. The veterinarian making treatment decisions was unaware of ultrasonographic findings. Forty-six (17%) foals developed clinical signs of pneumonia and were treated; all 46 had ultrasonographic lesions.[68] Fifty-four foals (20%) remained clinically healthy and were exempt of pulmonary lesions, whereas 170 foals (63%) remained clinically healthy but had pulmonary lesions of various degrees of severity.[68] Ultrasonography was relatively sensitive (89%) but poorly specific (62%) for the diagnosis of clinical pneumonia.[68] By being more selective and treating only foals with larger lesion scores (eg, 8–20 cm), some farms have decreased antimicrobial drug use by approximately 75% without an apparent increase in mortality.[66]

However, because it is impossible to know which specific foals might not recover spontaneously from subclinical disease, and because *R equi* infections can cause severe disease, other breeding farms still elect to treat all foals with ultrasonographic lesions. In an attempt to find an alternative therapy that would result in a decrease in the use of macrolides and rifampin on those farms, a controlled randomized noninferiority trial comparing oral gallium maltolate (30 mg/kg every 24 hours for 30 days) to standard therapy with a combination of clarithromycin (7.5 mg/kg every 12 hours) and rifampin (5 mg/kg every 12 hours) for the treatment of foals with subclinical *R equi* pneumonia was performed. Of 509 foals from 6 participating farms that were evaluated ultrasonographically, 54 foals were identified with lesion scores 1 cm or greater. The proportion of gallium-treated foals that resolved (70%; 14/20) was similar to that of foals treated with clarithromycin and rifampin (74%; 25/34).[69] A major limitation of the aforementioned study is the lack of a placebo control group. Thus, it could not be established whether the proportion of either treatment group was significantly different than what might be achieved using a placebo alone. Nevertheless, by using gallium rather than macrolides to treat foals with ultrasonographic evidence of presumed *R equi* pneumonia, it is plausible that selection pressure for macrolide resistance would be decreased.

ADVERSE EFFECTS

Although well tolerated by most foals, macrolides commonly cause diarrhea. The diarrhea is often self-limiting and does not necessitate cessation of therapy. However, affected foals should be monitored carefully because some may develop severe diarrhea, leading to dehydration and electrolyte losses that necessitate intensive fluid therapy and cessation of oral macrolides. The incidence of diarrhea in foals treated with erythromycin-rifampin has ranged between 17% and 36%.[47,70] In one study, foals treated with clarithromycin had a higher incidence of diarrhea (28%) than those treated with azithromycin (8%), although in most cases, diarrhea was mild and self-limiting.[47] In the same study, the incidence of severe diarrhea necessitating administration of intravenous fluids was not significantly different between groups of foals treated with azithromycin-rifampin, clarithromycin-rifampin, or erythromycin-rifampin.[47] During periods of very hot or humid weather, an idiosyncratic reaction characterized by severe hyperthermia and tachypnea has been described in foals treated with erythromycin.[70] Anecdotal reports suggest that these reactions may occasionally occur with newer macrolides as well. Drug-induced anhidrosis is the likely mechanism for hyperthermia in these foals. In one study, sweating in response to intradermal terbutaline was almost completely abolished within 2 days of starting oral erythromycin, and significant sweating impairment persisted for at least 10 days after treatment ended.[71] Azithromycin and clarithromycin also significantly reduce sweating responses but to a lower degree than erythromycin.[72] In contrast, rifampin does not impair sweating in foals.[73]

Severe enterocolitis also has been reported in mares whose foals are treated with erythromycin, presumably by disrupting the mare's normal colonic microflora following ingestion of small amounts of active drug during coprophagia or by contamination of feeders or water buckets with drug present on the foal's muzzle. This complication seems to be rare. Enterocolitis in mares has been reproduced experimentally by administration of subtherapeutic doses of erythromycin.[74] In some cases, the severe enterocolitis in the mares of treated foals is associated with *Clostridium difficile*.[75]

Adverse effects during therapy for *R equi* pneumonia have been reported with other drugs also. In one study, 3 of 13 foals treated with doxycycline and rifampin developed hemolytic anemia and icterus 17 to 20 days after initiating therapy, and a fourth foal developed increased liver enzymes on day 9 of therapy.[9] One foal with hemolytic anemia was subjected to euthanasia. In the same study, adverse effects were not noted with administration of doxycycline alone.[9] In another study, 23 of 40 foals (58%) treated with intramuscular gamithromycin displayed signs of adverse reactions to the drug, whereas adverse reactions were not noted in the other treatment groups.[66] Adverse effects consisted of signs of colic (n = 18; 45%) immediately after injection and lameness of the hind limb that was injected (n = 14; 35%). Signs of colic were mild in most foals and consisted of lying down and flank watching.[66] The transient hind limb lameness observed in many foals is likely the result of the irritating nature of the drug. The signs of colic observed in many foals in the aforementioned study might have been the result of gastrointestinal disturbances caused by gamithromycin. However, because signs of colic occurred almost immediately after injection and because none of the foals treated with gamithromycin developed diarrhea, it is more likely that these signs were due to pain at the site of injection rather than to abdominal pain. The lameness resolved over 48 to 72 hours in all foals.

PROGNOSIS

Before the introduction of the combination of erythromycin and rifampin as the treatment of choice in the early 1980s, the prognosis of R equi–infected foals was poor with survival rates as low as 20%.[76] Using erythromycin and rifampin, Hillidge[77] reported a successful outcome (as assessed by survival) in 50 (88%) of 57 foals with confirmed R equi pneumonia. Studies from referral centers, where severely affected cases are likely more prevalent, have revealed survival proportions ranging between 59% and 72%.[47,78,79] In contrast, farms using a screening program to identify and treat foals with subclinical lesions have reported survival proportions approaching 100%.[6,80] However, recent evidence summarized above indicates that many of these foals would have recovered without therapy.

The impact of R equi infections on future athletic performance has been examined in 3 studies. No significant differences in total earnings, average earning index, and age at the first race were observed when comparing 30 horses that previously had R equi pneumonia with either their dams' other progeny or the North American averages.[81] In a retrospective study of racing Standardbreds and Thoroughbreds in the United States, 54% of 83 foals that survived R equi pneumonia had at least 1 racing start compared with 65% of their birth cohort, suggesting that horses contracting R equi pneumonia as foals may be somewhat less likely to race as adults.[78] However, the racing performance of those foals that raced was not different from that of the US racing population.[78] In contrast, a retrospective cohort of 491 Thoroughbred horses in Australia (125 cases and 366 controls) provided opposite results. The probability of racing as a 2-year-old was similar between cases and controls.[82] However, cases had significantly less starts and won fewer races than controls.[82]

REFERENCES

1. Cohen ND. Causes of and farm management factors associated with disease and death in foals. J Am Vet Med Assoc 1994;204:1644–51.
2. Anonymous. Part I: baseline reference of 1998 equine health management. USDA-APHIS; 2008. Veterinary Services Report.
3. Giguère S, Gaskin JM, Miller C, et al. Evaluation of a commercially available hyperimmune plasma product for prevention of naturally acquired pneumonia caused by Rhodococcus equi in foals. J Am Vet Med Assoc 2002;220:59–63.

4. Reuss SM, Chaffin MK, Cohen ND. Extrapulmonary disorders associated with Rhodococcus equi infection in foals: 150 cases (1987-2007). J Am Vet Med Assoc 2009;235:855–63.

5. Zink MC, Yager JA, Smart NL. Corynebacterium equi infections in horses, 1958-1984: a review of 131 cases. Can J Vet Res 1986;27:213–7.

6. Slovis NM, McCracken JL, Mundy G. How to use thoracic ultrasound to screen foals for Rhodococcus equi at affected farms. Proc Am Assoc Equine Pract 2005;51:274–8.

7. Venner M, Kerth R, Klug E. Evaluation of tulathromycin in the treatment of pulmonary abscesses in foals. Vet J 2007;174:418–21.

8. Venner M, Rodiger A, Laemmer M, et al. Failure of antimicrobial therapy to accelerate spontaneous healing of subclinical pulmonary abscesses on a farm with endemic infections caused by Rhodococcus equi. Vet J 2012;192:293–8.

9. Venner M, Astheimer K, Lammer M, et al. Efficacy of mass antimicrobial treatment of foals with subclinical pulmonary abscesses associated with Rhodococcus equi. J Vet Intern Med 2013;27:171–6.

10. Peters J, Block W, Oswald S, et al. Oral absorption of clarithromycin is nearly abolished by chronic comedication of rifampicin in foals. Drug Metab Dispos 2011;39:1643–9.

11. Venner M, Peters J, Hohensteiger N, et al. Concentration of the macrolide antibiotic tulathromycin in broncho-alveolar cells is influenced by comedication of rifampicin in foals. Naunyn Schmiedebergs Arch Pharmacol 2010;381:161–9.

12. Giguère S, Lee EA, Guldbech KM, et al. In vitro synergy, pharmacodynamics, and postantibiotic effect of 11 antimicrobial agents against Rhodococcus equi. Vet Microbiol 2012;160:207–13.

13. Nordmann P, Ronco E. In-vitro antimicrobial susceptibility of Rhodococcus equi. J Antimicrob Chemother 1992;29:383–93.

14. Prescott JF, Nicholson VM. The effects of combinations of selected antibiotics on the growth of Corynebacterium equi. J Vet Pharmacol Ther 1984;7:61–4.

15. Blondeau JM. New concepts in antimicrobial susceptibility testing: the mutant prevention concentration and mutant selection window approach. Vet Dermatol 2009;20:383–96.

16. Berghaus LJ, Giguère S, Guldbech K. Mutant prevention concentration and mutant selection window for 10 antimicrobial agents against Rhodococcus equi. Vet Microbiol 2013;166:670–5.

17. Giguère S, Hondalus MK, Yager JA, et al. Role of the 85-kilobase plasmid and plasmid-encoded virulence-associated protein A in intracellular survival and virulence of Rhodococcus equi. Infect Immun 1999;67:3548–57.

18. Berghaus LJ, Giguère S, Sturgill TL, et al. Plasma pharmacokinetics, pulmonary distribution, and in vitro activity of gamithromycin in foals. J Vet Pharmacol Ther 2012;35:59–66.

19. Vivrette S, Bostian A, Bermingham E, et al. Quinolone induced arthropathy in neonatal foals. Proc Am Assoc Equine Pract 2001;47:376–7.

20. Drusano GL. Infection site concentrations: their therapeutic importance and the macrolide and macrolide-like class of antibiotics. Pharmacotherapy 2005;25:150S–8S.

21. Kiem S, Schentag JJ. Interpretation of antibiotic concentration ratios measured in epithelial lining fluid. Antimicrob Agents Chemother 2008;52:24–36.

22. Lakritz J, Wilson WD, Marsh AE, et al. Effects of prior feeding on pharmacokinetics and estimated bioavailability after oral administration of a single dose of

microencapsulated erythromycin base in healthy foals. Am J Vet Res 2000;61: 1011–5.

23. Davis JL, Gardner SY, Jones SL, et al. Pharmacokinetics of azithromycin in foals after i.v. and oral dose and disposition into phagocytes. J Vet Pharmacol Ther 2002;25:99–104.

24. Jacks S, Giguère S, Gronwall PR, et al. Pharmacokinetics of azithromycin and concentration in body fluids and bronchoalveolar cells in foals. Am J Vet Res 2001;62:1870–5.

25. Womble A, Giguère S, Murthy YV, et al. Pulmonary disposition of tilmicosin in foals and in vitro activity against Rhodococcus equi and other common equine bacterial pathogens. J Vet Pharmacol Ther 2006;29:561–8.

26. Suarez-Mier G, Giguère S, Lee EA. Pulmonary disposition of erythromycin, azithromycin, and clarithromycin in foals. J Vet Pharmacol Ther 2007;30:109–15.

27. Scheuch E, Spieker J, Venner M, et al. Quantitative determination of the macrolide antibiotic tulathromycin in plasma and broncho-alveolar cells of foals using tandem mass spectrometry. J Chromatogr B Analyt Technol Biomed Life Sci 2007;850:464–70.

28. Kohn CW, Sams R, Kowalski JJ, et al. Pharmacokinetics of single intravenous and single and multiple dose oral administration of rifampin in mares. J Vet Pharmacol Ther 1993;16:119–31.

29. Burrows GE, MacAllister CG, Ewing P, et al. Rifampin disposition in the horse: effects of age and method of oral administration. J Vet Pharmacol Ther 1992;15: 124–32.

30. Peters J, Eggers K, Oswald S, et al. Clarithromycin is absorbed by an intestinal uptake mechanism that is sensitive to major inhibition by rifampicin: results of a short-term drug interaction study in foals. Drug Metab Dispos 2012;40:522–8.

31. Berlin S, Spieckermann L, Oswald S, et al. Pharmacokinetics and pulmonary distribution of clarithromycin and rifampicin after concomitant and consecutive administration in foals. Mol Pharm 2016;13:1089–99.

32. Garver E, Hugger ED, Shearn SP, et al. Involvement of intestinal uptake transporters in the absorption of azithromycin and clarithromycin in the rat. Drug Metab Dispos 2008;36:2492–8.

33. Womble A, Giguère S, Lee EA. Pharmacokinetics of oral doxycycline and concentrations in body fluids and bronchoalveolar cells of foals. J Vet Pharmacol Ther 2007;30:187–93.

34. Burton AJ, Giguère S, Arnold RD. Pharmacokinetics, pulmonary disposition and tolerability of liposomal gentamicin and free gentamicin in foals. Equine Vet J 2015;47:467–72.

35. Javsicas LH, Giguère S, Womble AY. Disposition of oral telithromycin in foals and in vitro activity of the drug against macrolide-susceptible and macrolide-resistant Rhodococcus equi isolates. J Vet Pharmacol Ther 2010;33:383–8.

36. Nordmann P, Kerestedjian JJ, Ronco E. Therapy of Rhodococcus equi disseminated infections in nude mice. Antimicrob Agents Chemother 1992;36:1244–8.

37. Burton AJ, Giguère S, Berghaus LJ, et al. Activity of clarithromycin or rifampin alone or in combination against experimental Rhodococcus equi infection in mice. Antimicrob Agents Chemother 2015;59:3633–6.

38. Burton AJ, Giguère S, Berghaus LJ, et al. Efficacy of liposomal gentamicin against Rhodococcus equi in a mouse infection model and colocalization with R. equi in equine alveolar macrophages. Vet Microbiol 2015;176:292–300.

39. Caston SS, McClure SR, Martens RJ, et al. Effect of hyperimmune plasma on the severity of pneumonia caused by Rhodococcus equi in experimentally infected foals. Vet Ther 2006;7:361–75.

40. Martens RJ, Martens JG, Fiske RA. Rhodococcus equi foal pneumonia: pathogenesis and immunoprophylaxis. Proc Am Assoc Equine Pract 1989;35:189–213.

41. Perkins GA, Yeagar A, Erb HN, et al. Survival of foals with experimentally induced Rhodococcus equi infection given either hyperimmune plasma containing R. equi antibody or normal equine plasma. Vet Ther 2001;3:334–46.

42. Sanz M, Loynachan A, Sun L, et al. The effect of bacterial dose and foal age at challenge on Rhodococcus equi infection. Vet Microbiol 2013;167:623–31.

43. Horohov DW, Loynachan AT, Page AE, et al. The use of streptolysin O (SLO) as an adjunct therapy for Rhodococcus equi pneumonia in foals. Vet Microbiol 2011; 154:156–62.

44. Cohen ND, Giguère S, Burton AJ, et al. Use of liposomal gentamicin for treatment of 5 foals with experimentally induced Rhodococcus equi pneumonia. J Vet Intern Med 2016;30:322–5.

45. Sweeney CR, Sweeney RW, Divers TJ. Rhodococcus equi pneumonia in 48 foals: response to antimicrobial therapy. Vet Microbiol 1987;14:329–36.

46. Ainsworth DM, Erb HN, Eicker SW, et al. Effects of pulmonary abscesses on racing performance of horses treated at referral veterinary medical teaching hospitals: 45 cases (1985-1997). J Am Vet Med Assoc 2000;216:1282–7.

47. Giguère S, Jacks S, Roberts GD, et al. Retrospective comparison of azithromycin, clarithromycin, and erythromycin for the treatment of foals with Rhodococcus equi pneumonia. J Vet Intern Med 2004;18:568–73.

48. Chaffin MK, Cohen ND, Martens RJ, et al. Foal-related risk factors associated with development of Rhodococcus equi pneumonia on farms with endemic infection. J Am Vet Med Assoc 2003;223:1791–9.

49. Chaffin MK, Cohen ND, Martens RJ. Chemoprophylactic effects of azithromycin against Rhodococcus equi-induced pneumonia among foals at equine breeding farms with endemic infections. J Am Vet Med Assoc 2008;232:1035–47.

50. Giguère S, Cohen ND, Keith CM, et al. Diagnosis, treatment, control, and prevention of infections caused by Rhodococcus equi in foals. J Vet Intern Med 2011;25: 1209–20.

51. Cohen ND. Rhodococcus equi foal pneumonia. Vet Clin North Am Equine Pract 2014;30:609–22.

52. Giguère S, Jordan LM, Glass K, et al. Relationship of mixed bacterial infection to prognosis in foals with pneumonia caused by Rhodococcus equi. J Vet Intern Med 2012;26:1443–8.

53. Giguère S, Lee E, Williams E, et al. Determination of the prevalence of antimicrobial resistance to macrolide antimicrobials or rifampin in Rhodococcus equi isolates and treatment outcome in foals infected with antimicrobial-resistant isolates of R. equi. J Am Vet Med Assoc 2010;237:74–81.

54. Burton AJ, Giguère S, Sturgill TL, et al. Macrolide- and rifampin-resistant Rhodococcus equi on horse breeding farm, Kentucky, USA. Emerg Infect Dis 2013;19: 282–5.

55. Anastasi E, Giguère S, Berghaus LJ, et al. Novel transferable erm(46) determinant responsible for emerging macrolide resistance in Rhodococcus equi. J Antimicrob Chemother 2015;70:3184–90.

56. Fines M, Pronost S, Maillard K, et al. Characterization of mutations in the rpoB gene associated with rifampin resistance in Rhodococcus equi isolated from foals. J Clin Microbiol 2001;39:2784–7.

57. Riesenberg A, Fessler AT, Erol E, et al. MICs of 32 antimicrobial agents for Rhodococcus equi isolates of animal origin. J Antimicrob Chemother 2014;69: 1045–9.

58. Takai S, Takeda K, Nakano Y, et al. Emergence of rifampin-resistant Rhodococcus equi in an infected foal. J Clin Microbiol 1997;35:1904–8.

59. Asoh N, Watanabe H, Fines-Guyon M, et al. Emergence of rifampin-resistant Rhodococcus equi with several types of mutations in the rpoB gene among AIDS patients in northern Thailand. J Clin Microbiol 2003;41:2337–40.

60. Carlson K, Kuskie K, Chaffin K, et al. Antimicrobial activity of tulathromycin and 14 other antimicrobials against virulent Rhodococcus equi in vitro. Vet Ther 2010;11: E1–9.

61. Berghaus LJ, Giguère S, Guldbech K, et al. Comparison of etest, disk diffusion, and broth macrodilution for in vitro susceptibility testing of Rhodococcus equi. J Clin Microbiol 2015;53:314–8.

62. Falcon J, Smith BP, O'Brien TR, et al. Clinical and radiographic findings in Corynebacterium equi pneumonia of foals. J Am Vet Med Assoc 1985;186:593–9.

63. Hoffman AM, Viel L. A percutaneous transtracheal catheter system for improved oxygenation in foals with respiratory distress. Equine Vet J 1992;24:239–41.

64. Valdes A, Johnson JR. Septic pleuritis and abdominal abscess formation caused by Rhodococcus equi in a foal. J Am Vet Med Assoc 2005;227:960–3, 919.

65. McCracken JL, Slovis NM. Use of thoracic ultrasound for the prevention of Rhodococcus equi pneumonia on endemic farms. Proc Am Assoc Equine Pract 2009;55:38–44.

66. Hildebrand F, Venner M, Giguère S. Efficacy of gamithromycin for the treatment of foals with mild to moderate bronchopneumonia. J Vet Intern Med 2015;29:333–8.

67. Venner M, Credner N, Lammer M, et al. Comparison of tulathromycin, azithromycin and azithromycin-rifampin for the treatment of mild pneumonia associated with Rhodococcus equi. Vet Rec 2013;173:397.

68. Chaffin MK, Cohen ND, Blodgett GP, et al. Evaluation of ultrasonographic screening methods for early detection of Rhodococcus equi pneumonia in foals. J Equine Vet Sci 2012;32:S20–1.

69. Cohen ND, Slovis NM, Giguère S, et al. Gallium maltolate as an alternative to macrolides for treatment of presumed Rhodococcus equi pneumonia in foals. J Vet Intern Med 2015;29:932–9.

70. Stratton-Phelps M, Wilson WD, Gardner IA. Risk of adverse effects in pneumonic foals treated with erythromycin versus other antibiotics: 143 cases (1986-1996). J Am Vet Med Assoc 2000;217:68–73.

71. Stieler AL, Sanchez LC, Mallicote MF, et al. Macrolide-induced hyperthermia in foals: role of impaired sweat responses. Equine Vet J 2016;48(5):590–4.

72. Stieler A, Sanchez LC, Mallicote M, et al. A comparison of the effects on sweating of three macrolide antibiotics used in foals. J Vet Intern Med 2015;29:1248–9.

73. Stieler A, Sanchez LC, Mallicote M, et al. Effects of rifampin on erythromycin-induced anhidrosis in foals. J Vet Intern Med 2015;27:1238.

74. Gustafsson A, Baverud V, Gunnarsson A, et al. The association of erythromycin ethylsuccinate with acute colitis in horses in Sweden. Equine Vet J 1997;29: 314–8.

75. Baverud V, Franklin A, Gunnarsson A, et al. Clostridium difficile associated with acute colitis in mares when their foals are treated with erythromycin and rifampicin for Rhodococcus equi pneumonia [see comments]. Equine Vet J 1998;30: 482–8.

76. Elissalde GS, Renshaw HW, Walberg JA. Corynebacterium equi: an interhost review with emphasis on the foal. Comp Immunol Microbiol Infect Dis 1980;3: 433–45.

77. Hillidge CJ. Use of erythromycin-rifampin combination in treatment of Rhodococcus equi pneumonia. Vet Microbiol 1987;14:337–42.

78. Ainsworth DM, Eicker SW, Yeagar AE, et al. Associations between physical examination, laboratory, and radiographic findings and outcome and subsequent racing performance of foals with Rhodococcus equi infection: 115 cases (1984-1992). J Am Vet Med Assoc 1998;213:510–5.

79. Chaffin MK, Martens RJ. Extrapulmonary disorders associated with Rhodococcus equi pneumonia in foals: retrospective study of 61 cases (1988-1996). Proc Am Assoc Equine Pract 1997;43:79–80.

80. Venner M, Reinhold B, Beyerbach M, et al. Efficacy of azithromycin in preventing pulmonary abscesses in foals. Vet J 2009;179:301–3.

81. Bernard B, Dugan J, Pierce S, et al. The influence of foal pneumonia on future racing performance. Proc Am Assoc Equine Pract 1991;37:17–8.

82. Treloar SK, Dhand NK, Muscatello G. Rhodococcus equi pneumonia and future racing performance of the Thoroughbred. J Equine Vet Sci 2012;32:S16–7.

83. Jacks S, Giguère S, Nguyen A. In vitro susceptibilities of Rhodococcus equi and other common equine pathogens to azithromycin, clarithromycin and 20 other antimicrobials. Antimicrob Agents Chemother 2003;47:1742–5.

84. Womble AY, Giguère S, Lee EA, et al. Pharmacokinetics of clarithromycin and concentrations in body fluids and bronchoalveolar cells of foals. Am J Vet Res 2006;67:1681–6.

Therapeutics for Equine Protozoal Myeloencephalitis

Nicola Pusterla, DVM, PhD[a],*, Thomas Tobin, MVB, MSC, PhD, MRCVS[b]

KEYWORDS

- Equine protozoal myeloencephalitis (EPM) • *Sarcocystis neurona*
- *Neospora hughesi* • Treatment • Prevention

KEY POINTS

- Equine protozoal myeloencephalitis (EPM) is a diagnosis of exclusion and relies on the presence of neurologic signs, ruling out other neurologic disorders, and the detection of antibodies to *Sarcocystis neurona* or *Neospora hughesi* in serum and cerebrospinal fluid using quantitative immunodiagnostic tests.
- Three treatment formulations approved by the US Food and Drug Administration are commercially available for the treatment of EPM and these formulations are broadly equivalent in therapeutic efficacy. Two of these formulations are specifically antiapicomplexan and a positive response to these agents strongly supports an EPM diagnosis. Treatment should be continued until no further clinical improvement is observed. Relapse following cessation of treatment may occur in a percentage of cases and is not an insignificant clinical problem.
- Nonempiric treatment recommendations have been proposed to treat relapsing horses. These include prolonging the standard treatment course, combining various classes of antiprotozoal agents, using higher doses of triazine antiprotozoal agents, instituting maintenance therapy following the initial treatment course, and administering immunomodulators.
- Intermittent use of antiprotozoal agents has shown promise in the prevention of EPM. Such protocols have been able to reduce clinical signs, delay seroconversion, and decrease intrathecal anti–*S neurona* antibody response under experimental conditions. Seroprevalence of anti–*S neurona* antibodies has been shown to significantly decline in horses continuously exposed to *S neurona* through the daily extended use of antiprotozoal agents.

[a] Department of Medicine and Epidemiology, School of Veterinary Medicine, University of California, Davis, One Shields Avenue, Davis, CA 95616, USA; [b] Department of Toxicology and Cancer Research, The Maxwell H. Gluck Equine Research Center, College of Agriculture, University of Kentucky, 1400 Nicholasville Road, Lexington, KY 40506, USA
* Corresponding author.
E-mail address: npusterla@ucdavis.edu

INTRODUCTION

Equine protozoal myeloencephalitis (EPM) is an important infectious disease of the central nervous system (CNS) that is typically caused by infection with *Sarcocystis neurona* and less frequently by *Neospora hughesi*.[1] The biology of *S neurona* relies on a 2-host life cycle, with the Virginia opossum as the definitive host and skunks, raccoons, armadillos, and cats serving as intermediate hosts. *Sarcocystis neurona* forms latent sarcocysts in the muscle tissue of the intermediate host and the sarcocysts-containing tissue of these hosts serves as the infection source for scavenging opossums. Horses become infected following the accidental ingestion of sporozoite-containing sporocysts of *S neurona* from feed or water contaminated with opossum feces. Although horses are regarded as aberrant hosts in the life cycle of *S neurona*, there is recent evidence suggesting that they can occasionally become intermediate hosts.[2] Although the life cycle of *N hughesi* in horses is still unresolved, many comparisons have been drawn with *Neospora caninum*, the causative agent of ascending neuromuscular disease in dogs and abortion in cattle worldwide. Similar to the epidemiology of bovine neosporosis, recently published work showed that *N hughesi* persisted in horse populations through endogenous transplacental infection.[3] By contrast, congenital *S neurona* infection has rarely been reported in the literature.[4–6]

Clinical signs associated with EPM are seldom characteristic. EPM routinely presents as progressive and asymmetrical neurologic deficits of the CNS. Due to the lack of a definitive antemortem diagnostic test for EPM, the diagnosis of EPM relies on the presence of neurologic signs, ruling out other infectious and noninfectious neurologic disorders and the detection of intrathecally-derived antibodies to either *S neurona* and/or *N hughesi*. For treatment of EPM, it is recommended that 1 of the 3 FDA-approved anticoccidial drug formulations should be used to control infection. Additional medical and supportive treatment should be provided based on the severity of neurologic deficits and complications arising from them. This review article focuses on the recent data related to diagnosis, pharmacologic treatment, and prevention of EPM.

PATIENT EVALUATION OVERVIEW

The first step in the evaluation of a patient with possible EPM is completion of a comprehensive neurologic examination to determine the neuroanatomical localizations of the disease process. Clinical signs of EPM vary from acute to chronic with insidious onset of focal or multifocal signs of neurologic disease involving the brain, brainstem, and/or spinal cord.[7] The variability of clinical signs is due to infection of both white and gray matter at multiple sites in the CNS. Signs of gray matter involvement include focal muscle atrophy and severe muscle weakness, whereas damage to white matter frequently results in ataxia and weakness in limbs caudal to the site of infection. EPM often presents with progressive and asymmetrical signs, such as weakness, ataxia, spasticity involving all 4 limbs, and focal muscle atrophy. Less frequent signs include depression, behavioral changes, cranial nerve paralysis, head tilt, seizure, and gait abnormality.

Although a definitive diagnosis of EPM requires postmortem detection of *S neurona* or *N hughesi* infection of the CNS, a suspected diagnosis of EPM can be established based on the following parameters: (1) the presence of neurologic signs compatible with EPM, (2) ruling out other neurologic disorders, and (3) detection of specific antibodies to either *S neurona* or *N hughesi* with quantitative immunodiagnostics using serum and cerebrospinal fluid (CSF) (**Box 1**). Additionally, a positive therapeutic response to diclazuril or toltrazuril sulfone is very strong evidence in support of a diagnosis of EPM.

Box 1
Criteria to establish a suspected equine protozoal myeloencephalitis diagnosis

- Perform a comprehensive neurologic examination
- Presence of neurologic deficits compatible with EPM
- Rule out other frequent neurologic disorders using imaging and laboratory diagnostic modalities
- Establish infection based on serum antibodies to *Sarcocystis neurona* or *N hughesi*
- Document intrathecal antibodies to *S neurona* or *N hughesi* using serum to CSF ratio or antibody indices

---

Although it is not the scope of this article to expand on the various immunodiagnostics, the reader is referred to the recently updated consensus statement of the American College of Veterinary Internal Medicine.[8] The consensus on the use of quantitative immunodiagnostics is that they be used on serum and CSF to confirm intrathecal antibody production against *S neurona* or *N hughesi*.

PHARMACOLOGIC TREATMENT OPTIONS

There are currently 3 commercially available US Food and Drug Administration (FDA) approved therapies for EPM. In order of FDA approval, they are: Merial Marquis, approved 2001; PRN Pharmacal ReBalance, approved 2004; and Merck Protazil, approved 2011.[9] Use of FDA-approved products in the prevention and treatment of EPM is strongly recommended.

Sulfonamide/Pyrimethamine Combinations

Sulfonamide/pyrimethamine combinations have long been used in the treatment of apicomplexan diseases and constituted the first therapeutic approaches to EPM.[10] In 2004, the FDA-approved ReBalance Antiprotozoal Oral Suspension, a carefully optimized sulfadiazine/pyrimethamine anticoccidial combination formulation. In these combinations, sulfonamides/sulfadiazine and pyrimethamine act by sequentially inhibiting tetrahydrofolate synthesis and thus purine, pyrimidine, and nucleic acid synthesis. When both substances are present together in the parasite at greater than the required inhibitory concentrations, their combined actions are synergistic.[11] Sulfadiazine is the optimal sulfonamide for use in EPM formulations because of its superior ability to maintain effective CNS tissue concentrations.[9] Hay feeding optimally should be withheld for 2 hours before and after dosing, to maximize bioavailability.

As initially applied, these sulfonamide/pyrimethamine combination therapies had certain limitations. For optimal synergistic response, the CNS levels of both medications must be consistently maintained above the required minimal inhibitory concentrations. However, given the relatively short plasma half-lives of these compounds in the horse, it can be challenging to consistently maintain full effective CNS concentrations of these agents.[12] Additionally, this is all the more so given that treatment schedules with these combinations may be relatively prolonged, usually in the order of about 90 days but can be significantly longer.[9] That said, experimental work with the FDA-approved ReBalance formulation has shown that a 90-day course of treatment yielded clinical improvement of 2 or more grades in neurologic function in 60% to 70% of treated horses, close to, if not equivalent to, the results reported with other FDA-approved therapies. Overall, it seems that the success rate of treatment with the sulfonamide/pyrimethamine combination was in the area of 60% to 70% of animals treated, with a relapse rate in the order of 10%.[13]

A significant concern with sulfonamide/pyrimethamine combinations is their potential for adverse reactions.[14] These adverse reactions are often directly related to their inhibitory actions on purine, pyrimidine, and nucleic acid metabolism; these are the required actions on S neurona but may also give rise to adverse reactions in the horse. Adverse reactions to sulfonamide/pyrimethamine combinations may include anorexia, intestinal disturbances, urticaria, and bone marrow suppression. Bone marrow suppression may manifest as anemia, neutropenia, and/or thrombocytopenia.[14] Pyrimethamine is also known to be teratogenic and, therefore, should not be used in pregnant mares and there are also similar concerns about its use in stallions.[15,16]

Although trimethoprim was at one time recommended for use along with pyrimethamine, this combination is no longer recommended. This is because pyrimethamine is a substantially more effective inhibitor of dihydrofolate reductase than trimethoprim. The inclusion of trimethoprim in the formulation simply acts to reduce the efficacy of pyrimethamine in inhibiting dihydrofolate reductase.[9]

Benzeneacetonitrile Agents: Diclazuril and Toltrazuril

Starting in 1996, diclazuril and the related benzeneacetonitrile substances toltrazuril and toltrazuril sulfone have been shown to be highly effective in the treatment of EPM.[17–19] These agents are remarkably specific for S neurona and related apicomplexans, apparently acting directly on chloroplast-related material acquired by these organisms 800 million or so years ago and not represented in mammalian systems.[20] These agents are chemically related to the herbicide atrazine; as such, they are highly specific for apicomplexans and, for all practical purposes, relatively nontoxic for mammalian systems.[9,18] Diclazuril and toltrazuril sulfone are commercially available as 2 FDA-approved formulations, diclazuril as Protazil, a pelleted top dressing, and ponazuril/toltrazuril sulfone as Marquis, an oral paste formulation.

As well as being specifically antiapicomplexan, these agents also have very favorable equine pharmacokinetics, Diclazuril and toltrazuril sulfone are well absorbed orally and have relatively long plasma half-lives, at least 48 to 96 hours and at times longer.[18,21,22] As such, daily oral dosage schedules readily maintain effective plasma and CNS concentrations of these agents. In fact, the plasma half-lives of these agents are sufficiently long that it can take up to 7 or more days of daily dosing to attain the full steady-state plasma and CNS concentrations of these agents. Given this long half-life, a useful therapeutic maneuver with some formulations is to accelerate the attainment of effective blood concentrations by administration of a double or triple dose on the first treatment day, followed by the manufacturer's daily recommended dose.[9,23] The advantage of a loading dose is that it allows more rapid attainment of full therapeutic plasma and CNS concentrations of these agents and equivalently rapid attainment of their therapeutic action.

Therapeutically, these agents are highly effective and their antiapicomplexan specificity means that a positive clinical response to treatment strongly supports an EPM diagnosis.[9,18] The first clinical report on the use of diclazuril in the treatment of EPM cases reported a 5% relapse rate at 6 months after a 28-day treatment protocol. It was administered at a dose of 5.5 mg/kg of diclazuril, administered as Clinacox under an FDA Investigational New Animal Drug protocol.[24,25] These early clinical investigations were soon followed by FDA approval in 2001 of the Bayer oral toltrazuril sulfone (ponazuril) paste formulation, Marquis, and later by the

FDA-approved diclazuril oral pellet formulation, Merck Protazil, approved in 2011. Work with these formulations suggests a therapeutic efficacy in the order of 62% to 67% based on either improvement of 1 grade on a neurologic examination or becoming negative to antibodies against *S neurona* in CSF; this second criterion is a much more challenging one.[26]

Although virtually all EPM horses will respond to chemotherapy, the quality of the therapeutic response is to some extent unpredictable and likely related to the quality of the immune deficit that allowed the appearance of clinical signs of EPM in the first place. Given this circumstance, therapy should be maintained until there is no further clinical improvement in the animal's status. Relapse following withdrawal of therapy is a consistent risk and even the best therapeutic protocols carry a significant (approximately 10%) risk of relapse. Relapsing animals generally respond well to renewed therapy and the concern then becomes choosing the type and level of maintenance therapy required to prevent a second relapse.

Other Pharmacologic Treatments: Decoquinate/Levamisole

Decoquinate, a quinoline carboxylic acid anticoccidial drug, is available as a compounded combination product with levamisole, termed Orogin (Pathogenes) for treatment of EPM.[27] Decoquinate is a well-established antiapicomplexan agent that has been demonstrated to prevent *Toxoplasma gondii* abortions in sheep[28]; the role of levamisole in the Orogin formulation is to improve the anti–*S neurona* immune response.[29] Levamisole, however, has been shown to be metabolized to aminorex, a CNS-stimulant substance banned in performance horses, and apparently also to the closely related and also banned stimulant, pemoline.[30] Administration of levamisole to horses likely to be subjected to drug testing, therefore, gives rise to the possibility of regulatory problems if levamisole is administered to such horses.

Supportive and Other Treatments

Because of the significant contribution of inflammatory responses to the clinical presentation of EPM, the use of anti-inflammatory medications can be effective and appropriate adjunctive treatments. A current standard recommendation is the administration of flunixin meglumine to moderately or severely affected horses during the first 3 to 7 days of therapy, after which time the antiapicomplexan chemotherapy should begin to be effective.[9] If the presented animal is showing severe signs of EPM, and is in danger of becoming recumbent and unable to rise, corticosteroid therapy may be appropriate, usually administered for not more than 3 days. Other approaches include administration of dimethyl sulfoxide (DMSO), either intravenously or orally, and vitamin E supplementation with the goal of reducing oxidative damage associated with the inflammatory component of EPM.[8]

The possible contributions of combination therapy, immune supplementation, and the prophylactic use of currently available therapies need to be further explored. Although the currently available therapies can produce good clinical responses, relapses following withdrawal of therapy remain a significant concern. At this time, the only available approach to relapses is to renew therapy along with formulating a practical therapeutic maintenance program, which is usually a variant of 1 or more of the current recommended therapies. The potential role of these medications in prophylaxis was recognized early[19] and research is now being presented in this area.[31–34] Additionally, the role of combination therapy remains to be explored; it may well turn out that combinations of various antiapicomplexan agents will be more therapeutically effective than these agents used as monotherapy.

EVALUATION OF OUTCOME AND LONG-TERM RECOMMENDATIONS

The FDA-approved treatments for EPM have shown similar clinical improvement rates, ranging from 57% to 62%.[13,33,35] In these studies successful treatment was defined as improvement by at least 1 clinical grade on neurologic examination and reversion to a negative S neurona antibody status in the CSF. In light of these published studies, the treatment of EPM seems only modestly effective when used at the label recommended duration of therapy.

It is reasonable to estimate that at least 10% of horses successfully treated with any of the FDA-approved EPM treatments will relapse within 1 to 3 years of discontinuation of treatment. Relapse is generally considered when horses develop neurologic deficits similar to the original presentation. The reasons for relapses are unknown but there are some hypotheses. They may be caused by a failure to achieve therapeutic concentrations of the treatment drugs in the CSF, as a result of either poor blood-brain-barrier penetration or relatively short elimination half-lives. Another hypothesis for relapses with EPM includes the inability of the immune system of affected horses to effectively eliminate S neurona following antiprotozoal treatment. Such immunologic dysfunction may relate to a deficient cell-mediated immunity; protective immunity to intracellular parasites generally depends on the ability of the host to mount specific type 1-like responses.[36]

Nonempiric treatment recommendations have been proposed to treat relapsing horses (**Box 2**). One strategy has been to double the initial treatment duration, which generally means treating a relapsing horse for at least 56 days with a triazine antiprotozoal agent and for at least 90 days with a sulfonamide/pyrimethamine formulation. Administration of combinations of different antiprotozoal agents has also been proposed. In such a scenario, 1 of the 2 FDA-approved triazine antiprotozoal agents is combined with the FDA-approved formulation of sulfonamide/pyrimethamine.

Failure of maintaining concentrations of antiprotozoal drugs in the CNS when used at the standard treatment dose may be another possible explanation for relapses. Variations in individual absorption and lack of ability of these agents to pass through the blood-brain barrier in some horses may allow for the use of higher, extra-labeled doses of antiprotozoal agents in these cases. In this regard, both FDA-approved triazine antiprotozoal agents have been shown to be safe at higher doses.[37,38] Ponazuril has been shown to be safe at doses 6 times the FDA-approved dose, causing only mild uterine edema on postmortem examination.[37] When diclazuril was given at 5, 15, 25, and 50 times the clinical dose, no clinical abnormalities were noticed.[38] At doses of 50 times the recommended therapeutic dose, test subjects did not gain their expected amount of weight. This means that diclazuril given at 2 or 5 times the

---

Box 2
Proposed nonempiric treatment options for relapsing horses

- Extend the treatment protocol with an FDA-approved antiprotozoal drug to at least twice the initial treatment time
- Combine a triazine antiprotozoal agent with the FDA-approved formulation of pyrimethamine and sulfadiazine
- Use of higher doses of triazine antiprotozoal agents
- Institute maintenance therapy following initial treatment course
- Administration of immunomodulators concurrently with an antiprotozoal drug

recommended dose seems to be safe, with the benefit of yielding higher therapeutic concentrations within the central nervous tissue. Because of the narrower safety margin for sulfonamide/pyrimethamine, the clinician should not increase the dose of these drugs above the manufacturers approved doses.

Another proposed strategy to maintain clinical remission following initial treatment is to institute a maintenance antiprotozoal drug therapy protocol (see later discussion on preventive treatment options for specific protocols). Immunomodulators have anecdotally been included by some clinicians in the treatment of refractory or relapsing cases. These include levamisole and commercially available immunomodulating products that contain killed *Propionibacterium acnes*, mycobacterial wall extract, and inactivated parapox ovis virus. The clinician must keep in mind that the effectiveness of any of these protocols is unproven for the treatment of relapsing EPM cases and their justification is theoretic.

PREVENTIVE TREATMENT OPTIONS

Preventative approaches to EPM can be achieved by decreasing stress along with reducing exposure to scat from opossums. Practical approaches to prevention include feeding off the ground, providing separate sources of fresh water, and preventing wildlife access to horse pastures, paddocks, and stalls to help reduce the incidence of protozoal infections in horses.

Intermittent use of coccidiostatic or coccidiocidal drugs is another approach used to prevent EPM (**Table 1**). Two prophylactic studies have looked at the use of ponazuril

Table 1
Studies investigating the use of antiprotozoal drugs to prevent infection with *Sarcocystis neurona*

Drug	Drug Regimen	Challenge	Measured Parameters	Outcome
Ponazuril[31]	2.5 mg/kg for 28 d 5.0 mg/kg for 28 d	Transport and experimental infection with *S neurona* sporocysts	Neurologic examination, serum, and CSF antibodies to *S neurona* (Western blot)	Treatment reduced neurologic signs and reduced seroconversion
Ponazuril[33]	20 mg/kg every 7 or 14 d for 12 wk	Experimental infection with *S neurona* sporocysts	Neurologic examination, serum and CSF antibodies to *S neurona* (Western blot)	Reduction of intrathecal anti–*S neurona* antibody response
Nitazoxanide[32]	25 mg/kg 2 d per week for 10 mo	Natural infection	Neurologic examination, CSF antibodies to *S neurona*, response to treatment	Protection against the development of clinical EPM
Diclazuril[39]	0.5 mg/kg every day for 11 mo	Natural infection	Neurologic examination, serum antibodies to *S neurona*	Significant reduction of seroprevalence in treated horses by the end of the study

following an experimental challenge.[31,33] In the study by Furr and colleagues,[31] treatment at either 2.5 or 5.0 mg/kg by mouth, every 24 hours, of ponazuril was administered beginning 7 days before experimental challenge and continued for 28 days. In that study, administration of ponazuril reduced clinical signs and delayed seroconversion. In the second study, by MacKay and colleagues,[33] intermittent ponazuril paste administration at 20 mg/kg by mouth, every 7 days, was associated with a significantly decreased intrathecal anti–S neurona antibody response in horses experimentally inoculated with S neurona sporocysts. Together, these 2 studies showed that daily or intermittent treatment with ponazuril minimized, but did not eliminate, infection in horses experimentally infected with S neurona. A nonrandomized study looked at the incidence of EPM following the treatment of 2-year to 3-year-old training horses with nitazoxanide (NZT).[32] In that study, 43 horses received NZT at 25 mg/kg by mouth, 2 days a week (Saturday and Sunday), for a 10-month period. The incidence of EPM of the treatment group was compared with the historical EPM incidence in 147 horses at the farm diagnosed during the 5 years preceding the administration of NZT. In that study, twice-weekly prophylactic administration of NZT was able to reduce the development of clinical EPM from 12% (18/147 untreated horses) to 0% (0/43 treated horses).[32]

Recently, Hunyadi and colleagues[34] investigated the pharmacokinetics of daily low-dose diclazuril (0.5 mg/kg PO, q 24h) given to adult healthy horses. The results of that study show that diclazuril pellets given at a low-dose attained plasma and CSF concentrations known to inhibit S neurona and N caninum in cell culture. The daily administration of a low-dose diclazuril pellet topdressing to healthy foals from a farm with a high exposure rate to S neurona significantly reduced the monthly seroprevalence to S neurona when compared to untreated foals.[39] The investigators suggested that the reported difference in temporal seroprevalence between treated and untreated foals was likely due to the successful reduction of S neurona infection in foals receiving a daily low-dose diclazuril. This preventive strategy has the potential to be used in high-risk horses in an attempt to reduce the incidence of EPM, although future longitudinal studies will be required before establishing a standard protocol.

SUMMARY

EPM is a diagnosis of exclusion and relies on the presence of neurologic signs, ruling out other neurologic disorders and the detection of antibodies to S neurona or N hughesi in serum and CSF using quantitative immunodiagnostic tests. Three FDA-approved treatment formulations are commercially available for the treatment of EPM and these are broadly equivalent in therapeutic efficacy. Two of these formulations are specifically antiapicomplexan and a positive response to these agents strongly supports an EPM diagnosis. Treatment should be continued until no further clinical improvement is observed. Relapse following cessation of treatment may occur and is not an insignificant clinical problem. Nonempiric treatment recommendations have been proposed to treat relapsing horses. These include prolonging standard treatment courses, combining various classes of antiprotozoal agents, using higher doses of triazine antiprotozoal agents, instituting maintenance therapy following initial treatment course, and administering immunomodulators. Intermittent use of antiprotozoal agents has shown promise in the prevention of EPM. Such protocols have been able to reduce clinical signs, delay seroconversion, and decrease intrathecal anti–S neurona antibody response under experimental conditions. Seroprevalence of anti–S neurona antibodies has been shown to significantly decline in horses continuously exposed to S neurona through the daily extended use of antiprotozoal agents.

REFERENCES

1. Dubey JP, Howe DK, Furr M, et al. An update on *Sarcocystis neurona* infections in animals and equine protozoal myeloencephalitis (EPM). Vet Parasitol 2015; 209(1–2):1–42.
2. Mullaney T, Murphy AJ, Kiupel M, et al. Evidence to support horses as natural intermediate hosts for *Sarcocystis neurona*. Vet Parasitol 2005;133:27–36.
3. Pusterla N, Conrad PA, Packham AE, et al. Endogenous transplacental transmission of *Neospora hughesi* in naturally infected horses. J Parasitol 2011;97(2): 281–5.
4. Gray LC, Magdesian KG, Sturges BK, et al. Suspected protozoal myeloencephalitis in a two-month-old colt. Vet Rec 2001;149(9):269–73.
5. Dubey JP, Black SS, Verma SK, et al. *Sarcocystis neurona* schizonts-associated encephalitis, chorioretinitis, and myositis in a two-month-old dog simulating toxoplasmosis, and presence of mature sarcocysts in muscles. Vet Parasitol 2014; 202(3–4):194–200.
6. Pivoto FL, de Macêdo AG Jr, da Silva MV, et al. Serological status of mares in parturition and the levels of antibodies (IgG) against protozoan family Sarcocystidae from their pre colostral foals. Vet Parasitol 2014;199(1–2):107–11.
7. MacKay RJ, Davis SW, Dubey JP. Equine protozoal myeloencephalitis. Compend Contin Educ Pract Vet 1992;14:1359–67.
8. Reed SM, Furr M, Howe DK, et al. Equine protozoal myeloencephalitis: an updated consensus statement with a focus on parasite biology, diagnosis, treatment, and prevention. J Vet Intern Med 2016;30(2):491–502.
9. Dirikolu L, Foreman JH, Tobin T. Current therapeutic approaches to equine protozoal myeloencephalitis. J Am Vet Med Assoc 2013;242(4):482–91.
10. Kisthardt K, Lindsay DS. Equine protozoal myeloencephalitis. Equine Pract 1997; 19:8–13.
11. Lindsay SD, Dubey JP. Determination of activity of pyrimethamine, trimethoprim, sulfonamides, and combinations of pyrimethamine and sulfonamides against *Sarcocystis neurona* in cell cultures. Vet Parasitol 1999;82:205–10.
12. Brown MP, Kelly RH, Stover SM, et al. Trimethoprim-sulfadiazine in the horse: serum, synovial, peritoneal, and urine concentrations after single-dose intravenous administration. Am J Vet Res 1983;44:540–3.
13. Reed SM, Saville WJ. Equine protozoal encephalomyelitis. Proceedings of 1996 Veterinary Symposium. American Association of Equine Practitioners. Denver, December 8–11, 1996.
14. Welsch BB. Treatment of equine protozoal myeloencephalitis. Compend Contin Educ Pract Vet 1991;13:1599–602.
15. Toribio RE, Bain FT, Mrad DR, et al. Congenital defects in newborn foals of mares treated for equine protozoal myeloencephalitis during pregnancy. J Am Vet Med Assoc 1998;212:697–701.
16. Bedford SJ, McDonnell SM. Measurements of reproductive function in stallions treated with trimethoprim-sulfamethoxazole and pyrimethamine. J Am Vet Med Assoc 1999;215:1317–9.
17. Granstrom DE, McCrillis S, Wulff-Strobel C, et al. Diclazuril and equine protozoal myeloencephalitis. Proceedings of 1997 Veterinary Symposium. American Association of Equine Practitioners. Phoenix, December 7–10, 1997.
18. Tobin T, Dirikolu L, Harkins JD, et al. Preliminary pharmacokinetics of diclazuril and toltrazuril in the horse. Proceedings of 1997 Veterinary Symposium. American Association of Equine Practitioners. 1996.

19. Granstrom DE, Tobin T. Formulations and methods to treat and prevent equine protozoal myeloencephalitis. US patent 5,883,095. March 16, 1999.
20. Hackstein JHP, Meijerink PPJ, Schubert H, et al. Parasitic apicomplexans harbor a chlorophyll a-D1 complex, the potential target for therapeutic triazines. Parasitol Res 1995;81:207–16.
21. Dirikolu L, Lehner AF, Nattrass C, et al. Diclazuril in the horse: its identification detection and preliminary pharmacokinetics. J Vet Pharmacol Ther 1999;22: 374–9.
22. Furr M, Kennedy T. Cerebrospinal fluid and serum concentrations of ponazuril in horses. Vet Ther 2001;2:232–7.
23. Reed SM, Wendel M, King S, et al. Pharmacokinetics of ponazuril in horses. Proceedings of 2012 Veterinary Symposium. American Association of Equine Practitioners. Anaheim (CA): December 1–5, 2012.
24. Bentz BG, Carter WG, Tobin T. Equine protozoal myeloencephalitis (EPM): Review of a diagnostic approach. Compend Contin Educ Pract Vet 1999;21: 975–81.
25. Bentz BG, Dirikolu L, Carter WG, et al. Diclazuril and equine protozoal myeloencephalitis (EPM): a clinical report. Equine Vet Educ 2000;2:258–63.
26. Dirikolu L, Bentz BG, Lehner AF, et al. New therapeutic approaches to equine protozoal myelo-encephalitis: pharmacokinetics of diclazuril sodium salts in the horse. Vet Ther 2006;7:52–63.
27. Ellison SP, Lindsay DS. Decoquinate combined with levamisole reduce the clinical signs and serum SAG 1,5,6 antibodies in horses with suspected equine protozoal myeloencephalitis. Intern J App Res Vet Med 2012;10:1–7.
28. Buxton D, Brebner J, Wright S, et al. Decoquinate and the control of experimental ovine toxoplasmosis. Vet Rec 1996;138(18):434–6.
29. Sajid MS, Iqbal Z, Muhammad G, et al. Immunomodulatory effect of various antiparasitics: a review. Parasitol 2006;132:301–13.
30. Gutierrez J, Eisenberg RL, Koval NJ, et al. Pemoline and tetramisole 'positives' in English racehorses following levamisole administration. Ir Vet J 2010;63(8): 498–500.
31. Furr M, McKenzie H, Saville WJ, et al. Prophylactic administration of ponazuril reduces clinical signs and delays seroconversion in horses challenged with *Sarcocystis neurona*. J Parasitol 2006;92:637–43.
32. Easter L, Coles TB. Prevention of equine protozoal myeloencephalitis. Vet Forum 2007;24(8):54–60.
33. Mackay RJ, Tanhauser ST, Gillis KD, et al. Effect of intermittent oral administration of ponazuril on experimental *Sarcocystis neurona* infection of horses. Am J Vet Res 2008;69:396–402.
34. Hunyadi L, Papich MG, Pusterla N. Pharmacokinetics of a low dose and FDA-labeled dose of diclazuril administered orally as a pelleted topdressing in adult horses. J Vet Pharmacol Ther 2015;38(3):243–8.
35. Furr M, Kennedy T, Mackay R, et al. Efficacy of ponazuril 15% oral paste as a treatment for equine protozoal myeloencephalitis. Vet Ther 2001;2:215–22.
36. Witonsky SG, Gogal RM Jr, Duncan RB, et al. Protective immune response to experimental infection with *Sarcocystis neurona* in 57BL/6 mice. J Parasitol 2003;89(5):924–31.
37. Kennedy T, Campbell J, Selzer V. Safety of ponazuril 15% oral paste in horses. Vet Ther 2001;2:223–31.
38. US FDA. Protazil antiprotozoal pellets. 1.56% diclazuril. Freedom of Information Summary. Original new animal drug application. NADA 141–268. Available

at: www.fda.gov/downloads/AnimalVeterinary/Products/ApprovedAnimalDrug Products/FOIADrugSummaries/ucm02320.pdf. Accessed July 7, 2016.

39. Pusterla N, Packham A, Mackie S, et al. Daily feeding of diclazuril top dress pellets in foals reduces seroconversion to *Sarcocystis neurona*. Vet J 2015;206(2): 236–8.

Antiherpetic Drugs in Equine Medicine

Lara K. Maxwell, DVM, PhD

KEYWORDS

- Equine • Herpesvirus • EHV-1 • EHV-5 • Antiviral • Nucleoside analogs • Acyclovir
- Valacyclovir

KEY POINTS

- Equine herpesvirus (EHV)-1 differentially affects different classes of horses but can be particularly devastating to neonatal foals, pregnant mares, and adult performance horses.
- Recent high-profile outbreaks of EHV myeloencephalopathy (EHM) have had an impact on the equine industry and stimulated interest in antiherpetic interventions.
- Several antiherpetic drugs that are active against EHV-1 in the laboratory have been investigated both clinically and experimentally in horses and foals.
- The recent association between equine pulmonary multinodular fibrosis (EMPF) and EHV-5 has resulted in the empiric use of antiherpetic drugs for this condition.
- Little is currently known about resistance patterns of EHV-1 or EHV-5 for antiherpetic drugs in horses.

INTRODUCTION

Herpesviruses comprise a large, ancient family of viruses that infect most if not all vertebrates and even lower organisms.[1] The herpesviruses are specialists that have coevolved with their host species over many years, evading multiple steps of immunity.[2] Perhaps as a consequence of this immune evasion, current equine vaccines can decrease the replication and clinical signs associated with several herpesvirus infections but cannot completely prevent infection.[3–6] Currently, 9 herpesviruses have been described from equids and are appropriately named EHV-1 through EHV-9.[1] These 9 herpesviruses belong to 2 separate subfamilies, either the Alphaherpesvirinae (EHV-1, EHV-3, EHV-4, EHV-6, EHV-8, and EHV-9) or the Gammaherpesvirinae (EHV-2, EHV-5, and EHV-7). Several of these viruses, such as EHV-1, EHV-2, EHV-3, EHV-4, and EHV-5, are associated with clinical disease in horses. Whereas in vitro antiherpetic drug susceptibility testing (**Table 1**) has been performed with EHV-1, EHV-3,

The author has nothing to disclose.
Department of Physiological Sciences, Center for Veterinary Health Sciences, Oklahoma State University, 264 McElroy Hall, Stillwater, OK 74078, USA
E-mail address: lk.maxwell@okstate.edu

Table 1
In vitro half-maximal inhibitory concentration values of antiherpetic drugs for equine herpesviruses

Virus	Drug	Virus Strain	Cell Type	Half-maximal Inhibitory Concentration (μg/mL)	Reference
EHV-1	Acyclovir	Rac-H, H-45	PK13	0.45	Rollinson & White,[85] 1983
		Kentucky D	PRK	7	De Clerq et al,[109] 1986
		Quai Hais	R13	2.6	Boyd et al,[60] 1987
		94P247, 97P70, and 99P96; 97P82, 99P136, and 03P37	EEL	1.7–3	Garre et al,[84] 2007
		89c25	RK13	2.3–3.1	Azab et al,[82] 2010
		T953 (Findlay OH 2003)	ELF	11.4 ± 1.5	(Maxwell LK, Bentz BG, Gilliam LL, et al. Efficacy of the early administration of valacyclovir for the therapy of neuropathogenic EHV-1 in horses. Submitted for publication.)
		T953 (Findlay OH 2003)	PBMC	0.8	(Maxwell LK, Bentz BG, Gilliam LL, et al. Efficacy of the early administration of valacyclovir for the therapy of neuropathogenic EHV-1 in horses. Submitted for publication.)
	Penciclovir	Quai Hais	R13	1.6	Boyd et al,[60] 1987
		AB4	RK13	1.3–1.9	de la Fuente et al,[76] 1992
		T953 (Findlay OH 2003)	ELF	4.8 ± 0.7	(Maxwell LK, Bentz BG, Gilliam LL, et al. Efficacy of the early administration of valacyclovir for the therapy of neuropathogenic EHV-1 in horses. Submitted for publication.)
	Ganciclovir	Rac-H, H-45	PK13	0.02	Rollinson and White,[85] 1983
		Kentucky D	E Derm	0.03	Smith et al,[110] 1983
		Rac-H, H-45	RK13	0.02–0.1	Rollinson,[111] 1987
		94P247, 97P70, and 99P96; 97P82, 99P136, and 03P37	EEL	0.1–4	Garre et al,[84] 2007
		89c25	RK13	0.1–0.7	Azab et al,[82] 2010

	Drug	Strain	Cell	IC	Reference
		T953 (Findlay OH 2003)	ELF	0.1 ± 0.1	(Maxwell LK, Bentz BG, Gilliam LL, et al. Efficacy of the early administration of valacyclovir for the therapy of neuropathogenic EHV-1 in horses. Submitted for publication.)
	Cidofovir	AB4	RK13	0.01–0.2	Gibson et al,[10] 1992
		94P247, 97P70, and 99P96; 97P82, 99P136, and 03P37	EEL	1.1–6.7	Garre et al,[84] 2007
	Adefovir	94P247, 97P70, and 99P96; 97P82, 99P136, and 03P37	EEL	2.8–5.6	Garre et al,[84] 2007
	Foscarnet	94P247, 97P70, and 99P96; 97P82, 99P136, and 03P37	EEL	6.6–16.2	Garre et al,[84] 2007
EHV-3	Ganciclovir	118 (ATCC)	E Derm	0.16	Smith et al,[110] 1983
EHV-4	Acyclovir	TH20p	RK13	>50	Azab et al,[82] 2010
	Ganciclovir	TH20p	RK13	1.5–3.5	Azab et al,[82] 2010

Abbreviations: E Derm, equine dermal cells; EEL, equine embryonic lung; ELF, equine fetal lung; PBMC, peripheral blood mononuclear cell viremia as determined in horses in vivo during drug administration; PK13, porcine kidney; PRK, primary rabbit kidney; RK13, rabbit kidney cells.

and EHV-4, only EHV-1 and EHV-5 infections are routinely treated with antiherpetic drugs, so this review focuses on these 2 viral diseases, with a brief description of EHV-2.

Neurologic impairment due to EHV-1 infection results in EHM, whereas EHV-5 is associated with equine multinodular pulmonary fibrosis (EMPF). Because vaccination may not prevent disease, antiherpetic therapies are used for both prophylaxis and treatment of viral disease. Like vaccination, current antiherpetic therapies seem unable to completely prevent herpesvirus infections. Therefore, the primary goal of antiherpetic therapy is to decrease viral replication until the immune system mounts an appropriate response and controls active infection. In humans, the link between herpesvirus reactivation and immunosuppression is both multifactorial and well established, especially in cases with physiologic stress and pharmacologically immunosuppressed transplant recipients.[7–9] In horses, supraphysiological doses of exogenous glucocorticoids also stimulate reactivation of EHV-1, with limited viral replication and mild disease.[10–12] Little is known, however, about the role of normal immune function in the maintenance of herpesvirus latency and control of active viral replication in horses; an association between common sources of stress and EHV-1 infection has not been demonstrated.[13–15] A case report describing EHV-5 infection in a horse after cytotoxic therapy for lymphoma is intriguing,[16] because it suggests that pharmacologic immunosuppression may be a factor in EMPF.

In human medicine, tremendous strides have been made in the treatment HIV, a retrovirus. Many of the newest strides in antiviral therapy have occurred as a result of intense study of this pathogen. The commercial availability of antiherpetic drugs, however, actually predated the advent of antiretroviral agents. Still, the use of antiviral drugs is unfamiliar to many veterinary practitioners, who often equate antiviral therapy with antibacterial therapy. There are similarities between antiviral and antibacterial drugs, but there are also substantial differences. For example, because viruses use the host's cellular machinery for replication, selective toxicity of virally infected cells can be difficult to achieve. As a consequence, there are fewer drug targets for selective toxicity, so most antiviral agents target DNA replication, mechanistically resembling cytotoxic anticancer drugs. The side effects associated with some of these antiviral agents can, therefore, resemble those of cytotoxic drugs. Another unique characteristic of antiviral drugs is that they tend to much more narrowly inhibit a specific viral subfamily or species than do most antibacterial drugs. As a result, antiherpetic drugs are not uniformly effective against all herpesviruses in horses or against the different alphaherpesviruses affecting cats and horses. When antiherpetic drugs are effective, that activity is expected to be virostatic, because no systemically administered antiviral drug is capable of "killing" viruses. Only a disinfectant can truly exert a virocidal effect. As a consequence, a host's immune system must be competent to clear the viral infection, even when effective antiviral therapy is administered. Because antiherpetic drugs prevent viral replication, they are also ineffective against virus in the latent, or nonreplicating, state. These virostatic effects contribute to the critical importance of the timing of antiviral therapy, because well-established herpesvirus infections are generally not ameliorated pharmacologically, and latent virus is not affected.[17–19] Instead, antiviral therapy is most effective when begun prophylactically or early in the course of infection.[19]

As with antibacterial drugs, the efficacy and potency of antiviral drugs can be determined in vitro, but this determination differs in that it requires viral replication to occur within a primary or immortalized cell line. The drug concentration that reduces viral plaques by 50% is termed the half-maximal inhibitory concentration (IC_{50}) and is analogous to the familiar minimum inhibitory concentration (MIC) of antibacterial drugs.

Although the plaque reduction assay is considered the gold standard of measuring antiviral susceptibility, the IC_{50} is not as well standardized as is the MIC, because many factors, such as the cell line, incubation time, and laboratory reagents, have an impact on the IC_{50} and affect the definition of clinically meaningful breakpoints.[20] Whereas pharmacokinetic and pharmacodynamic relationships are well defined for most antibacterial drugs, such relationships are poorly defined for most antiviral drugs. Plasma drug concentrations and IC_{50} may correlate poorly with drug efficacy, due partially to poor correlation between plasma and intracellular drug concentrations. Although the antiherpetic nucleoside analogs are fairly polar, they accumulate in virally infected cells in a thymidine kinase (TK)-dependent manner and result in more prolonged intracellular half-lives than expected from plasma drug concentrations.[21,22] Some antiherpetic drugs, such as penciclovir and cidofovir, have particularly prolonged intracellular half-lives, contributing to their efficacy when plasma drug concentrations drop below inhibitory concentrations.[23,24] Therefore, although in vitro testing is useful for screening likely antiviral drugs, testing in live animals may produce wholly different results.[25] For example, when the IC_{50} of acyclovir was determined both in vitro and in horses for the same strain of EHV-1, the in vitro IC_{50} was more than 10 times higher than the in vivo IC_{50}. (Maxwell LK, Bentz BG, Gilliam LL, et al. Efficacy of the early administration of valacyclovir for the therapy of neuropathogenic EHV-1 in horses. Submitted for publication.)

PATIENT POPULATION OVERVIEW
Equine Herpesvirus 1

EHV-1 is genetically related to bovine herpesvirus 1, herpes simplex virus (HSV)-1 and HSV-2, varicella-zoster virus, and pseudorabies virus.[26,27] EHV-1 is transmitted between horses by the respiratory route, occurs throughout the world, and causes significant economic loss due to respiratory disease, abortion, and neurologic signs.[28,29] The incomplete protection that vaccination currently offers against clinical disease associated with EHV-1 infection has led to the investigation of several antiherpetic drug strategies to protect vulnerable populations of horses. Pulmonary inflammation secondary to EHV-1 infection can cause substantial morbidity and mortality in neonatal foals and upper respiratory signs in weanlings.[30,31] Vaccination can decrease clinical signs of disease in weanling foals and upper respiratory signs are generally not severe, but no such protection exists for neonatal foals.[5] In pregnant mares, EHV-1 is primarily an abortigenic virus that can cause abortion storms, or clusters of abortions within a farm.[5,31] Vaccination can prevent abortion storms but does not protect all animals. EHM occurs when EHV-1 infection produces neurologic signs, ranging from mild ataxia to severe paresis. These signs are reported to be primarily caused by damage to the endothelium of vessels in the spinal cord and brain.[6,32,33] High-profile outbreaks of EHM have stimulated interest in interventions that mitigate neurologic signs in horses, because no vaccine is currently labeled to prevent EHM.[34,35]

Equine Herpesvirus 5

Equine pulmonary multinodular fibrosis (EMPF) compromises lung function in adult horses and has been associated with the ubiquitous gammaherpesvirus, EHV-5, both by association in clinically affected animals and by induction of the disease by experimental inoculation of horses.[36–39] Little is definitively known about the factors that underlie development of EMPF, but there is a possible link between EHV-5, EHV-2, and lymphoma or leukemia.[16,40–42] Currently, antiherpetic drugs, in conjunction with other therapies, are often administered to horses with EMPF in hopes of clinical improvement, although their efficacy in this setting is still unclear.

Equine Herpesvirus 2

Like EHV-5, EHV-2 is widely present throughout the equine population. Weanling foals with conjunctivitis, epiphora, and keratopathy attributed to the gammaherpesvirus EHV-2 have been described in large case series.[43,44] Keratoconjunctivitivs and keratopathy have also been associated with EHV-2 in adult horses, but a causal relationship is difficult to demonstrate because the virus is present in both healthy horses and those with conjunctivitis.[45]

ANTIVIRAL TREATMENT OPTIONS

Multiple antiherpetic therapies have been tested against EHVs. Several of these agents are novel but currently unavailable to practitioners as a manufactured product, so they are not discussed further in this review.[46–48] The antiherpetic drugs that are most commonly used for therapy for EHVs are acyclovir and its prodrug, valacyclovir. Therefore, discussion focuses on the use of these drugs in horses. A variety of supportive and anti-inflammatory therapies are also commonly administered to horses with EHM, including flunixin meglumine, dimethyl sulfoxide, and dexamethasone, and have been recently described.[29]

Acyclovir

Over the past few decades, the greatest strides in antiviral therapy have been made in treating HIV with sophisticated multidrug protocols. It was the development of acyclovir, however, as a specific and potent inhibitor of human herpesviruses (HHVs) that led to a Nobel prize and first generated widespread enthusiasm for antiviral therapeutics.[49] Acyclovir is a nucleoside analog that ultimately resembles and substitutes for GTP in DNA synthesis. Although other antiherpetic drugs were known before acyclovir, acyclovir was the first to be selectively toxic to herpesviruses, like HSV. That selectivity hinges on the first phosphorylation step by the enzyme TK, followed by subsequent phosphorylation until the acyclovir is triply phosphorylated and can be incorporated into the viral DNA strand by DNA polymerase. Selective toxicity of acyclovir is primarily achieved by its higher affinity for viral TK, compared with cellular (host) TK, and coupled with the higher affinity of triply phosphorylated acyclovir for viral DNA polymerase, compared with cellular DNA polymerase.

Side effects generally attributed to acyclovir administration include nephrotoxicity and bone marrow suppression, with hepatotoxicity also described.[50] Nephrotoxicity is the most common side effect in most species and occurs when high concentrations of acyclovir in the renal tubules precipitate, resulting in obstructive nephropathy.[51] Because acyclovir is primarily excreted through glomerular filtration and tubular secretion, nephrotoxicity is more likely with preexisting renal compromise.[52] Additionally, acyclovir must be cautiously administered by the intravenous (IV) route, because the resulting plasma and renal concentrations are higher than those associated with oral administration and can potentiate precipitation in the renal tubule. Injectable acyclovir (pioneer product Zovirax, GlaxoSmithKline, Greenville, North Carolina) is rarely administered to horses but has been diluted in an isotonic crystalloid solution, such as normal saline solution, to a concentration of 5 mg/mL to 15 mg/mL, and administered as an infusion over at least 1 hour.[53–55] The Zovirax brand of acyclovir has been discontinued, but several injectable acyclovir sodium products are available in the United States. Although the manufacturer of injectable acyclovir states that infusion concentrations should not exceed 7 mg/mL,[56] the length of infusion seems to be the key factor affecting safety in horses, because 5 mg/mL administered over a shorter, 15-minute infusion rapidly produced sweating, tremors, and colic in 1 of 6 treated horses.[57] Injectable acyclovir should not be given subcutaneously or intramuscularly, due to its high pH of 11.[56] Oral administration of acyclovir seems safe in horses, with few side effects reported despite weeks or months of therapy.[30,34,38,58] As a consequence of the high selectivity of acyclovir for herpesviruses, it may even be administered to pregnant women, even though the drug crosses the placenta.[59] Oral acyclovir has also been administered to neonatal foals for the treatment of EHV-1 infections with apparent safety.[30]

Acyclovir is the least expensive antiherpetic drug administered to horses, a major factor when considering weeks to months of treatment (**Table 2**). There are 2 critical characteristics of acyclovir that limit its utility in horses, however. First, although HSV is highly sensitive to acyclovir, with an IC_{50} generally less than 1 μg/mL, most other herpesviruses, including EHV-1, are considerably less sensitive (see **Table 1**).[60] Differences in herpesvirus sensitivities to acyclovir are usually due to variability in viral TK, with EHV-1 generally less sensitive to acyclovir than is HSV-1, although EHV-1 does phosphorylate acyclovir with moderate efficiency.[61] Although the affinity of EHV-1 TK for acyclovir is less than that of HSV-1, it is still superior to the binding of feline herpesvirus 1 (FHV-1), an important distinction because acyclovir and related drugs do not protect cats from FHV-1.[50,61] A second disadvantage is that acyclovir is poorly absorbed after oral administration to adult horses, so that oral bioavailability is poor (<5%) (see **Table 2**).[54,55,57] Acyclovir also does not readily distribute into the central nervous system, resulting in low acyclovir concentrations in equine cerebrospinal fluid. (Maxwell LK, Bentz BG, Gilliam LL, et al. Efficacy of the early administration of valacyclovir for the therapy of neuropathogenic EHV-1 in horses. Submitted for publication.)[62]

Despite these disadvantages, acyclovir is the best studied of the antiviral drugs used in horses due to its low cost, high safety profile, and long historical availability (see **Tables 1** and **2**, **Table 3**). Several pharmacokinetic studies have examined both oral and IV routes of administration in horses, with an emphasis on investigation of oral administration of tablets for clinical use. Unfortunately, the oral availability of acyclovir in horses is so low as to be negligible (approximately 3%), even when administered by nasogastric tube to fasted horses.[54,55,57] Although low oral bioavailability is a common feature of acyclovir (approximately 20% in humans) and related nucleoside analogs, the abysmal oral absorption in horses is much lower than it is in other species and calls into question the utility of oral acyclovir in horses.[52,63] Nonetheless, oral acyclovir has been administered clinically to foals and horses infected with EHV-1 with some reports of success (discussed later). Because acyclovir absorption is much higher in suckling rats compared with weaned rats, neonatal foals might absorb orally administered acyclovir to a greater extent than do adult horses, but pharmacokinetic studies in foals are not currently available.[64] Another explanation for the potential efficacy of oral acyclovir resides in the prolonged elimination half-life of acyclovir in horses, resulting in drug accumulation over the 2-day to 5-day period required to reach steady state conditions.[63] Because the primary elimination pathway for acyclovir is through glomerular filtration and tubular secretion in the kidney, the elimination half-life of acyclovir in most species is short, approximately 3 hours.[65] The elimination half-life of acyclovir is considerably longer in horses, however, with single-dose IV acyclovir studies estimating elimination half-lives of 5 hours to 53 hours, along with marked interindividual variability.[53–55,57] Although renal elimination has not been quantified in horses, the prolonged elimination phase in this species is theorized

Table 2
Dosing regimens recommended from the cited study and current cost of therapy for antiherpetic drugs in horses

Drug	Route	Bioavailability	Target Half-maximal Inhibitory Concentration (μg/mL)	Dose and Interval	Cost/day ($)	Unit	$/Unit	Reference
Acyclovir	1-h IV infusion	NA	0.3	10 mg/kg q12h	252	1 g vial	25.20	Wilkins et al,[55] 2005
	0.25-h IV infusion	NA	0.3–7	NA				Bentz et al,[57] 2006
	1-h IV infusion	NA	1.7–3	NA				Garré et al,[54] 2007
	1-h IV infusion	NA	2	NA				Maxwell et al,[53] 2008
	Oral	Negligible	0.3	10 mg/kg 5×/d?	11	800 mg	0.35	Wilkins et al,[55] 2005
	Oral	3% ± 1%	1.7–3	NA				Garré et al,[54] 2007
	Intragastric	2.8%–4%	0.3–7	NA				Bentz et al,[57] 2006
Valacyclovir	Intragastric	26% ± 5%[a]	1.7–3	40 mg/kg q8h	86	1000 mg	1.43	Garré et al,[54] 2007
	Oral	48%–60%[b]	2	LD: 27 mg/kg q8h, 2d; Maint: 18 mg/kg q12h	58; 26	1000 mg	1.43	Maxwell et al,[53] 2008
	Oral	ND	1.7	40 mg/kg q8h	86	1000 mg	1.43	Garre et al,[62] 2009
	Oral	ND	0.8	LD: 27 mg/kg q8h, 2 d; Maint: 18–36 mg/kg q12h	58; 26–52	1000 mg	1.43	(Maxwell LK, Bentz BG, Gilliam LL, et al. Efficacy of the early administration of valacyclovir for the therapy of neuropathogenic EHV-1 in horses. Submitted for publication.)
Famciclovir	Intragastric	ND	1.6	Similar to valacyclovir?	116–184	500 mg	2.50	Tsujimura et al,[80] 2010
Ganciclovir	IV	NA	0.1–0.4	LD: 2.5 mg/kg q8h, 1 d; Maint: 2.5 mg/kg q12h	600; 400	50 mg/mL	8.00	Carmichael et al,[90] 2013
Valganciclovir	Oral	41% ± 20%[b]	0.1–0.4	3.6 g q12h	365	450 mg	45.61	Carmichael et al,[90] 2013

Abbreviations: LD, loading dosing regimen; Maint, maintenance dosing regimen; NA, not applicable; ND, not determined; ?, No definitive recommended dosing regimen in cited reference.
[a] Calculated from the weight-based dose of the prodrug and active form.
[b] Calculated from the molar dose of the prodrug and active form.

Table 3
Clinical and experimental efficacy of antiherpetic drugs in horses

Virus	Drug	Strain	Clinical Signs	Signalment	Horses Treated (Number)	Origin	Time Therapy Initiated	Dosing Regimen	Outcome	Reference
EHV-1	Acyclovir	ND	Pulmonary	TB foal	3	Natural	At diagnosis	8–16 mg/kg PO q8h for 1–2 wk	2 survived, 1 died	Murray et al,[30] 1998
		ND	EHM	Adult riding horses	7	Natural	3–4 d after ataxia	20 mg/kg PO q8h for 5 d	Difficult to assess	Friday et al,[58] 2000
		T953	EHM	>3 y riding horses	99	Natural	9–12 d after outbreak began	20 mg/kg PO q8h for 5 d	Positive impression but difficult to assess	Henninger et al,[34] 2007
	Valacyclovir	03P37	Upper respiratory	8 mo–2 y Shetland pony	4	Exper	At inoculation	40 mg/kg PO q8h for 5–7 d	No beneficial effects	Garre et al,[73] 2009
		T953	EHM	Mares >20 y	12	Exper	−1 to +2 d from inoculation	27 mg/kg q8h PO for 2 d, then 18 mg/kg q12h for 1–2 wk	Decreased viral replication and ataxia	(Maxwell LK, Bentz BG, Gilliam LL, et al. Efficacy of the early administration of valacyclovir for the therapy of neuropathogenic EHV-1 in horses. Submitted for publication.)
		ND	EHM	7 y QH mare	1	Natural	On ataxia	30 mg/kg PO q12h for 10d	Survived	Goehring et al,[95] 2010

(continued on next page)

Table 3
(continued)

Virus	Drug	Strain	Clinical Signs	Signalment	Horses Treated (Number)	Origin	Time Therapy Initiated	Dosing Regimen	Outcome	Reference
		T953	EHM	Mares >20 y	9	Exper	4–6 d after inoculation	27 mg/kg q8h PO for 2d, then 18 mg/kg q12h for 1–2 wk	Did not decrease ataxia	Maxwell et al,[88] 2011
		ND	EHM	3–15 y QH, SB	7	Natural	At admission	30 mg/kg q8h PO for 2 d, then 20 mg/kg q12h for 10 d	5/7 survived	Estell et al,[71] 2015
	Ganciclovir	T953	EHM	Mares >20 y	9	Exper	4–6 d after inoculation	2.5 mg/kg q8h IV for 1 d, then q12h for 1 wk	Decreased viral replication and ataxia	Maxwell et al,[88] 2011
		Ogden 2011	EHM	4–15 y QH or WB mares	2	Natural	On encephalopathy	2.5 mg/kg IV q8h	2/2 died	Estell et al,[71] 2015
	Cidofovir	AB4	Upper respiratory	SPF 3–4 mo foal	2	Exper	At inoculation	20 mg/kg SC 1×, or 1 mg/kg SC q3d 2×	Reduced clinical signs in high dose foal	Gibson et al,[92] 1992

Virus/Drug	Origin	System	Signalment	n	Type	Timing	Dose	Outcome	Reference
EHV-5 Acyclovir	ND	Pulmonary	8–24 y gelding TB or Olden	4	Natural	At diagnosis	20 mg/kg PO q8h for 2–3 mo	Survival in 2/4 horses	Wong et al,[38] 2008
	ND	Pulmonary	12 TB mare	1	Natural	At diagnosis	20 mg/kg PO q8h for 1 mo	Mare died	Spelta et al,[37] 2013
	ND	Pulmonary	12 y QH mare	1	Natural	7 mo after lymphoma therapy	20 mg/kg PO q8h for 4 mo	Survival	Vander Werf and Davis,[16] 2013
	ND	Pulmonary	6–8 y Olden, Holsteiner	2	Natural	At diagnosis	20 mg/kg PO q8h until death	Both died	Schwartz et al,[36] 2013
Valacyclovir	ND	Pulmonary	22 y Trakehner stallion	1	Natural	At diagnosis	40 mg/kg PO q8h for 1 wk	Survival	Schwartz et al,[72] 2013

Note that the numbers of horses present in case series may have been larger, but that only horses that received specific antiviral therapy are included.

Abbreviations: Exper, experimental inoculation; Olden, oldenburg; Origin, source of viral infection; QH, quarter horse; SB, standardbred; SC, subcutaneous; SPF, specific pathogen free; TB, thoroughbred.

to be due to the presence of a deep compartment, from which acyclovir is slowly released to the plasma.[53]

Valacyclovir

The 3 primary antiherpetic drugs, acyclovir, ganciclovir, and penciclovir, developed for routine and long-term systemic use in humans, all suffer from poor oral bioavailability. In response, corresponding prodrugs, valacyclovir, valganciclovir, and famciclovir, have been synthesized and formulated for enhanced oral absorption. Valacyclovir is the L-valyl ester prodrug of acyclovir, which enhances enteral absorption of acyclovir through activity of dipeptide transporters on the apical surface of enterocytes.[66] Once absorbed, valacyclovir is rapidly hydrolyzed to its active form, acyclovir, such that plasma concentrations of the prodrug are very low or absent in horses.[53] Although valacyclovir was not found in equine plasma, acyclovir appeared rapidly, with maximal concentrations occurring 45 minutes to 60 minutes after oral valacyclovir administration and an absorption half-life of 0.5 hours to 0.7 hours.[53–55] Oral absorption of valacyclovir in horses is considerably better (41%–60%) than that of acyclovir and did not substantially change with doses between 5 g and 15 g (8–34 mg/kg) of valacyclovir (discussed later).[53,54] Note that the 2 studies cited delivery of valacyclovir using a nasogastric tube and that 1 study fasted the horses before drug administration. Additional data suggested, however, that fasting did not affect valacyclovir absorption.[54] Subsequent studies confirmed the pharmacokinetic profile in horses using multiple orally administered doses of valacyclovir.[62] (Please also see Maxwell LK, Bentz BG, Gilliam LL, et al. Efficacy of the early administration of valacyclovir for the therapy of neuropathogenic EHV-1 in horses. Submitted for publication.) Although dose rates of valacyclovir ranging from 8 mg/kg to 40 mg/kg did not substantially affect oral bioavailability, a trend toward decreasing bioavailability was present, with values of 60% at 8 mg/kg and 48% at 34 mg/kg. A decrease in oral absorption is expected at higher doses due to saturable, carrier-mediated transport, as noted with oral absorption of valacyclovir in other species.[66] Data in humans and rodents suggest that valacyclovir absorption may also be inhibited by some antibiotics, anions, and cations. There are also studies indicating that the coadministration of valacyclovir and nonsteroidal anti-inflammatory drugs may increase the risk of acute kidney disease and that cimetidine and probenecid increase acyclovir exposure in humans.[66–68] Because valacyclovir drug interactions have not been investigated in horses, cautious coadministration of other oral drugs is warranted. The stability of valacyclovir in extemporaneously prepared solutions should also be considered, because tablets must be pulverized or dissolved prior to administration to horses. Because tablets have a protective coating and seemed unpalatable to some horses, the author prefers to grind tablets prior to mixing with maple-flavored syrup. (Maxwell LK, Bentz BG, Gilliam LL, et al. Efficacy of the early administration of valacyclovir for the therapy of neuropathogenic EHV-1 in horses. Submitted for publication.) Other investigators have mixed valacyclovir with apple sauce with acceptable palatability.[62] Tablets should not be dissolved and stored prior to administration without following proved protocols, because the ester bond of valacyclovir is subject to degradation in neutral to alkaline aqueous solutions.[69,70] The resulting degraded solution contains L-valine and acyclovir in the place of the much more bioavailable and expensive valacyclovir, with a commensurate drop in activity and efficacy.

As with IV acyclovir, the elimination half-life of acyclovir after oral valacyclovir administration is prolonged and variable, with initial single-dose studies estimating elimination half-lives of 2 hours to 53 hours.[53,54] Because the elimination half-life of acyclovir is prolonged, multiple-dose pharmacokinetic studies can more definitively estimate the elimination half-life of acyclovir from oral valacyclovir administration, where a mean value of 20 hours ± 22 hours was obtained. (Maxwell LK, Bentz BG, Gilliam LL, et al. Efficacy of the early administration of valacyclovir for the therapy of neuropathogenic EHV-1 in horses. Submitted for publication.) Various valacyclovir dosing regimens have been recommended for use in horses. Because plasma acyclovir is expected to accumulate slowly after valacyclovir administration, and horses at risk for developing EHM require rapid attainment of therapeutic concentrations, 1 protocol involves the use of a loading-dose regimen of 27 mg/kg orally every 8 hours for the first 2 days to rapidly achieve steady state, followed by a maintenance dose regimen of 18 mg/kg orally every12 hours.[53] Some equine clinicians have rounded these doses to 30 mg/kg and 20 mg/kg orally, respectively, for convenience.[71] In multiple-dose efficacy studies, the proposed dosing regimen reached effective concentrations in most horses, but, due to wide interindividual variability, maintenance doses of up to 36 mg/kg every 12 hours were required to maintain therapeutic acyclovir concentrations in some horses. (Maxwell LK, Bentz BG, Gilliam LL, et al. Efficacy of the early administration of valacyclovir for the therapy of neuropathogenic EHV-1 in horses. Submitted for publication.) No changes in serum biochemistry, complete blood cell counts, or bone marrow were observed after administration of oral valacyclovir to horses for 1 to 2 weeks. (Maxwell LK, Bentz BG, Gilliam LL, et al. Efficacy of the early administration of valacyclovir for the therapy of neuropathogenic EHV-1 in horses. Submitted for publication.) A higher valacyclovir dosing regimen of 40 mg/kg every 8 hours has also been proposed and was able to maintain concentrations above a goal concentrations of 1.7 to 3 μg/mL for at least half of the dosing interval.[54,62] Although no health effects were noted when oral valacyclovir, 40 mg/kg every 8 hours, was administered to horses and ponies for 4 to 7 days, specific testing for toxicity was not reported and safety of this high-dose rate (120 mg/kg/d) beyond 1 week has not been well investigated.[62,72,73] Although toxicity of valacyclovir is poorly defined in horses, toxicity is expected to depend on plasma and renal acyclovir concentrations; therefore, it would have the same potential spectrum of side effects discussed previously for acyclovir. A daily dose rate of 120 mg/kg of valacyclovir approaches the daily dose rate, 240 mg/kg/d, that produced renal and bone marrow toxicity in cats.[50] Human high-dose valacyclovir therapy ranges from 40 mg/kg/d to 110 mg/kg/d for several days, for HSV therapy, and up to several months, in the case of transplant recipients.[74,75] Therefore, high-dose valacyclovir is at the upper limit of that tolerated well by humans and should be used cautiously in horses over an extended time period.

Although initial studies in horses were performed when valacyclovir tablets were expensive, the pioneer product (Valtrex, GlaxoSmithKline) is no longer under patent in the United States, so the availability of generic tablets has profoundly decreased the price per tablet (see **Table 2**). Current prices of generic valacyclovir are highly variable in the United States, differing day by day between the many generic manufacturers and pharmacies. Although the pharmacokinetics of these generic formulations have not been examined in horses, they have been found bioequivalent to Valtrex in humans, as part of the standard data submitted to the Food and Drug Administration for generic drugs.

Substitution of Intravenous Acyclovir for Oral Valacyclovir

Currently, oral valacyclovir therapy in horses is much more commonly used and better understood than is IV acyclovir. As an oral drug, valacyclovir is usually more convenient to administer than IV acyclovir, which must be administered as a 1-hour infusion. In addition, valacyclovir is currently much less expensive than even generic injectable acyclovir (see **Table 2**), because IV acyclovir is a drug that is needed for life-threatening human infections. Nonetheless, IV acyclovir therapy may be preferred to oral valacyclovir in horses that are too compromised for oral drug administration or that have concurrent anterior enteritis. Given that IV acyclovir is administered as a 1-hour infusion and that valacyclovir is rapidly absorbed and converted to acyclovir after oral administration, the plasma acyclovir concentration versus time curves after pharmacokinetically equivalent doses of IV acyclovir and oral valacyclovir are similar. Higher peak concentrations occur with IV administration, but they have similar profiles after distribution (**Fig. 1**). Because trough concentrations are more indicative of efficacy than peak concentrations, this similarity in dispositional profiles suggests that IV acyclovir can be readily substituted for oral valacyclovir when necessary. (Maxwell LK, Bentz BG, Gilliam LL, et al. Efficacy of the early administration of valacyclovir for the therapy of neuropathogenic EHV-1 in horses. Submitted for publication.)

To make this substitution, equivalent doses of injectable acyclovir and oral valacyclovir can be calculated from the bioavailability of valacyclovir. One report[54] calculated the dose from the weight of valacyclovir administered, whereas the other[53] corrected for the molar ratio (0.624) of the molecular weights of acyclovir:valacyclovir because valacyclovir is a larger molecule than is acyclovir. Because drug doses are calculated on a weight/kilogram basis, rather than a molar basis, an equivalent dose of injectable valacyclovir can be calculated as: dose acyclovir = dose valacyclovir × weight-based bioavailability. If the average molar oral bioavailability of valacyclovir was 48%, then the weight-based bioavailability is 30%, and a 30-mg/kg dose of oral valacyclovir could be substituted by a 9-mg/kg dose of IV acyclovir. Because the postabsorptive disposition of acyclovir after the oral administration of valacyclovir is similar to that of IV acyclovir at the end of a 1-hour infusion, similar dosing intervals could be used for both IV acyclovir and oral valacyclovir dosing regimens. A dose of 10 mg/kg IV acyclovir has been examined in single-dose equine studies, because 10 mg/kg every 8 hours is a common dose administered to humans as an IV infusion.[56] This IV dose

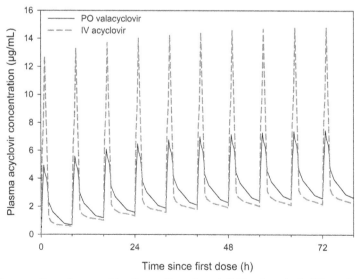

Fig. 1. Comparative pharmacokinetic profiles of oral (PO) valacyclovir (27 mg/kg every 8 hours) and IV acyclovir (10 mg/kg every 8 hours) in horses.

rate of 10 mg/kg every 8 hours is predicted to be a suitable substitution for the oral loading dose regimen of valacyclovir of 27 mg/kg every 8 hours in horses, because an acyclovir infusion produces higher peak concentrations, but slightly lower troughs, than an equivalent dose of oral valacyclovir (see **Fig. 1**). An approximate half-carton or five 1-g vials of acyclovir sodium, therefore, are needed per dose for a 500-kg horse, at a cost of approximately $378 per day.

Penciclovir/Famciclovir

Penciclovir is used in humans as an alternative to acyclovir to treat HSV and related infections. Penciclovir is similar to acyclovir in terms of its structure, selectivity, and mechanism of action, requiring viral TK for activation to its triply phosphorylated form.[76,77] Penciclovir differs, however, from acyclovir in its prolonged intracellular half-life, enhancing its efficacy even when plasma penciclovir concentrations drop below concentrations required for viral inhibition.[21,78] In cats with ocular lesions attributed to FHV-1, famciclovir has become a popular therapeutic agent that is substantially more potent and effective against FHV-1 than is acyclovir or valacyclovir.[79] EHV-1 differs from FHV-1, however, in that the IC_{50} values of penciclovir and acyclovir against EHV-1 are more similar to one another (see **Table 1**). (Maxwell LK, Bentz BG, Gilliam LL, et al. Efficacy of the early administration of valacyclovir for the therapy of neuropathogenic EHV-1 in horses. Submitted for publication.)[60,76] Penciclovir has a safety profile that is comparable to that of acyclovir but is unlikely to cause nephrotoxicity and is not formulated for parenteral administration. Instead, penciclovir itself is only applied topically, whereas its prodrug, famciclovir, is administered orally. The single-dose pharmacokinetics of famciclovir have been investigated in horses, and although bioavailability was not determined, its disposition seems similar to that of other antiherpetic drugs in horses, with a prolonged terminal phase half-life.[80] The intracellular persistence and somewhat lower IC_{50} values of penciclovir are expected to offer similar therapeutic advantages to famciclovir compared with valacyclovir for therapy of EHV-1 infection in horses. Multiple-dose pharmacokinetic and efficacy studies of famciclovir in horses are lacking, however, possibly due to the high expense of famciclovir and lack of available injectable products. Because the cost of famciclovir has recently dropped to approximately twice the cost of valacyclovir with the availability of US generics, future studies may rectify this knowledge gap (see **Table 2**).

Ganciclovir/Valganciclovir

Ganciclovir and valganciclovir are licensed for therapy for the human cytomegalovirus (CMV), a betaherpesvirus. Like acyclovir and penciclovir, ganciclovir must be triply phosphorylated within the cell before it is active, but because CMV does not express TK, phosphorylation instead occurs through the viral protein UL97 kinase.[81] EHV-1 and HSV-1 TK, however, are able to phosphorylate ganciclovir, similar to their activation of acyclovir and penciclovir.[21,61,82] In general, ganciclovir is a more potent inhibitor of most herpesviruses than are either acyclovir or penciclovir, with a commensurate increase in cytotoxic profile.[17,83] Several studies have shown that ganciclovir is at least 10 times more potent than acyclovir and penciclovir against EHV-1, with activity both in vitro and in mice. (Maxwell LK, Bentz BG, Gilliam LL, et al. Efficacy of the early administration of valacyclovir for the therapy of neuropathogenic EHV-1 in horses. Submitted for publication.)[84,85] In humans and rodents, ganciclovir is much less likely to be nephrotoxic compared with acyclovir.[86] Instead, the most prominent side effect associated with IV ganciclovir administration in humans is neutropenia.[87] When multiple doses of IV ganciclovir were administered to 9 horses for 1 week in a preliminary report, no neutropenia was noted.[88] Consistent with its more cytotoxic profile compared with acyclovir, carcinogenicity, teratogenicity, and aspermatogenesis are possible adverse effects of ganciclovir and should be considered carefully before administration to pregnant or breeding animals.[89]

Because orally administered ganciclovir is poorly absorbed in humans, an L-valyl ester prodrug has been developed for ganciclovir, valganciclovir, similar to the development of valacyclovir as a prodrug for acyclovir. The single-dose pharmacokinetics of oral valganciclovir and IV ganciclovir have been reported in horses, with oral bioavailability of valganciclovir similar to that of valacyclovir (see **Table 2**).[90] The elimination half-life of ganciclovir in horses was again prolonged compared with that in other species, showing that the related nucleoside analogs, acyclovir, penciclovir, and ganciclovir, all follow a similar, uniquely prolonged elimination phase in horses.[53,80,90]

Although ganciclovir more potently inhibits EHV-1 than acyclovir or penciclovir, was well-tolerated in horses, and enjoys a similarly favorable pharmacokinetic profile, the expense of injectable ganciclovir makes this drug cost-prohibitive for most equine patients (see **Table 2**). Because injectable ganciclovir sodium (Cytovene, Genentech, San Francisco, California) must generally be purchased as a carton of 25 vials, 500 mg each, a strategy is to purchase and administer 1 case of injectable ganciclovir for its potent antiherpetic effects, followed by the use of oral valacyclovir for the remainder of therapy. Oral valganciclovir hydrochloride (Valcyte, Genentech) is even more expensive than injectable ganciclovir, so likely will remain cost-prohibitive until generic products become available in the future. The manufacturer suggests handling ganciclovir as a cytotoxic substance, due to its cytotoxic profile.[89] Because valganciclovir is coated in an acid-soluble layer, tablets may be dissolved in lemon juice, then mixed with syrup just prior to administration, because crushing of tablets could expose personnel to cytotoxic drug.[90] In humans, ganciclovir sodium vials are reconstituted in water to 50 mg/mL, then diluted in crystalline solutions for administration at concentrations of 10 mg/mL as a 1-hour infusion, similar to the administration of IV acyclovir. The 50-mg/mL ganciclovir sodium solution, however, has been administered directly to horses through a jugular catheter as a slow (2-minute) bolus, approximately 15 doses administered over a 1-week period, without apparent adverse effects.[88] Due to the high pH (11) of ganciclovir sodium, it should be administered through an indwelling catheter, rather than by venipuncture, to prevent extravasation and should only be administered by the IV route.

Cidofovir

Like ganciclovir, cidofovir is licensed for use against human CMV but is only available as an injectable formulation (Vistide, Gilead Sciences, Foster City, California). Also like ganciclovir, cidofovir is thought to be carcinogenic and teratogenic and can induce hypospermia in some animal tests, so humans are advised to refrain from pregnancy for 1 month to 3 months after treatment.[91] Its most substantial side effects in humans, however, are neutropenia and renal impairment that can be partially mitigated by the coadministration of probenicid.[91] Unlike ganciclovir, cidofovir is a nucleotide analog that is doubly phosphorylated by cellular enzymes to its active form, cidofovir diphosphate, and thus does not require a viral kinase. This difference serves to increase the spectrum of activity of cidofovir, including activity against otherwise resistant herpesviruses, but also contributes to its poorer, more cytotoxic safety profile compared with the nucleoside analogs. One of the benefits of cidofovir is its unique 1-week dosing interval in humans, which is attributed to the prolonged intracellular half-life of cidofovir diphosphate.[23] Only a few divergent IC_{50} values for cidofovir have been reported against EHV-1 isolates, although it effectively protected mice from EHV-1 infection.[84,92] Although cidofovir is administered as a 1-hour infusion in humans, its neutral pH has allowed for subcutaneous administration in other species. Consequently, cidofovir has also been administered subcutaneously to several foals, but pharmacokinetic studies in horses are lacking.[92]

Idoxuridine and Trifluridine

Idoxuridine and trifluridine are structurally related thymidine analogs that inhibit DNA synthesis. Trifluridine (1% solution) is licensed for ophthalmic use in therapy for HSV keratitis, but idoxuridine is no longer commercially produced in the United States. Compounded formulations of idoxuridine are available as a 0.1% solution and a 0.5% ointment; these are popular choices for the treatment of herpetic keratitis and conjunctivitis in cats.[93] Antiherpetic drugs administered as solutions are cleared rapidly from the eye, which is problematic for a virostatic drug.

THERAPY FOR SPECIFIC VIRAL INFECTIONS
Equine Herpesvirus 1

The safety profile of oral acyclovir makes this drug an attractive antiherpetic in neonatal foals suffering from EHV-1 infections, with cautious optimism for therapeutic efficacy.[30] Oral acyclovir has also been administered to adult horses during several outbreaks of EHM.[34,58] Seven adult riding horses received acyclovir, beginning several days after EHM was diagnosed.[58] The investigators of this report[58] were unable, however, to determine whether acyclovir administration was helpful due to the chaotic nature of investigating multiple therapeutic interventions during an EHM outbreak. During the subsequent Findlay, Ohio, outbreak of EHM associated with a neuropathogenic strain of EHV-1, a large number (99) of horses were administered oral acyclovir, and those horses had better survival than the 36 untreated horses, with an odds ratio of 14 (CI, 4–54). Despite this impressive difference in survival, the existence of extraneous factors obscures definitive assessment of efficacy, because acyclovir was primarily administered to horses later in the course of the outbreak, at 9 days to 12 days after the likely index case was affected and 7 days to 9 days after the majority of the remaining horses became febrile. Because 11 of the 135 resident horses had already become recumbent at this time and were not eligible for acyclovir therapy, acyclovir may have been primarily administered to the least susceptible horses, obscuring the analysis of its true therapeutic efficacy.[63]

In light of the moderately high IC_{50} of acyclovir for EHV-1 and the low plasma acyclovir concentrations associated with oral administration, oral acyclovir is unlikely to effectively treat or prevent EHM in adult horses. The possibility of a discrepancy between the in vitro and in vivo inhibitory activities should be considered, however. The pharmacokinetics of oral acyclovir in foals has not been investigated, so its bioavailability could be higher in foals than in adults.[64] Given that 1 case series reported survival in neonatal foals infected with EHV-1 with oral acyclovir administration, examination of its bioavailability in foals is warranted. Because acyclovir and its derivatives are administered to pregnant women and neonates with apparent safety, these drugs might also be beneficial to prevent abortions due to EHV-1 or EHV-4 infection in pregnant mares. The safety and efficacy of antiviral therapy administered to pregnant mares has not yet been investigated, however, and the single tested EHV-4 isolate was deemed resistant to acyclovir (see **Table 1**).[63,82]

Two separate studies have examined the use of oral valacyclovir to protect horses experimentally inoculated with EHV-1 (see **Table 3**). The first study administered a high-dose rate of valacyclovir for 5 days to 3 weanling and 1 adult Shetland ponies that were inoculated intranasally with EHV-1.[73] Despite the high-dose rate, valacyclovir administration did not decrease viral replication or fever in these ponies. In contrast, a second study showed that lower dose rates of oral valacyclovir administered within 2 days of inoculation with a neuropathogenic strain of EHV-1 did protect aged mares from viral replication and EHM, although therapy did not completely prevent infection or ataxia.[88] The discordant results between these 2 valacyclovir efficacy studies might be explained by the difference in disease presentations and viral kinetics between foals and aged mares. Because young horses have lower viral loads and are less susceptible to EHM compared with geriatric horses, valacyclovir administration could potentially have a greater effect in more susceptible horses with more rapidly expanding viral loads.[94] That these separate experimental studies reached contradictory results regarding the efficacy of valacyclovir against EHV-1 further underscores the low likelihood that oral acyclovir, with its much lower plasma acyclovir concentrations, is effective against EHM.

Oral valacyclovir has been administered to ataxic horses with naturally acquired EHM during several outbreaks of EHV-1, with a total of 6 of 8 total treated horses surviving.[71,95] In an experimental study, oral valacyclovir was administered to aged mares later in the course of EHV-1 infection at 4 days to 6 days after inoculation, when EHM was imminent.[88] With this delayed therapy, valacyclovir administration did not decrease ataxia, but administration of the more potent antiherpetic nucleoside drug, ganciclovir, did rapidly decrease viremia and protected horses from EHM.[88] In a case series of naturally affected horses with EHM, valacyclovir was initiated on hospital admission, but ganciclovir therapy was only begun on recumbency.[71] In those horses treated with ganciclovir only when neurologic signs became severe, ganciclovir therapy was not successful in preventing death.

Cidofovir has been administered subcutaneously at 1 high-dose rate and 1 low-dose rate to 2 foals that were experimentally inoculated with EHV-1.[92] In the foal that received the high dose of cidofovir, clinical signs of EHV-1 infection seemed reduced. Despite this encouraging result, the sample size was quite small, and further evidence of the safety and efficacy of cidofovir in horses is currently lacking.

Equine Herpesvirus 5

Although no drugs are currently licensed to treat human gammaherpesvirus infections, the nucleoside analogs acyclovir, ganciclovir, and cidofovir have been tested in vitro against Epstein-Barr virus and HHV-8, with acyclovir potently inhibiting Epstein-Barr virus but not HHV-8, whereas both ganciclovir and cidofovir inhibited both viruses.[96] These drugs may be similarly active against EHV-5, but there are currently no in vitro data to support this hypothesis. Nonetheless, acyclovir and valacyclovir have been administered to horses with EMPF in hopes of reducing EHV-5 replication and the resulting fibrosis and compromise of the affected lung (see **Table 3**). Because most case reports describing the successful use of antiherpetic drugs for therapy for EMPF administered the drug for months of therapy, oral acyclovir has most commonly been chosen over valacyclovir due its lower cost. Four separate case reports or case series have described the administration of oral acyclovir over a 2-month to 4-month period, over which 3 of 8 horses diagnosed with EMPF survived.[16,36–38] Although EHV-5 needs to be exquisitely sensitive to acyclovir for the low plasma acyclovir concentrations associated with these dosing regimens to be effective, accumulation of oral acyclovir over days or longer does produce low but consistent concentrations of plasma acyclovir that might inhibit EHV-5.[63] An additional case report also discusses the use of a high-dose rate of oral valacyclovir over a much shorter period with apparent success against EMPF.[72]

Equine Herpesvirus 2

Ophthalmic instillation of idoxuridine and trifluridine has been administered to horses and foals with ocular signs suggestive of EHV-2, with reports of therapeutic success.[43–45] Although differing frequencies of administration of topical antiherpetic drugs have been used in horses, one suggestion is to administer drugs every 2 to 4 hours while lesions are present, before decreasing the frequency to every 4 to 6 hours for another 3 days to 4 days.[97]

TREATMENT RESISTANCE

Because antiherpetic drugs are routinely used in humans for therapy of HSV and CMV, most data regarding drug resistance originate from these settings. Viral resistance to the nucleoside and nucleotide analogs occur by mutation of the genes encoding viral thymidine kinase, UL97 kinase, or, more rarely, DNA polymerase.[81,98–101] The mechanism of viral resistance depends on the mechanism of action of the antiviral drug. Most drug-resistant HSV and CMV isolates have mutations in the genes that encode their drug metabolizing enzymes, TK and UL97 kinase, respectively, that are responsible for phosphorylation and, therefore, activation of these antiherpetic drugs.[100–102] As with the selection of antibiotic-resistant bacteria, drug-resistant herpesviruses can be readily selected for in the laboratory by serial passage of virus in the presence of the antiherpetic drug or by genetic modification.[76,101,103] Accordingly, multiple TK-deficient mutants of EHV-1 or EHV-4, with the expected cross-resistance to acyclovir, penciclovir, and ganciclovir, have been characterized in vitro.[61,76,82,103–105] Although TK mutant EHV strains have been developed and selected for in the laboratory, antiherpetic drug-resistant strains of EHV have not yet been isolated from equine patients. This is likely due to the relative paucity of data regarding the clinical use of antiherpetic drugs in horses; because EHV-1 and HSV-1 share similar mechanisms of drug resistance, the large volume of data available regarding drug resistance of HSV in human patients can inform the theoretic assessment of resistance in horses.

Humans with HSV-1 and HSV-2 infections are routinely treated with continuous or intermittent oral acyclovir, valacyclovir, or famciclovir for prophylaxis. Despite the chronic, widespread use and recurrent reactivation of HSV that can occur with infection, resistance of HSV to acyclovir occurs in less than 0.5% of immunocompetent people, and in vitro sensitivity patterns in these patients remain unchanged.[102,106] Sequential isolation of HSV from immunocompetent human patients treated with acyclovir for 6 years showed no evidence of acquired resistance.[107] Instead, the main concerns about antiherpetic resistance in human medicine reside in immunocompromised patients, populations of which have experienced an increase in HSV or CMV resistance over time (eg, rising from a prevalence of acyclovir-resistant HSV from 4% to 16% over a 9-year period).[106,108] Unfortunately, specific subsets of the most immunocompromised patients, such as hematopoietic stem cell transplant patients, may have a much higher prevalence of resistance (approximately 50%).[106] Immunocompetent patients from the same geographic area who were monitored in parallel with the immunocompromised patients did not experience an increase in HSV resistance.[106] The stability of HSV resistance patterns in the immunocompetent populace despite years of extensive exposure to acyclovir and penciclovir is probably due to the altered pathogenicity of HSV when the TK gene produces a nonfunctional enzyme, because the resulting viral strain is nearly incapable of reactivating from a latent state.[102] Patients with resistant herpesvirus infections are treated by switching to a second choice drug with a different mechanism of drug metabolism, such as replacing ganciclovir with cidofovir to treat a ganciclovir-resistant CMV infection.

Extrapolating antiherpetic drug resistance population data from humans to horses is a speculative exercise, because no similar data exist for horses. Such speculation, however, suggests the following:

- For both HSV and EHV, acyclovir-resistant, TK-deficient mutants can be selected for in vitro and could, therefore, spontaneously occur in patients.
- Nonetheless, antiherpetic drug resistance develops rarely in immunocompetent people.
- In immunocompromised people, antiherpetic resistance develops slowly, over months of therapy.
- Antiherpetic therapy for EHV-1 infection in horses is usually only administered for 1 to 2 weeks, because viral replication is controlled by the horse within that time period.
- Therefore, TK-resistant EHV-1 mutants are unlikely to be selected for in horses over that short time frame.
- Factors known to increase drug resistance, such as immunocompromise or subtherapeutic doses of acyclovir, could increase the chance of resistance, making oral acyclovir more likely to select for drug-resistant EHV-1 compared with oral valacyclovir.
- In therapy for EHV-5, oral acyclovir may be administered over several months of time.
- Little is known about drug susceptibility of EHV-5, but oral acyclovir is likely to produce suboptimal plasma acyclovir concentrations due to its poor bioavailability.
- EMPF might be associated with immunocompromise in some horses.
- The combination of a long duration of low plasma acyclovir concentrations and possible immunocompromised state suggests that viral resistance might be more likely in the setting of therapy for EMPF compared with EHM.

EVALUATION OF OUTCOME AND LONG-TERM RECOMMENDATIONS

Taken together, case series and experimental studies support the importance of the timing of antiherpetic therapy in effectively protecting horses from the most devastating sequelae of EHM. As with herpesvirus infections in other species, antiherpetic therapy that is initiated well before the onset of neurologic signs has the best chance of efficacy. When initiated early, there is some evidence that oral valacyclovir can limit viral replication, although results are contradictory. Given the virostatic action of antiviral drugs, it is likely that antiherpetic drugs primarily function to give the immune system time to mount a sufficient response to control viral replication. As a consequence, horses can survive EHM without the use of antiviral drugs, because the immune system is ultimately responsible for controlling the replication of EHV-1. When therapy is delayed until ataxia is present, neurologic damage has already occurred and cannot be reversed by the actions of antiherpetic drugs. The use of potent and effective antiviral agents, however, such as ganciclovir, may still be indicated in ataxic horses, especially if active viral replication is ongoing or if immunosuppressive anti-inflammatory drugs are administered. Alternatively, valacyclovir might also present some efficacy late in infection, although lower efficacy is expected compared with the more potent drug, ganciclovir, which more rapidly inhibits viral replication. Other antiherpetic drugs, including famciclovir and cidofovir, have experimental support for further study against EHV-1. Other classes of horses affected by EHV-1, such as neonatal foals and pregnant mares, would also potentially benefit from the further study of antiherpetic therapies.

Only case series exist to support a therapeutic benefit from the administration of oral acyclovir or valacyclovir to horses with EMPF. By their nature, such case series have multiple extraneous factors that complicate the definitive assessment of drug efficacy. Importantly, some horses diagnosed with EMPF spontaneously resolve without specific therapy, whereas others treated with antiviral drugs fail to respond.[37] Therefore, although there is some evidence to suggest that oral antiherpetic drugs may enhance survival of horses with EMPF, the use of antiviral drugs in this setting has not yet been shown to be beneficial and requires further study.

SUMMARY

- Oral acyclovir is unlikely to be effective in therapy for EHM, because it is poorly absorbed, whereas there is some evidence to support the use of valacyclovir and ganciclovir in this setting.
- Because antiviral drugs are virostatic, antiherpetic drugs can at best limit viral replication whereas the immune system mounts a response to active viral infection; latent viral infections are not affected by antiviral therapy.
- The timing of antiherpetic therapy is important, with earlier intervention more likely to protect horses from the most devastating sequelae of EHM compared with therapy that occurs after neurologic damage has occurred.
- Oral acyclovir and valacyclovir have been administered to horses with EMPF in hopes of decreasing the replication of EHV-5 that is associated with this condition, but further study is required to determine the most effective therapies for EMPF.
- Viral keratitis may be empirically treated with topical idoxuridine or trifluridine.

REFERENCES

1. Davison AJ, Eberle R, Ehlers B, et al. The order Herpesvirales. Arch Virol 2009; 154(1):171–7.
2. Ma G, Azab W, Osterrieder N. Equine herpesviruses type 1 (EHV-1) and 4 (EHV-4)–masters of co-evolution and a constant threat to equids and beyond. Vet Microbiol 2013;167(1–2):123–34.
3. Goehring LS, Wagner B, Bigbie R, et al. Control of EHV-1 viremia and nasal shedding by commercial vaccines. Vaccine 2010;28(32):5203–11.
4. Goodman LB, Wagner B, Flaminio MJ, et al. Comparison of the efficacy of inactivated combination and modified-live virus vaccines against challenge infection with neuropathogenic equine herpesvirus type 1 (EHV-1). Vaccine 2006;24(17):3636–45.
5. Heldens JG, Hannant D, Cullinane AA, et al. Clinical and virological evaluation of the efficacy of an inactivated EHV1 and EHV4 whole virus vaccine (Duvaxyn EHV1,4). Vaccination/challenge experiments in foals and pregnant mares. Vaccine 2001;19(30):4307–17.
6. Patel JR, Heldens J. Equine herpesviruses 1 (EHV-1) and 4 (EHV-4)–epidemiology, disease and immunoprophylaxis: a brief review. Vet J 2005;170(1):14–23.
7. Shiley K, Blumberg E. Herpes viruses in transplant recipients: HSV, VZV, human herpes viruses, and EBV. Hematol Oncol Clin North Am 2010;25(1):171–91.
8. Strachan E, Saracino M, Selke S, et al. The effects of daily distress and personality on genital HSV shedding and lesions in a randomized, double-blind, placebo-controlled, crossover trial of acyclovir in HSV-2 seropositive women. Brain Behav Immun 2011;25(7):1475–81.

9. Uchakin PN, Parish DC, Dane FC, et al. Fatigue in medical residents leads to reactivation of herpes virus latency. Interdiscip Perspect Infect Dis 2011;2011: 571340.

10. Gibson JS, Slater JD, Awan AR, et al. Pathogenesis of equine herpesvirus-1 in specific pathogen-free foals - primary and secondary infections and reactivation. Arch Virol 1992;123(3–4):351–66.

11. Pusterla N, Hussey SB, Mapes S, et al. Molecular investigation of the viral kinetics of equine herpesvirus-1 in blood and nasal secretions of horses after corticosteroid-induced recrudescence of latent infection. J Vet Intern Med 2010;24(5):1153–7.

12. Edington N, Bridges CG, Huckle A. Experimental reactivation of equid herpesvirus 1 (EHV 1) following the administration of corticosteroids. Equine Vet J 1985;17(5):369–72.

13. Carr E, Schott H, Pusterla N. Absence of equid herpesvirus-1 reactivation and viremia in hospitalized critically ill horses. J Vet Intern Med 2011;25(5):1190–3.

14. Badenhorst M, Page P, Ganswindt A, et al. Detection of equine herpesvirus-4 and physiological stress patterns in young Thoroughbreds consigned to a South African auction sale. BMC Vet Res 2015;11:126.

15. Schulman M, Becker A, Ganswindt S, et al. The effect of consignment to broodmare sales on physiological stress measured by faecal glucocorticoid metabolites in pregnant Thoroughbred mares. BMC Vet Res 2014;10:25.

16. Vander Werf K, Davis E. Disease remission in a horse with EHV-5-associated lymphoma. J Vet Intern Med 2013;27(2):387–9.

17. Goldthorpe SE, Boyd MR, Field HJ. Effects of penciclovir and famciclovir in a murine model of encephalitis induced by intranasal inoculation of herpes-simplex virus type-1. Antivir Chem Chemother 1992;3(1):37–47.

18. Sawtell NM, Bernstein DI, Stanberry LR. A temporal analysis of acyclovir inhibition of induced herpes simplex virus type 1 in vivo reactivation in the mouse trigeminal ganglia. J Infect Dis 1999;180(3):821–3.

19. Sawtell NM, Thompson RL, Stanberry LR, et al. Early intervention with high-dose acyclovir treatment during primary herpes simplex virus infection reduces latency and subsequent reactivation in the nervous system in vivo. J Infect Dis 2001;184(8):964–71.

20. Weinberg A, Leary JJ, Sarisky RT, et al. Factors that affect in vitro measurement of the susceptibility of herpes simplex virus to nucleoside analogues. J Clin Virol 2007;38(2):139–45.

21. Bae PK, Kim JH, Kim HS, et al. Intracellular uptake of thymidine and antiherpetic drugs for thymidine kinase-deficient mutants of herpes simplex virus type 1. Antiviral Res 2006;70(3):93–104.

22. Furman PA, de Miranda P, St Clair MH, et al. Metabolism of acyclovir in virus-infected and uninfected cells. Antimicrob Agents Chemother 1981;20(4): 518–24.

23. Cundy KC, Li ZH, Hitchcock MJM, et al. Pharmacokinetics of cidofovir in monkeys - evidence for a prolonged elimination phase representing phosphorylated drug. Drug Metab Dispos 1996;24(7):738–44.

24. Hodge RA, Perkins RM. Mode of action of 9-(4-hydroxy-3-hydroxymethylbut-1-yl)guanine (BRL 39123) against herpes simplex virus in MRC-5 cells. Antimicrob Agents Chemother 1989;33(2):223–9.

25. Brush LA, Black DH, McCormack KA, et al. Papiine herpesvirus 2 as a predictive model for drug sensitivity of Macacine herpesvirus 1 (monkey B virus). Comp Med 2014;64(5):386–93.

26. Telford EA, Watson MS, McBride K, et al. The DNA sequence of equine herpes-virus-1. Virology 1992;189(1):304–16.
27. Studdert MJ. Restriction endonuclease DNA fingerprinting of respiratory, foetal and perinatal foal isolates of equine herpesvirus type 1. Arch Virol 1983;77(2–4): 249–58.
28. Dunowska M. A review of equid herpesvirus 1 for the veterinary practitioner. Part B: pathogenesis and epidemiology. N Z Vet J 2014;62(4):179–88.
29. Dunowska M. A review of equid herpesvirus 1 for the veterinary practitioner. Part A: clinical presentation, diagnosis and treatment. N Z Vet J 2014;62(4):171–8.
30. Murray MJ, del Piero F, Jeffrey SC, et al. Neonatal equine herpesvirus type 1 infection on a thoroughbred breeding farm. J Vet Intern Med 1998;12(1):36–41.
31. Brown JA, Mapes S, Ball BA, et al. Prevalence of equine herpesvirus-1 infection among Thoroughbreds residing on a farm on which the virus was endemic. J Am Vet Med Assoc 2007;231(4):577–80.
32. Edington N, Bridges CG, Patel JR. Endothelial cell infection and thrombosis in paralysis caused by equid herpesvirus-1: equine stroke. Arch Virol 1986; 90(1–2):111–24.
33. Whitwell KE, Blunden AS. Pathological findings in horses dying during an outbreak of the paralytic form of equid herpesvirus type-1 (Ehv-1) infection. Equine Vet J 1992;24(1):13–9.
34. Henninger RW, Reed SM, Saville WJ, et al. Outbreak of neurologic disease caused by equine herpesvirus-1 at a university equestrian center. J Vet Intern Med 2007;21(1):157–65.
35. Pronost S, Legrand L, Pitel PH, et al. Outbreak of equine herpesvirus myeloen-cephalopathy in France: a clinical and molecular investigation. Transbound Emerg Dis 2012;59(3):256–63.
36. Schwarz B, Klang A, Bezdekova B, et al. Equine multinodular pulmonary fibrosis (EMPF): five case reports. Acta Vet Hung 2013;61(3):319–32.
37. Spelta CW, Axon JE, Begg A, et al. Equine multinodular pulmonary fibrosis in three horses in Australia. Aust Vet J 2013;91(7):274–80.
38. Wong DM, Belgrave RL, Williams KJ, et al. Multinodular pulmonary fibrosis in five horses. J Am Vet Med Assoc 2008;232(6):898–905.
39. Williams KJ, Robinson NE, Lim A, et al. Experimental induction of pulmonary fibrosis in horses with the gammaherpesvirus equine herpesvirus 5. PLoS One 2013;8(10):e77754.
40. Hartley CA, Dynon KJ, Mekuria ZH, et al. Equine gammaherpesviruses: perfect parasites? Vet Microbiol 2013;167(1–2):86–92.
41. Bawa B, Vander K, Beard L, et al. Equine multinodular pulmonary fibrosis and lymphoma in a horse associated with equine herpesvirus-5. J Equine Vet Sci 2014;34(5):694–700.
42. Schwarz B, Gruber A, Benetka V, et al. Concurrent T cell leukaemia and equine multinodular pulmonary fibrosis in a Hanoverian Warmblood mare. Equine Vet Education 2012;24(4):187–92.
43. Collinson PN, O'Rielly JL, Ficorilli N, et al. Isolation of equine herpesvirus type 2 (equine gammaherpesvirus 2) from foals with keratoconjunctivitis. J Am Vet Med Assoc 1994;205(2):329–31.
44. Thein P, Bohm D. Etiology and clinical aspects of a viral keratoconjunctivitis in foals. Zentralbl Veterinarmed B 1976;23(5–6):507–19 [in German].
45. Kershaw O, von Oppen T, Glitz F, et al. Detection of equine herpesvirus type 2 (EHV-2) in horses with keratoconjunctivitis. Virus Res 2001;80(1–2):93–9.

46. Brosnahan MM, Damiani A, van de Walle G, et al. The effect of siRNA treatment on experimental equine herpesvirus type 1 (EHV-1) infection in horses. Virus Res 2010;147(2):176–81.

47. Glorieux S, Vandekerckhove AP, Goris N, et al. Evaluation of the antiviral activity of (1 ' S,2 ' R)-9-[[1 ',2 '-bis(hydroxymethyl)cycloprop-1 '-yl]methyl]guanine (A-5021) against equine herpesvirus type 1 in cell monolayers and equine nasal mucosal explants. Antiviral Res 2012;93(2):234–8.

48. Perkins GA, Van de Walle GR, Pusterla N, et al. Evaluation of metaphylactic RNA interference to prevent equine herpesvirus type 1 infection in experimental herpesvirus myeloencephalopathy in horses. Am J Vet Res 2013;74(2):248–56.

49. Elion GB, Furman PA, Fyfe JA, et al. Selectivity of action of an antiherpetic agent, 9-(2-hydroxyethoxymethyl) guanine. Proc Natl Acad Sci U S A 1977;74(12): 5716–20.

50. Nasisse MP, Dorman DC, Jamison KC, et al. Effects of valacyclovir in cats infected with feline herpesvivus 1. Am J Vet Res 1997;58(10):1141–4.

51. Sawyer MH, Webb DE, Balow JE, et al. Acyclovir-induced renal failure. Clinical course and histology. Am J Med 1988;84(6):1067–71.

52. de Miranda P, Blum MR. Pharmacokinetics of acyclovir after intravenous and oral administration. J Antimicrob Chemother 1983;12(Suppl B):29–37.

53. Maxwell LK, Bentz BG, Bourne DW, et al. Pharmacokinetics of valacyclovir in the adult horse. J Vet Pharmacol Ther 2008;31(4):312–20.

54. Garré B, Shebany K, Gryspeerdt A, et al. Pharmacokinetics of acyclovir after intravenous infusion of acyclovir and after oral administration of acyclovir and its prodrug valacyclovir in healthy adult horses. Antimicrob Agents Chemother 2007;51(12):4308–14.

55. Wilkins PA, Papich M, Sweeney RW. Pharmacokinetics of acyclovir in adult horses. J Vet Emerg Crit Care 2005;15(3):174–8.

56. Zovirax(R) [prescribing information]. Greenville (NC): GlaxoSmithKline; 2003. Available at: http://www.accessdata.fda.gov/drugsatfda_docs/label/2004/18603slr027_zovirax_lbl.pdf. Accessed July 1, 2016.

57. Bentz BG, Maxwell LK, Erkert RS, et al. Pharmacokinetics of acyclovir after single intravenous and oral administration to adult horses. J Vet Intern Med 2006; 20(3):589–94.

58. Friday PA, Scarratt WK, Elvinger F, et al. Ataxia and paresis with equine herpesvirus type 1 infection in a herd of riding school horses. J Vet Intern Med 2000; 14(2):197–201.

59. Spangler JG, Kirk JK, Knudson MP. Uses and safety of acyclovir in pregnancy. J Fam Pract 1994;38(2):186–91.

60. Boyd MR, Bacon TH, Sutton D, et al. Antiherpesvirus activity of 9-(4-hydroxy-3-hydroxy-methylbut-1-yl)guanine (BRL 39123) in cell culture. Antimicrob Agents Chemother 1987;31(8):1238–42.

61. Kit S, Ichimura H, De Clercq E. Phosphorylation of nucleoside analogs by equine herpesvirus type 1 pyrimidine deoxyribonucleoside kinase. Antiviral Res 1987;7(1):53–67.

62. Garre B, Baert K, Nauwynck H, et al. Multiple oral dosing of valacyclovir in horses and ponies. J Vet Pharmacol Ther 2009;32(3):207–12.

63. Wong DM, Maxwell LK, Wilkins PA. Use of antiviral medications against equine herpes virus associated disorders. Equine Vet Education 2010;22(5):244–52.

64. Fujioka Y, Mizuno N, Morita E, et al. Effect of age on the gastrointestinal absorption of acyclovir in rats. J Pharm Pharmacol 1991;43(7):465–9.

65. Whitley RJ, Blum MR, Barton N, et al. Pharmacokinetics of acyclovir in humans following intravenous administration - a model for the development of parenteral antivirals. Am J Med 1982;73(1A):165–71.

66. Sinko PJ, Balimane PV. Carrier-mediated intestinal absorption of valacyclovir, the L-valyl ester prodrug of acyclovir: 1. Interactions with peptides, organic anions and organic cations in rats. Biopharm Drug Dispos 1998;19(4):209–17.

67. De Bony F, Tod M, Bidault R, et al. Multiple interactions of cimetidine and probenecid with valaciclovir and its metabolite acyclovir. Antimicrob Agents Chemother 2002;46(2):458–63.

68. Yue Z, Shi J, Jiang P, et al. Acute kidney injury during concomitant use of valacyclovir and loxoprofen: detecting drug-drug interactions in a spontaneous reporting system. Pharmacoepidemiol Drug Saf 2014;23(11):1154–9.

69. Fish DN, Vidaurri VA, Deeter RG. Stability of valacyclovir hydrochloride in extemporaneously prepared oral liquids. Am J Health Syst Pharm 1999;56(19):1957–60.

70. Granero GE, Amidon GL. Stability of valacyclovir: Implications for its oral bioavailability. Int J Pharm 2006;317(1):14–8.

71. Estell KE, Dawson DR, Magdesian KG, et al. Quantitative molecular viral loads in 7 horses with naturally occurring equine herpesvirus-1 infection. Equine Vet J 2015;47(6):689–93.

72. Schwarz B, Schwendenwein I, van den Hoven R. Successful outcome in a case of equine multinodular pulmonary fibrosis (EMPF) treated with valacyclovir. Equine Vet Education 2013;25(8):389–92.

73. Garré B, Gryspeerdt A, Croubels S, et al. Evaluation of orally administered valacyclovir in experimentally EHV1-infected ponies. Vet Microbiol 2009;135:214–21.

74. Johnston C, Saracino M, Kuntz S, et al. Standard-dose and high-dose daily antiviral therapy for short episodes of genital HSV-2 reactivation: three randomised, open-label, cross-over trials. Lancet 2012;379(9816):641–7.

75. Ljungman P, de La Camara R, Milpied N, et al. Randomized study of valacyclovir as prophylaxis against cytomegalovirus reactivation in recipients of allogeneic bone marrow transplants. Blood 2002;99(8):3050–6.

76. de la Fuente R, Awan AR, Field HJ. The acyclic nucleoside analogue penciclovir is a potent inhibitor of equine herpesvirus type 1 (EHV-1) in tissue culture and in a murine model. Antiviral Res 1992;18(1):77–89.

77. Hussein IT, Miguel RN, Tiley LS, et al. Substrate specificity and molecular modelling of the feline herpesvirus-1 thymidine kinase. Arch Virol 2008;153(3):495–505.

78. Sutton D, Boyd MR. Comparative activity of penciclovir and acyclovir in mice infected intraperitoneally with herpes-simplex virus type-1 Sc16. Antimicrob Agents Chemother 1993;37(4):642–5.

79. Thomasy SM, Lim CC, Reilly CM, et al. Evaluation of orally administered famciclovir in cats experimentally infected with feline herpesvirus type-1. Am J Vet Res 2011;72(1):85–95.

80. Tsujimura K, Yamada M, Nagata S, et al. Pharmacokinetics of penciclovir after oral administration of its prodrug famciclovir to horses. J Vet Med Sci 2010;72(3):357–61.

81. Littler E, Stuart AD, Chee MS. Human cytomegalovirus UL97 open reading frame encodes a protein that phosphorylates the antiviral nucleoside analogue ganciclovir. Nature 1992;358(6382):160–2.

82. Azab W, Tsujimura K, Kato K, et al. Characterization of a thymidine kinase-deficient mutant of equine herpesvirus 4 and in vitro susceptibility of the virus to antiviral agents. Antiviral Res 2010;85(2):389–95.

83. Focher F, Lossani A, Verri A, et al. Sensitivity of monkey B virus (Cercopithecine herpesvirus 1) to antiviral drugs: role of thymidine kinase in antiviral activities of substrate analogs and acyclonucleosides. Antimicrob Agents Chemother 2007; 51(6):2028–34.

84. Garré B, van der Meulen K, Nugent J, et al. In vitro susceptibility of six isolates of equine herpesvirus 1 to acyclovir, ganciclovir, cidofovir, adefovir, PMEDAP and foscarnet. Vet Microbiol 2007;122(1–2):43–51.

85. Rollinson EA, White G. Relative activities of acyclovir and BW759 against Aujeszky's disease and equine rhinopneumonitis viruses. Antimicrob Agents Chemother 1983;24(2):221–6.

86. DosSantos MDF, DosSantos OFP, Boim MA, et al. Nephrotoxicity of acyclovir and ganciclovir in rats: evaluation of glomerular hemodynamics. J Am Soc Nephrol 1997;8(3):361–7.

87. Jabs DA, Newman C, De Bustros S, et al. Treatment of cytomegalovirus retinitis with ganciclovir. Ophthalmology 1987;94(7):824–30.

88. Maxwell L, Gilliam L, Pusterla N, et al. Efficacy of delayed antiviral therapy against EHV-1 challenge. Paper presented at: Proceedings of the American College of Veterinary Internal Medicine Forum. Denver (CO), June 15–18, 2011.

89. Cytovene(R)-IV [prescribing information]. San Francisco (CA): Genentech, Inc; Roche Group; 2010. Available at: www.gene.com/download/pdf/cytovene_prescribing.pdf. Accessed July 1, 2016.

90. Carmichael RJ, Whitfield C, Maxwell LK. Pharmacokinetics of ganciclovir and valganciclovir in the adult horse. J Vet Pharmacol Ther 2013;36(5):441–9.

91. Vistide(R) [prescribing information]. Foster City (CA): Gilead Sciences, Inc; 2010. Available at: http://www.gilead.com/~/media/files/pdfs/medicines/other/vistide/vistide.pdf. Accessed July 1, 2016.

92. Gibson JS, Slater JD, Field HJ. The activity of (S)-1-[(3-hydroxy-2-phosphonyl methoxy) propyl] cytosine (Hpmpc) against equine herpesvirus-1 (Ehv-1) in cell-cultures, mice and horses. Antiviral Res 1992;19(3):219–32.

93. Stiles J. Treatment of cats with ocular disease attributable to herpesvirus infection: 17 cases (1983-1993). J Am Vet Med Assoc 1995;207(5):599–603.

94. Allen GP. Risk factors for development of neurologic disease after experimental exposure to equine herpesvirus-1 in horses. Am J Vet Res 2008;69(12): 1595–600.

95. Goehring LS, Landolt GA, Morley PS. Detection and management of an outbreak of equine herpesvirus type 1 infection and associated neurological disease in a veterinary teaching hospital. J Vet Intern Med 2010;24(5):1176–83.

96. Friedrichs C, Neyts J, Gaspar G, et al. Evaluation of antiviral activity against human herpesvirus 8 (HHV-8) and Epstein-Barr virus (EBV) by a quantitative real-time PCR assay. Antiviral Res 2004;62(3):121–3.

97. Matthews AG. Ophthalmic antimicrobial therapy in the horse. Equine Vet Education 2009;21(5):271–80.

98. Andrei G, Snoeck R, Balzarini J, et al. Combination of azidothymidine (Azt) and (E)-5-(2-bromovinyl)-2'-deoxyuridine (Bvdu) inhibits the replication of herpes-simplex virus type-1 (Hsv-1) and type-2 (Hsv-2) and varicella-zoster virus (Vzv) strains that are deficient in the expression of the viral thymidine kinase (Tk). Nucleosides Nucleotides 1995;14(3–5):559–62.

99. McLaren C, Chen MS, Ghazzouli I, et al. Drug resistance patterns of herpes simplex virus isolates from patients treated with acyclovir. Antimicrob Agents Chemother 1985;28(6):740–4.

100. Boivin G, Chou S, Quirk MR, et al. Detection of ganciclovir resistance mutations quantitation of cytomegalovirus (CMV) DNA in leukocytes of patients with fatal disseminated CMV disease. J Infect Dis 1996;173(3):523–8.

101. Field HJ, Darby G, Wildy P. Isolation and characterization of acyclovir-resistant mutants of herpes simplex virus. J Gen Virol 1980;49(1):115–24.

102. Bacon TH, Levin MJ, Leary JJ, et al. Herpes simplex virus resistance to acyclovir and penciclovir after two decades of antiviral therapy. Clin Microbiol Rev 2003; 16(1):114–28.

103. Field HJ, Awan AR, Delafuente R. Isolation of equine herpesvirus-1 mutants in the presence of (S)-9-(3-hydroxy-2-phosphonylmethoxypropyl)adenine - demonstration of resistance invitro and invivo. Antiviral Res 1991;16(1):29–39.

104. Cornick J, Martens J, Martens R, et al. Safety and efficacy of a thymidine kinase negative equine herpesvirus-1 vaccine in young horses. Can J Vet Res 1990; 54(2):260–6.

105. Slater JD, Gibson JS, Field HJ. Pathogenicity of a thymidine kinase-deficient mutant of equine herpesvirus 1 in mice and specific pathogen-free foals. J Gen Virol 1993;74(Pt 5):819–28.

106. Frobert E, Burrel S, Ducastelle-Lepretre S, et al. Resistance of herpes simplex viruses to acyclovir: an update from a ten-year survey in France. Antiviral Res 2014;111:36–41.

107. Fife KH, Crumpacker CS, Mertz GJ, et al. Recurrence and resistance patterns of herpes simplex virus following cessation of > or = 6 years of chronic suppression with acyclovir. Acyclovir Study Group. J Infect Dis 1994;169(6):1338–41.

108. Young PG, Rubin J, Angarone M, et al. Ganciclovir-resistant cytomegalovirus infection in solid organ transplant recipients: a single-center retrospective cohort study. Transpl Infect Dis 2016;18(3):390–5.

109. De Clercq E, Holy A, Rosenberg I, et al. A novel selective broad-spectrum anti-DNA virus agent. Nature 1986;323(6087):464–7.

110. Smith KO, Galloway KS, Hodges SL, et al. Sensitivity of equine herpesviruses 1 and 3 in vitro to a new nucleoside analogue, 9-[[2-hydroxy-1-(hydroxymethyl) ethoxy] methyl] guanine. Am J Vet Res 1983;44(6):1032–5.

111. Rollinson EA. Comparative efficacy of three 2'-fluoropyrimidine nucleosides and 9-(1,3-dihydroxy-2-propoxymethyl)guanine (BW B759U) against pseudorabies and equine rhinopneumonitis virus infection in vitro and in laboratory animals. Antiviral Res 1987;7(1):25–33.

Therapeutics for Equine Endocrine Disorders

Andy E. Durham, BSc, BVSc, CertEP, DEIM, MRCVS

KEYWORDS

- Equine • Endocrine • PPID • EMS • Diabetes • Therapeutics

KEY POINTS

- Endocrine disease is commonly encountered in equine practice.
- Pergolide remains the most popular drug for treating PPID although some alternatives exist if required.
- Equine metabolic syndrome control requires compliance with strict management measures although these may be supplemented by medical therapy in some cases.
- Rarer endocrinopathies such as diabetes mellitus, diabetes insipidus, hyperthyroidism and critical illness-related corticosteroid insufficiency present some therapeutic options but are frequently challenging to manage.

Endocrinopathic causes of laminitis have attracted considerable research interest over the last decade alongside a parallel surge in caseload seen in general equine practice.[1,2] The justification for medical intervention in cases of pituitary pars intermedia dysfunction (PPID) seems to be relatively straightforward, in contrast with the potential danger that equine metabolic syndrome (EMS) cases are medicated as an easier alternative to implementing essential management changes. Such reliance on medical treatment of EMS cases is likely to fail unless administered alongside strict dietary and exercise management.[3] Indeed, dietary management may also play an important role in other rarer endocrine diseases, such as diabetes mellitus (DM) and diabetes insipidus (DI), but such recommendations are beyond the scope of this article.

PITUITARY PARS INTERMEDIA DYSFUNCTION

PPID is suspected to arise after a loss of dopaminergic neuronal input to the pars intermedia, thus freeing the secretory melanotrope cells from tonic inhibition.[4] This pathophysiology forms the basis for preferential selection of dopaminergic agents in PPID

Disclosure Statement: A.E. Durham has acted on a few occasions as a consultant for Boehringer Ingelheim Vetmedica, the manufacturer of Prascend, and has performed laboratory testing services for the same company.
Liphook Equine Hospital, Liphook, Hampshire GU30 7JG, UK
E-mail address: andy.durham@theleh.co.uk

cases to moderate excessive pars intermedia secretion.[5,6] There is currently no evidence that medical treatment (**Table 1**) can reduce or reverse the pathologic changes in the affected pars intermedia of PPID cases,[7] although this is a variable but realistic expectation in association with treatment of human prolactinomas with dopamine agonists.[8]

The dopamine agonist pergolide mesylate was first approved for the treatment of Parkinson's disease in humans more than 30 years ago and remains the only equine-licensed drug for the treatment of PPID in horses (Prascend, Boerhinger Ingelheim). The drug acts as a potent agonist of dopamine D2 receptors, but has additional effects on other classes of dopamine receptors as well as adrenergic and 5-hydroxytryptamine receptors. The drug was withdrawn as a human medicine from the United States and Canadian market in 2007 owing to increased risk of cardiac valvulopathy. Similar adverse effects are not recognized in horses, although temporary inappetence is not uncommon after commencement of medication or after dosage increases.[9,10] Pergolide is generally administered at a starting dose of 0.002 mg/kg orally (PO) every 24 hours with clinical and endocrine improvement expected within 1 to 3 months.[9–14] Improvements in signs such as lethargy, hypertrichosis, and polydipsia may be readily noticeable, although it is less easy to judge treatment success based on reduced likelihood of further attacks of laminitis or susceptibility to infections. Hence, there may be value in monitoring endocrine test results, although it should be stated that clinical and endocrine improvements do not always concur. Similarly, in human studies of prolactinomas, there may be poor correlation between clinical signs, prolactin concentrations, and adenoma size after treatment with dopamine agonists.[8] Unpublished data from this author (AE Durham, 2014) monitored endocrine changes between 1 and 2 months after the treatment of 402 PPID cases with 0.002 mg/kg pergolide every 24 hours. This revealed that 30% of cases showed a return of plasma adrenocorticotrophic hormone (ACTH) concentrations to the reference interval. A further 41% of horses showed a greater than 50% decrease in basal ACTH concentrations, but

Table 1
Drug dosages for PPID and EMS in horses

	Drug	Dosage	Comments
PPID	Pergolide	0.002–0.010 mg/kg PO q24h	Begin at lower end of dose range and increase gradually if required. Inappetence not uncommon.
	Cyproheptadine	0.25 mg/kg PO q12–24h	May be used alone or in combination with pergolide.
	Bromocriptine	0.1 mg/kg PO q12h	Alternative dopamine agonist to pergolide.
	Trilostane	0.4–1 mg/kg PO q24h	Only indicated if evidence of hyperadrenocorticism.
EMS	Levothyroxine	0.1 mg/kg PO q24h for 3–6 mon, then taper to 0.05 mg/kg PO q24h for 2 wk, then 0.025 mg/kg PO q24h for 2 wk	Must be used alongside dietary control.
	Metformin	30 mg/kg PO q12h	Ideally, immediately before grazing/feeding

Abbreviations: EMS, equine metabolic syndrome; PO, per os; PPID, pituitary pars intermedia dysfunction.

they failed to return to the reference interval. There was no notable change in post-treatment plasma ACTH in 11% of cases (**Fig. 1**), which is similar to the 15% nonre-sponse rate reported in pergolide treatment of prolactinomas in humans.[8,15]

The reason for variable responsiveness of treated cases is unknown but could relate to interindividual differences in pergolide pharmacokinetics/pharmacodynamics and/or an inherent variability in the exact nature of the disease process. PPID is clearly a heterogeneous disease with a spectrum from hyperplasia and hypertrophy to micro-adenoma and macroadenoma formation[16,17] and, intuitively, the dose–response might differ between these pathologic categories. Human studies of drug-resistant prolactinomas have indicated similar plasma dopamine agonist concentrations in responsive versus unresponsive patients,[18] although there is a significant decrease in dopaminergic D2 binding sites, as well as dysregulated intracellular transduction pathways, in the pituitary glands of the latter group.[15,19,20]

Gradual dosage increases are probably the most common approach in nonre-sponders to pergolide, with some horses eventually receiving doses as high as 0.01 mg/kg per day.[10] Pharmacokinetic studies of pergolide in horses are inconclu-sive[21–23] and although twice daily dosing has been reported,[24] there is no evidence of additional benefit versus once daily dosing.[25] Nevertheless this seems a reasonable approach to try in nonresponders because there is no apparent therapeutic disadvan-tage.[25] The final therapeutic tactic with pergolide in apparent nonresponders is patience, because it has been observed that good treatment responses can be delayed for as long as 3 to 4 years in some cases (H.C. Schott, personal communication, 2014).

Switching dopamine agonists has been shown to be another effective approach in several human studies of drug-resistant hyperprolactinemia, with a change to caber-goline seeming to be most successful.[26–28] The dopaminergic agonists bromocriptine and cabergoline have been used in horses, although neither drug has been extensively investigated in PPID cases. Bromocryptine is a selective D2 dopamine agonist with a shorter half-life than pergolide, but it has been shown to be effective in controlling PPID at a dose of 0.1 mg/kg PO every 12 hours.[29] Anecdotal reports exist of the use of cabergoline, an especially long-acting D2 receptor agonist, in PPID cases. This author is not aware of clinical studies of cabergoline in PPID cases, although pars intermedia responsiveness has been shown to be decreased in normal horses by administration of 0.01 mg/kg cabergoline intramuscularly every 10 days.[30]

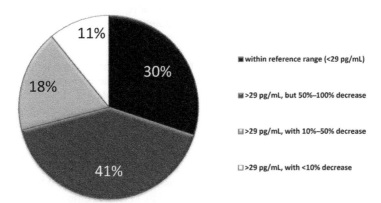

Fig. 1. Endocrine responses, judged by changes in plasma adrenocorticotrophic hormone concentrations, in 402 pituitary pars intermedia dysfunction cases after 1 to 2 months of per-golide treatment at 0.002 mg/kg orally every 24 hours (AE Durham, 2014).

Cyproheptadine hydrochloride is a further product with multiple modes of action, primarily listed as a serotonin, cholinergic, and histamine antagonist. The origin of its use in PPID likely lies in reports of decreased ACTH secretion from pars distalis corticotrophs in humans,[31] although there is no established mode of action in PPID cases. Reports have described inconsistent efficacy of cyproheptadine in PPID,[12,13,32] although the most favorable study used a higher dosage of 0.25 mg/kg every 12 hours.[12] Anecdotally, treatment responses have been reported in PPID using a combination of pergolide and cyproheptadine where 1 drug alone seemed to be ineffective.

Adrenal corticosteroid biosynthesis inhibitors have also been administered to PPID cases with favorable responses reported for trilostane, administered at 0.4 to 1.0 mg/kg PO every 24 hours.[33,34] Although increased basal plasma ACTH concentration is clearly associated with the presence of PPID,[35] the frequent absence of secondary adrenal hyperplasia and hypercortisolemia[36,37] suggests that most PPID cases do not suffer from hyperadrenocorticism, and that trilostane and similar drugs are unlikely to benefit the majority of cases.

EQUINE METABOLIC SYNDROME

EMS was initially recognized and named in recognition of analogy with the metabolic syndrome in humans,[38] although it is evident that there are also numerous fundamental differences between the 2 conditions. Key therapeutic targets in humans with the metabolic syndrome include hyperglycemia, dyslipidemia, atherosclerosis, pancreatic beta cell failure, and chronic hypertension, none of which seem to be real concerns in equids. Thus, although pharmacotherapy of the metabolic syndrome is practiced commonly, interspecies differences mean that caution should be exercised when considering similar drugs in EMS cases.

To apply effective pharmacotherapy, it is important to have a clear idea of the pathophysiologic processes that we wish to moderate. The primary clinical concern in EMS cases is laminitis, which is commonly pasture or diet associated. Two linked elements of probable fundamental importance are that several studies have indicated sustained hyperinsulinemia will trigger laminitis,[39,40] whereas others have indicated that EMS cases demonstrate an excessive hyperinsulinemic response to oral sugars.[41] The underlying characteristics of EMS cases that lead to excessive hyperinsulinemia are not yet understood fully. They may represent a combination of genetic and acquired factors influencing several steps, potentially linking grazing with laminitis (**Fig. 2**). Management strategies play a key role in influencing many of these steps such as pasture management (restricted grass access, grazing muzzles, dry lots, etc), feeding diets with a reduced percentage of nonstructural carbohydrates, and obesity control through exercise programs. However, pharmacologic opportunities also exist and may play a role alongside good management (see **Table 1**).

The origins of levothyroxine administration to obese equids probably began with the misconception that hypothyroidism was prevalent in this population. However, clinical hypothyroidism, if it exists in equids, is clearly extremely rare and plays no role in EMS.[38] Nevertheless, metabolic benefits may still be attributable to an increased metabolic rate associated with levothyroxine supplementation in the absence of deficient endogenous secretory function. Obesity seems to be a significant but reversible contributing factor to insulin resistance (IR),[42] which, in turn, promotes compensatory hyperinsulinaemia[42] (see **Fig. 2**). Several studies have indicated enhanced weight loss[43–45] and proportionate improvements in insulin sensitivity[43] by 16 weeks when normal horses were treated with levothyroxine. Chronic therapy with levothyroxine

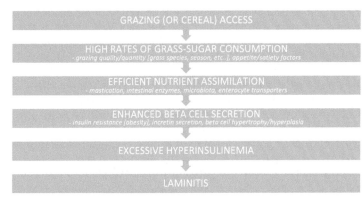

Fig. 2. Modifiable variables that might link grazing with predisposition to laminitis in individuals with equine metabolic syndrome.

has measurable cardiac effects as well as possible increased activity and mild hyperexcitability in treated horses, although none of the reported changes were judged to be of concern.[44]

In clinical practice levothyroxine sodium (Thyro-L, Lloyd Inc, Shenandoah, IA) may be indicated in individuals that seem to be particularly resistant to weight loss either owing to inherent metabolic characteristics[46] or perhaps owing to enforced exercise restriction as a result of chronic lameness. However, it is important that diet is controlled during treatment because an increased appetite may be a consequence of medication. A 3- to 6-month duration of treatment at a dosage of 0.1 mg/kg PO every 24 hours is recommended (approximately 48 mg [4 teaspoons] per day per 450–500 kg). A further increase in dosage by 50% (to 0.15 mg/kg) may be contemplated if there has been negligible impact on body condition by 3 months, although it is probably more important to closely scrutinize dietary management should this problem arise. When target body condition has been achieved, the dosage is decreased to 0.05 mg/kg for 2 weeks and then 0.025 mg/kg for a further 2 weeks before withdrawal to allow restoration of the suppressed thyroid axis.[45]

Unfortunately, commercially available levothyroxine products may be cost prohibitive in some countries, which has led to investigation of alternative pharmacologic aids for EMS. As a widely available, commonly prescribed, and affordable human generic product,[47] metformin hydrochloride was first used in a clinical study of EMS cases in the United Kingdom.[48] Given established modes of action in human subjects the authors of that study anticipated benefits in terms of improved insulin sensitivity, which was indeed consistent with the findings of decreased serum insulin and plasma glucose in metformin-treated subjects. However, further studies indicated very poor systemic absorption of metformin and no detectable effect on insulin sensitivity in treated horses,[49–51] leading to a reevaluation of the drug's potential mode of action.[52]

Metformin hydrochloride is well-known to have multiple modes of action, although its insulin-sensitizing and antihyperglycemic properties dominate its description in humans,[53] a species in which the drug is highly bioavailable.[54] However, metformin is also recognized to have important presystemic pharmacologic effects on enterocytes, which are found to preferentially accumulate the drug after oral or intravenous administration without any prerequisite systemic absorption.[55,56] First in rodents[57] and subsequently in horses,[58] it has been shown that metformin significantly blunts the glycemic and insulinemic response to orally ingested sugars, a property with potential therapeutic relevance to EMS given the proposed direct association of post-prandial hyperinsulinemia with laminitis.[39,40] Interestingly, it seems that metformin paradoxically increases the uptake of intestinal luminal glucose through increasing GLUT2 expression on enterocyte brush border membranes, with the absorbed glucose being largely "wasted" by anaerobic glycolysis within the enterocyte.

Thus, it seems unlikely that metformin has any insulin-sensitizing effect, or indeed any other direct peripheral effects in horses. However, a decrease in enteric glucose absorption and the subsequent insulinemic response seems to be likely. This was first implied in the initial study of its use in EMS cases, which showed decreased blood concentrations of glucose and insulin after treatment.[48] Clinical benefits of metformin have not yet been investigated in treated horses, although at least 2 potential benefits exist. First, weight loss might be promoted by decreased glucose absorption as has been described in humans[53] and, second, moderation of postprandial hyperinsuline-mia may reduce the likelihood of pasture-associated laminitis. Although both of these putative effects are intuitively beneficial in an individual prone to endocrinopathic lami-nitis, the ideal management of such horses should minimize dietary sugar content and grass access, thereby circumventing, or at least limiting, any possible beneficial effect of metformin.

It is important that clinical application of metformin should be considered in the context of the management and endocrine test results in the particular case. There may be a role for metformin where compliance with good dietary advice is compro-mised (eg, where owners insist on continued grazing), or perhaps as a longer term strategy in horses which have successfully lost weight but are found to retain an excessive insulinemic response to oral sugar tests. The dose regime for metformin is not currently established. The initial clinical study used a dose of 15 mg/kg PO every 12 hours and demonstrated a significant decrease in glucose and insulin concentra-tions.[48] A subsequent study demonstrating the enteric effects of metformin used a higher dose of 30 mg/kg PO.[58] Neither study cast any light on the duration of the drug's effects, although it is likely to be at least an hour.[58] In the absence of further pharmacokinetic data, where metformin is used to moderate postprandial hyperinsu-linemia in horses, it seems appropriate to target the drug administration according to the timing of anticipated sugar ingestion; that is, administration immediately before turnout or feeding.

Thiazolidinedione drugs are commonly used in humans as insulin sensitizers, either alone or alongside other drugs such as metformin. These drugs activate a nuclear re-ceptor called peroxisome proliferator activated receptor gamma, which regulates many genes involved in carbohydrate and lipid metabolism.[59] However, pioglitazone at 1 mg/kg PO attained relatively low plasma concentrations in horses[60] with little ev-idence of effects on insulin regulation[61] or inflammation.[62]

DIABETES MELLITUS

Occasional cases of DM are encountered in horses generally alongside signs of weight loss and polydipsia. Many cases of DM seem to be secondary to PPID,[35,63,64] although it is also reported in association with non–PPID-related chronic IR (type 2 DM)[63] and also primary pancreatic endocrine failure (type 1 DM).[65–68] Choice of therapy may depend on concentrations of endogenous insulin and the pres-ence and degree of β-cell dysfunction, IR, and predisposing conditions such as PPID.

Attempted long-term treatment of equine DM cases with exogenous insulin therapy has generally proved both costly and disappointing. Type 2 DM cases have not responded well owing to the presence of marked IR,[69] but limited success has been reported in cases of type 1 DM. Reasonable glycemic control was reported in a pony with DM secondary to pancreatitis treated with 1.0 IU/kg per day protamine zinc insulin as a single or divided dose administered intramuscularly.[66] Good clinical improvement was achieved over a 3-month period, although occasional hypoglycemic episodes arose. In a more recent case of type 1 DM in a horse, initial glycemic control was readily achieved with a constant rate intravenous infusion of 0.1 IU/kg per hour of regular insulin.[65] This was followed by long-term therapy using several different long acting insulins including Ultralente, Glargine, and Neutral Protamine Hagedorn at a dose of 0.4 IU/kg every 24 hours, with Neutral Protamine Hagedorn insulin seeming to be the most effective. Unfortunately, after 18 months, marked hyperglycemia recurred.

The effect of pergolide treatment on PPID-related DM is unclear. One study found that glucose concentrations did not change after pergolide treatment of PPID cases,[13] although other studies have demonstrated the contrary,[9] with 1 description of very prompt restoration of euglycemia within 12 hours of initiating pergolide treatment.[63] Despite apparently variable responses, it would seem advisable to at least attempt treatment with pergolide where PPID is identified in horses with DM. Other DM cases have been treated with insulin secretagogues in an attempt to regain glycemic control. Glyburide (glibenclamide) administration has been described in some reports[63,65,67] at up to 0.3 mg/kg PO every 12 hours. In the same reports, metformin was also administered, although given more recent evidence regarding the mode of action of this drug, including the absence of a peripheral insulin-sensitizing effect in horses (see above), it would seem unlikely to benefit equine DM cases.

DIABETES INSIPIDUS

Rarely, equine cases of polyuria and polydipsia as a result of DI are seen. Affected horses are essentially divisible into those failing to secrete vasopressin from their pituitary glands (central DI)[70,71] and those where their renal tubules fail to respond to vasopressin (peripheral DI).[72–74] Long-term pharmacologic treatment of equine DI cases is not reported, although several therapeutic options exist depending on which form is diagnosed.[75]

Only central DI cases are likely to be responsive to exogenous vasopressin therapy. This is usually in the form of desmopressin acetate,[76] but has only been reported as a short-term diagnostic measure in an equine case where a 10-mg dose administered as eye drops was effective in increasing urinary specific gravity in a 60-kg foal.[70] The anticonvulsant drug carbamazepine has been shown to have antidiuretic effects both through stimulation of central vasopressin release and by acting as an agonist of vasopressin receptors in the collecting ducts,[77] and may therefore be indicated in both central and peripheral DI. Its use or effectiveness in equid DI cases is unknown, although safety in horses is at least apparent from idiopathic headshaking cases.[78] Thiazide diuretics represent the main therapeutic modality for peripheral DI in other species.[79,80] These drugs decrease sodium (Na) and chloride (Cl) reabsorption in the distal convoluted tubule by inhibiting the Na–Cl cotransporter. The likely explanation for the paradoxic effect of reducing urinary output in DI cases is that increased Na losses lead to decreased extracellular fluid volume and decreased glomerular filtration rate, as well as increased Na and water reabsorption in the proximal tubule. Thiazides have not been reported in the treatment of equine DI, although hydrochlorothiazide (up to 3.3 mg/kg intravenously) is described for other purposes in horses.[81,82] Suspected central DI has been described in association with PPID in horses,[83] although the precise causes of polyuria and polydipsia in PPID cases are still not well-defined.[84] Nevertheless, attempted treatment of such cases with pergolide (or cyproheptadine) would seem to be a reasonable initial approach as improvement in polyuria and polydipsia is described after treatment.[9,11–14] Additional therapeutic choices used in human DI cases include the antikaliuretic drug amiloride and renal prostaglandin inhibitors such as indomethacin, which increase water reabsorption and reduce polyuria,[75] although these are likely to be cost prohibitive in horses.

THYROID DISEASE

Although many cases of suspected equine hypothyroidism have been treated with lev-othyroxine replacement therapy, firm establishment of this diagnosis is not straightfor-ward and serious doubts exist regarding its existence in adult horses.[38,85] Hyperthyroidism, although very rare, is less controversial and a few well-described cases are published.[86,87] Surgical treatment seems to be the favored approach, although a single report describes the additional medical treatment of one such case with propylthiouracil, an inhibitor of thyroid hormone synthesis, at a dose of 8 mg/kg PO every 24 to 48 hours.[88]

ADRENOCORTICAL DISEASE

Critical illness–related corticosteroid insufficiency describes a condition in which adre-nocortical glucocorticoid secretory response is considered to be abnormally sup-pressed, and is a possible complication of and contributor to critical illness in humans and other animals.[89] The condition has been described in foals,[90,91] with 1 study suggesting that as many as one-half of hospitalized foals could be affected.[90,91] Glucocorticoid replacement therapy is described in foals using intravenous and oral prednisone,[90] with a more recent therapeutic proposal to administer hydrocortisone at 0.22 mg/kg intravenously every 4 hours.[92] However, considerable controversy still surrounds this condition in all species and diagnostic and treatment recommendations remain far from clear.[93,94]

REFERENCES

1. Donaldson MT, Jorgensen AJ, Beech J. Evaluation of suspected pituitary pars in-termedia dysfunction in horses with laminitis. J Am Vet Med Assoc 2004;224(7): 1123–7.
2. Karikoski NP, Horn I, McGowan TW, et al. The prevalence of endocrinopathic laminitis among horses presented for laminitis at a first-opinion/referral equine hospital. Domest Anim Endocrinol 2011;41(3):111–7.
3. Morgan RA, Keen JA, McGowan CM. Treatment of equine metabolic syndrome: a clinical case series. Equine Vet J 2016;48(4):422–6.
4. Millington WR, Dybdal NO, Dawson R Jr, et al. Equine Cushing's disease: differ-ential regulation of beta-endorphin processing in tumors of the intermediate pitu-itary. Endocrinology 1988;123(3):1598–604.
5. Orth DN, Holscher MA, Wilson MG, et al. Equine Cushing's disease: plasma immunoreactive proopiolipomelanocortin peptide and cortisol levels basally and in response to diagnostic tests. Endocrinology 1982;110(4):1430–41.
6. Vazquez-Martinez R, Peinado JR, Cruz-Garcia D, et al. Melanotrope cells as a model to understand the (patho)physiological regulation of hormone secretion. J Endocrinol Invest 2005;28(10):949–58.
7. Pease AP, Schott HC 2nd, Howey EB, et al. Computed tomographic findings in the pituitary gland and brain of horses with pituitary pars intermedia dysfunction. J Vet Intern Med 2011;25(5):1144–51.

8. Molitch ME. Pharmacologic resistance in prolactinoma patients. Pituitary 2005; 8(1):43–52.
9. Andrews F, McFarlane D, Stokes A, et al. Freedom of information summary. Prascend tablets, pergolide mesylate, for the control of clinical signs associated with pituitary pars intermedia dysfunction (equine Cushing's disease) in horses. Original New Animal Drug Application, NADA; 2011. p. 141–331. Available at: http://www.fda.gov/downloads/AnimalV/UCM280354.pdf.
10. Durham AE, McGowan CM, Fey K, et al. Pituitary pars intermedia dysfunction: diagnosis and treatment. Equine Vet Educ 2014;26(4):216–23.
11. Rohrbach BW, Stafford JR, Clermont RS, et al. Diagnostic frequency, response to therapy, and long-term prognosis among horses and ponies with pituitary par intermedia dysfunction, 1993-2004. J Vet Intern Med 2012;26(4):1027–34.
12. Perkins GA, Lamb S, Erb HN, et al. Plasma adrenocorticotropin (ACTH) concentrations and clinical response in horses treated for equine Cushing's disease with cyproheptadine or pergolide. Equine Vet J 2002;34(7):679–85.
13. Donaldson MT, LaMonte BH, Morresey P, et al. Treatment with pergolide or cyproheptadine of pituitary pars intermedia dysfunction (equine Cushing's disease). J Vet Intern Med 2002;16(6):742–6.
14. Pongratz M, Graubner C, Eser M. Equine Cushing's syndrome. The effects of long-term therapy with pergolide. Pferdeheilkunde 2010;26:598–603.
15. Caccavelli L, Feron F, Morange I, et al. Decreased expression of the two D2 dopamine receptor isoforms in bromocriptine-resistant prolactinomas. Neuroendocrinology 1994;60(3):314–22.
16. Miller MA, Pardo ID, Jackson LP, et al. Correlation of pituitary histomorphometry with adrenocorticotrophic hormone response to domperidone administration in the diagnosis of equine pituitary pars intermedia dysfunction. Vet Pathol 2008; 45(1):26–38.
17. Leitenbacher J, Herbach N. Age-related qualitative histological and quantitative stereological changes in the equine pituitary. J Comp Pathol 2016;154(2–3): 215–24.
18. Thorner MO, Schran HF, Evans WS, et al. A broad spectrum of prolactin suppression by bromocriptine in hyperprolactinemic women: a study of serum prolactin and bromocriptine levels after acute and chronic administration of bromocriptine. J Clin Endocrinol Metab 1980;50(6):1026–33.
19. Pellegrini I, Rasolonjanahary R, Gunz G, et al. Resistance to bromocriptine in prolactinomas. J Clin Endocrinol Metab 1989;69(3):500–9.
20. Caccavelli L, Morange-Ramos I, Kordon C, et al. Alteration of G alpha subunits mRNA levels in bromocriptine resistant prolactinomas. J Neuroendocrinol 1996; 8(10):737–46.
21. Gehring R, Beard L, Wright A, et al. Single-dose oral pharmacokinetics of pergolide mesylate in healthy adult mares. Vet Ther 2010;11(1):E1–8.
22. Rendle DI, Hughes KJ, Doran GS, et al. Pharmacokinetics of pergolide after intravenous administration to horses. Am J Vet Res 2015;76(2):155–60.
23. Wright A. Pharmacokinetics of pergolide in normal mares. Master of Science Thesis. Manhattan (KS): Department of Clinical Sciences College of Veterinary Medicine, Kansas State University; 2009.
24. Peters D, Erfle J, Slobojan G. Low-dose pergolide mesylate treatment for equine hypophyseal adenomas (Cushing's syndrome). Proc. AAEP 1995;41:154–5.
25. Grotepaß D, Failing K, Fey K. Influence of once versus twice daily application of pergolide on ACTH levels in equines with PPID. 2nd European Equine Endocrinology Symposium. Windsor, UK: May 14–16, 2014.

26. Colao A, Di Sarno A, Sarnacchiaro F, et al. Prolactinomas resistant to standard dopamine agonists respond to chronic cabergoline treatment. J Clin Endocrinol Metab 1997;82(3):876–83.

27. Berezin M, Avidan D, Baron E. Long-term pergolide treatment of hyperprolactinemic patients previously unsuccessfully treated with dopaminergic drugs. Isr J Med Sci 1991;27(7):375–9.

28. Rohmer V, Freneau E, Morange I, et al. Efficacy of quinagolide in resistance to dopamine agonists: results of a multicenter study. Club de l'Hypophyse. Ann Endocrinol (Paris) 2000;61(5):411–7.

29. Beck D. Effective long-term treatment of a suspected pituitary adenoma with bromocryptine mesylate in a pony. Equine Vet Educ 1992;4(3):119–22.

30. Valencia N, Thompson D, Oberhaus E, et al. Long-term treatment of insulin-insensitive mares with cabergoline: effects on prolactin and melanocyte stimulating hormone responses to sulpiride and on indices of insulin sensitivity. J Equine Vet Sci 2014;34.

31. Ishibashi M, Yamaji T. Direct effects of thyrotropin-releasing hormone, cyproheptadine, and dopamine on adrenocorticotropin secretion from human corticotroph adenoma cells in vitro. J Clin Invest 1981;68(4):1018–27.

32. Schott H, Coursen C, Eberhart S, et al. The Michigan Cushing's project. Proc. AAEP 2001;47:22–4.

33. McGowan CM, Neiger R. Efficacy of trilostane for the treatment of equine Cushing's syndrome. Equine Vet J 2003;35(4):414–8.

34. McGowan CM, Frost R, Pfeiffer DU, et al. Serum insulin concentrations in horses with equine Cushing's syndrome: response to a cortisol inhibitor and prognostic value. Equine Vet J 2004;36(3):295–8.

35. Van der Kolk JH, Wensing T, Kalsbeek HC, et al. Laboratory diagnosis of equine pituitary pars intermedia adenoma. Domest Anim Endocrinol 1994;12:35–9.

36. Beech J, Boston R, Lindborg S. Comparison of cortisol and ACTH responses after administration of thyrotropin releasing hormone in normal horses and those with pituitary pars intermedia dysfunction. J Vet Intern Med 2011;25(6):1431–8.

37. McFarlane D, Beech J, Cribb A. Alpha-melanocyte stimulating hormone release in response to thyrotropin releasing hormone in healthy horses, horses with pituitary pars intermedia dysfunction and equine pars intermedia explants. Domest Anim Endocrinol 2006;30(4):276–88.

38. Johnson PJ. The equine metabolic syndrome peripheral Cushing's syndrome. Vet Clin North Am Equine Pract 2002;18(2):271–93.

39. Asplin KE, Sillence MN, Pollitt CC, et al. Induction of laminitis by prolonged hyperinsulinaemia in clinically normal ponies. Vet J 2007;174(3):530–5.

40. de Laat MA, McGowan CM, Sillence MN, et al. Equine laminitis: induced by 48 h hyperinsulinaemia in Standardbred horses. Equine Vet J 2010;42(2):129–35.

41. Schuver A, Frank N, Chameroy KA, et al. Assessment of Insulin and Glucose Dynamics by Using an Oral Sugar Test in Horses. J Equine Vet Sci 2014;34(4):465–70.

42. Ungru J, Bluher M, Coenen M, et al. Effects of body weight reduction on blood adipokines and subcutaneous adipose tissue adipokine mRNA expression profiles in obese ponies. Vet Rec 2012;171(21):528.

43. Frank N, Elliott SB, Boston RC. Effects of long-term oral administration of levothyroxine sodium on glucose dynamics in healthy adult horses. Am J Vet Res 2008;69(1):76–81.

44. Frank N, Buchanan BR, Elliott SB. Effects of long-term oral administration of levothyroxine sodium on serum thyroid hormone concentrations, clinicopathologic

variables, and echocardiographic measurements in healthy adult horses. Am J Vet Res 2008;69(1):68–75.

45. Sommardahl CS, Frank N, Elliott SB, et al. Effects of oral administration of levothyroxine sodium on serum concentrations of thyroid gland hormones and responses to injections of thyrotropin-releasing hormone in healthy adult mares. Am J Vet Res 2005;66(6):1025–31.

46. Argo CM, Curtis GC, Grove-White D, et al. Weight loss resistance: a further consideration for the nutritional management of obese Equidae. Vet J 2012; 194(2):179–88.

47. Inzucchi SE, Bergenstal RM, Buse JB, et al. Management of hyperglycemia in type 2 diabetes, 2015: a patient-centered approach: update to a position statement of the American Diabetes Association and the European Association for the Study of diabetes. Diabetes Care 2015;38(1):140–9.

48. Durham AE, Rendle DI, Newton JE. The effect of metformin on measurements of insulin sensitivity and beta cell response in 18 horses and ponies with insulin resistance. Equine Vet J 2008;40(5):493–500.

49. Tinworth KD, Edwards S, Noble GK, et al. Pharmacokinetics of metformin after enteral administration in insulin-resistant ponies. Am J Vet Res 2010;71(10):1201–6.

50. Tinworth KD, Boston RC, Harris PA, et al. The effect of oral metformin on insulin sensitivity in insulin-resistant ponies. Vet J 2012;191(1):79–84.

51. Hustace JL, Firshman AM, Mata JE. Pharmacokinetics and bioavailability of metformin in horses. Am J Vet Res 2009;70(5):665–8.

52. Durham AE. Metformin in equine metabolic syndrome: an enigma or a dead duck? Vet J 2012;191(1):17–8.

53. Inzucchi SE. Oral antihyperglycemic therapy for Type 2 diabetes. JAMA 2002; 287(3):360.

54. Pentikainen PJ, Neuvonen PJ, Penttila A. Pharmacokinetics of metformin after intravenous and oral administration to man. Eur J Clin Pharmacol 1979;16(3): 195–202.

55. Bailey CJ, Wilcock C, Scarpello JH. Metformin and the intestine. Diabetologia 2008;51(8):1552–3.

56. Wilcock C, Bailey CJ. Accumulation of metformin by tissues of the normal and diabetic mouse. Xenobiotica 1994;24(1):49–57.

57. Sakar Y, Meddah B, Faouzi MA, et al. Metformin-induced regulation of the intestinal D-glucose transporters. J Physiol Pharmacol 2010;61(3):301–7.

58. Rendle DI, Rutledge F, Hughes KJ, et al. Effects of metformin hydrochloride on blood glucose and insulin responses to oral dextrose in horses. Equine Vet J 2013;45(6):751–4.

59. Mudaliar S, Henry RR. New oral therapies for type 2 diabetes mellitus: the glitazones or insulin sensitizers. Annu Rev Med 2001;52:239–57.

60. Wearn JM, Crisman MV, Davis JL, et al. Pharmacokinetics of pioglitazone after multiple oral dose administration in horses. J Vet Pharmacol Ther 2011;34(3): 252–8.

61. Suagee JK, Corl BA, Wearn JG, et al. Effects of the insulin-sensitizing drug pioglitazone and lipopolysaccharide administration on insulin sensitivity in horses. J Vet Intern Med 2011;25(2):356–64.

62. Wearn JG, Suagee JK, Crisman MV, et al. Effects of the insulin sensitizing drug, pioglitazone, and lipopolysaccharide administration on markers of systemic inflammation and clinical parameters in horses. Vet Immunol Immunopathol 2012;145(1–2):42–9.

63. Durham AE, Hughes KJ, Cottle HJ, et al. Type 2 diabetes mellitus with pancreatic β cell dysfunction in 3 horses confirmed with minimal model analysis. Equine Vet J 2009;41(9):924–9.

64. Loeb WF, Capen CC, Johnson LE. Adenomas of the pars intermedia associated with hyperglycemia and glycosuria in two horses. Cornell Vet 1966;56(4):623–39.

65. Giri JK, Magdesian KG, Gaffney PM. Insulin-dependent diabetes mellitus associated with presumed autoimmune polyendocrine syndrome in a mare. Can Vet J 2011;52(5):506–12.

66. Jeffrey JR. Diabetes mellitus secondary to chronic pancreatitis in a pony. J Am Vet Med Assoc 1968;153(9):1168–75.

67. Johnson PJ, Scotty NC, Wiedmeyer C, et al. Diabetes mellitus in a domesticated Spanish mustang. J Am Vet Med Assoc 2005;226(4):584–8, 542.

68. Newman SJ. Equine pancreatic disease: a review and characterization of the lesions of four cases (2005-2014). J Vet Diagn Invest 2015;27(1):92–6.

69. Baker JR, Ritchie HE. Diabetes mellitus in the horse: a case report and review of the literature. Equine Vet J 1974;6(1):7–11.

70. Kranenburg LC, Thelen MH, Westermann CM, et al. Use of desmopressin eye drops in the treatment of equine congenital central diabetes insipidus. Vet Rec 2010;167(20):790–1.

71. Breukink HJ, Van Wegen P, Schotman AJ. Idiopathic diabetes insipidus in a Welsh pony. Equine Vet J 1983;15(3):284–7.

72. Brashier M. Polydipsia and polyuria in a weanling colt caused by nephrogenic diabetes insipidus. Vet Clin North Am Equine Pract 2006;22(1):219–27.

73. Morgan RA, Malalana F, McGowan CM. Nephrogenic diabetes insipidus in a 14-year-old gelding. N Z Vet J 2012;60(4):254–7.

74. Schott HC 2nd, Bayly WM, Reed SM, et al. Nephrogenic diabetes insipidus in sibling colts. J Vet Intern Med 1993;7(2):68–72.

75. Robertson GL. Diabetes insipidus: differential diagnosis and management. Best Pract Res Clin Endocrinol Metab 2016;30(2):205–18.

76. Ooi HL, Maguire AM, Ambler GR. Desmopressin administration in children with central diabetes insipidus: a retrospective review. J Pediatr Endocrinol Metab 2013;26(11–12):1047–52.

77. de Braganca AC, Moyses ZP, Magaldi AJ. Carbamazepine can induce kidney water absorption by increasing aquaporin 2 expression. Nephrol Dial Transplant 2010;25(12):3840–5.

78. Newton SA, Knottenbelt DC, Eldridge PR. Headshaking in horses: possible aetiopathogenesis suggested by the results of diagnostic tests and several treatment regimes used in 20 cases. Equine Vet J 2000;32(3):208–16.

79. Al Nofal A, Lteif A. Thiazide Diuretics in the Management of Young Children with Central Diabetes Insipidus. J Pediatr 2015;167(3):658–61.

80. Takemura N. Successful long-term treatment of congenital nephrogenic diabetes insipidus in a dog. J small Anim Pract 1998;39(12):592–4.

81. Beech J, Lindborg S. Prophylactic efficacy of phenytoin, acetazolamide and hydrochlorothiazide in horses with hyperkalaemic periodic paralysis. Res Vet Sci 1995;59(2):95–101.

82. Alexander F. The effect of diuretics on the faecal excretion of water and electrolytes in horses. Br J Pharmacol 1977;60(4):589–93.

83. Moses ME, Johnson PJ, Messer NT, et al. Antidiuretic response of a horse affected with pituitarypars intermedia dysfunction to desmopressin acetate. Equine Vet Educ 2013;25(3):111–5.

84. Schott HC. Water homeostasis and diabetes insipidus in horses. Vet Clin North Am Equine Pract 2011;27(1):175–95.
85. Breuhaus BA. Disorders of the equine thyroid gland. Vet Clin North Am Equine Pract 2011;27(1):115–28.
86. Ramirez S, McClure JJ, Moore RM, et al. Hyperthyroidism associated with a thyroid adenocarcinoma in a 21-year-old gelding. J Vet Intern Med 1998;12(6): 475–7.
87. Alberts MK, McCann JP, Woods PR. Hemithyroidectomy in a horse with confirmed hyperthyroidism. J Am Vet Med Assoc 2000;217(7):1051–4, 1009.
88. Tan RH, Davies SE, Crisman MV, et al. Propylthiouracil for treatment of hyperthyroidism in a horse. J Vet Intern Med 2008;22(5):1253–8.
89. Marik PE. Critical illness-related corticosteroid insufficiency. Chest 2009;135(1): 181–93.
90. Couetil LL, Hoffman AM. Adrenal insufficiency in a neonatal foal. J Am Vet Med Assoc 1998;212(10):1594–6.
91. Hart KA, Slovis NM, Barton MH. Hypothalamic-pituitary-adrenal axis dysfunction in hospitalized neonatal foals. J Vet Intern Med 2009;23(4):901–12.
92. Hart KA, Barton MH. Adrenocortical insufficiency in horses and foals. Vet Clin North Am Equine Pract 2011;27(1):19–34.
93. Creedon JM. Controversies surrounding critical illness-related corticosteroid insufficiency in animals. J Vet Emerg Crit Care (San Antonio) 2015;25(1):107–12.
94. Boonen E, Bornstein SR, Van den Berghe G. New insights into the controversy of adrenal function during critical illness. Lancet Diabetes Endocrinol 2015;3(10): 805–15.

Therapeutics for Equine Gastric Ulcer Syndrome

Fereydon Rezazadeh Zavoshti, DVM, DVSc[a], Frank M. Andrews, DVM, MS[b],*

KEYWORDS

- Horse • Equine • Gastric ulcer • Equine gastric ulcer syndrome • Therapeutics

KEY POINTS

- Equine gastric ulcer syndrome (EGUS) describes ulceration in the terminal esophagus, nonglandular and glandular stomach, and the proximal duodenum.
- Clinical signs in many cases do not clearly indicate the diagnosis of EGUS, thus a diagnosis should be confirmed by gastroscopy.
- Omeprazole, a potent proton pump inhibitor, is currently the drug of choice for treatment and prevention of recurrence; however, many other pharmaceutical agents, including antacids, H_2-receptor antagonists, sucralfate, and prostaglandin analogues, have been used alone or with omeprazole to treat and prevent EGUS.
- With the reduction of medications and the avocation of Clean Sport in racing and competitions, interest has grown in effective natural supplements and better nutrition to improve stomach health.

INTRODUCTION

Although gastric ulcers have been recognized for centuries, it was in 1999 that the term equine gastric ulcer syndrome (EGUS) was introduced to better characterize and describe lesions in the terminal esophagus, nonglandular and glandular stomach, and proximal duodenum.[1] Several recent reports were published to further explain the syndrome and highlight the differences in pathogenesis of lesions in the nonglandular versus glandular stomach. A better understanding of the differences in regional pathogenesis could lead to comprehensive therapeutic and preventive strategies.[2–5] EGUS is seen in all horse and breeds and is prevalent worldwide, leading to decreased productivity and economic loss to the horse industry. EGUS is seen in foals and adult horses and the relative risk for ulceration might increase with age in geldings, whereas stallions seem to be at greater risk than mares and geldings.[6] Recently, a consensus

Disclosure: The authors have nothing to disclose.
[a] University of Tabriz, 29th Bahman Boulevard, Tabriz 5166616471, Iran; [b] Equine Health Studies Program, Department of Veterinary Clinical Sciences, School of Veterinary Medicine, Louisiana State University, Baton Rouge, Skip Bertman Drive, LA 70803, USA
* Corresponding author.
E-mail address: fandrews@lsu.edu

statement was published to better explain the meaning of EGUS and highlight the differences in the pathogenesis of lesions in the horse stomach.[3] A better understanding of EGUS terminology might provide practitioners with clarity to better understand how to plan rational therapy.

Current therapeutic strategies for EGUS focus on blocking gastric acid secretion and increasing stomach pH. To date, there is only 1 registered pharmacologic agent for treatment and 1 pharmacologic agent for prevention of EGUS (GastroGard paste and Ulcergard paste; Merial Limited, Duluth, GA). However, a more comprehensive approach to therapy for EGUS includes determining and correcting the underlying cause, environmental management, dietary manipulation, and pharmacologic intervention. This article focuses on current terminology used to describe the pathogenesis of EGUS and presents a comprehensive therapeutic approach to maintain stomach health. In addition, current information on effective use of natural supplements is reviewed.

DEFINITION AND TERMINOLOGY

EGUS terminology was introduced in 1999 to describe ulceration in the terminal part of esophagus, nonglandular (squamous mucosa) and glandular gastric mucosa, and proximal duodenum.[1] After introduction, there was some confusion in the meaning,[7] because early pharmaceutical trials concentrated on treatment of nonglandular (squamous) ulcers, because glandular ulcers were not observed or recognized in Thoroughbred racehorses at a high prevalence in the United States.[8] The term EGUS was originally coined to be equivalent to the term peptic ulcer disease, which is the umbrella term used to describe erosive and ulcerative disease of the stomach and duodenum in humans.[9] The consensus statement introduced new terminology to describe EGUS and how lesions differ in the nonglandular squamous mucosa (equine squamous gastric disease [ESGD]) and in glandular mucosa (equine glandular gastric disease [EGGD]). ESGD can be primary and secondary. Secondary ESGD occurs in horses with delayed gastric emptying, secondary to pyloric stenosis, and results in erosions and ulcerations in the terminal esophagus. This condition is primarily seen in foals with pyloric stenosis.

Primary ESGD is associated with intensive and multiple management factors in horses with otherwise normal gastrointestinal tracts and are likely the result of increased exposure to hydrochloric acid (HCl) and organic acids. The squamous mucosa has an osmiophilic phospholipid surfactant–like layer that contributes to the mucosal barrier, but it lacks a significant mucus and bicarbonate layer, has poor blood supply, and has a variable ability to spontaneously heal at a high rate once injured.[10,11] Previous studies indicate that primary ESGD is likely caused by mucosal exposure to HCl alone or in combination with volatile fatty acids (VFAs; acetic, butyric, and propionic acids) and lactic acid, produced by resident stomach bacteria.[12–16] When gastric juice pH is less than or equal to 4, VFAs and, to a lesser extent, lactic acid are lipid soluble and enter the squamous mucosal cells, resulting in acid injury, cell swelling, and eventual ulceration.

EGGD refers to lesions in the glandular mucosa. The glandular stomach is diverse and consists of the cardia, adjacent to the margo plicatus, which is responsible for secreting mucus and bicarbonate to protect the glandular tissue from acid injury. The fundus or ventral glandular mucosa is the largest portion of the equine stomach and is made up of parietal cells, which secrete HCl; zymogen or chief cells, which secrete pepsinogen; and enterochromaffinlike (ECL) cells, which secrete histamine to stimulate HCL secretion by parietal cells and function to maintain gastric blood flow. The antrum and pyloric regions of the stomach are composed of G cells, which are a major source of gastrin; D cells, which secrete somatostatin; and ECL cells, which secrete serotonin.[17] Hormones from these cells control gastric emptying and maintain stomach motility function.

HCl and a low stomach pH contribute to acid injury in the glandular mucosa. However, the mucosal defense mechanisms are compromised first, which allows back flow of HCl and organic acids into and between glandular cells, resulting in sodium pump damage.[18] The reason for the breakdown in glandular defense mechanisms is unknown; however, experiments with laboratory rodents, humans, and horses showed lesions to be associated with stress, infection with bacteria, nonsteroidal anti-inflammatory drugs (NSAIDs), and inhibition of protective prostaglandins.[19–22] A study by Malmkvist and colleagues[19] (2012) implicates the role of stress in glandular ulceration in horses. Furthermore, true ulcers in the glandular mucosa of horses are rare and typical lesions are raised and inflammatory. The reason for inflammatory lesions is unknown, but they might be an extension of inflammatory bowel disease. Crohn disease, a form of human inflammatory bowel disease that affects the mucosa and deeper layer of the bowel wall, can cause duodenal strictures and may play a role in pyloric inflammatory changes. Hepatic duct stricture and pancreatic duct stricture have been reported in association with duodenitis in adult horses.

PREVALENCE AND CLINICAL SIGNS

The prevalence of ESGD varies from 40% in Quarter Horses participating in Western performance to 90% in Thoroughbreds actively racing and training.[23,24] The prevalence of EGGD varies from 8% in Thoroughbred racehorses in the United Kingdom to 63% of Thoroughbred racehorses in Australia.[25] Based on an abattoir in the United Kingdom, both ESGD and EGGD had high prevalence in domesticated horses (60.8%, 70.6%, respectively) compared with feral (22.2%, 29.6%, respectively) horses.[26] Rabuffo and colleagues[27] (2009) reported that gastric ulceration was determined to be the primary cause of colic in 31 of 111 cases (28%). The prevalence of EGUS in neonatal foals was estimated to be 25% to 50%.[28]

ESGD was evident in 68% and 72% of horses presented for colic and noncolic complaints, respectively; however, the difference was not statistically significant.[29,30] Some important risk factors for EGUS are age and gender, training, concurrent disease such as impaction colic, colonic tympany, intussusception and primary inflammatory bowel diseases such as duodenitis–proximal jejunitis, diet, environment, and psychological stress.[17] The induction of ESGD with exercise, high-concentrate/low-roughage diets, anorexia, transport, stall confinement, the administration of hypertonic electrolytes, and intermittent access to water can be rapid, occurring within 7 days in some studies and the risk of disease increasing with time in work.[31] It is taken for granted that horses housed in pasture have fewer ulcers, but a New Zealand study reported a high prevalence of gastric ulceration (>89%) in racehorses maintained at pasture for some part of the day, and another did so in pastured pregnant and nonpregnant broodmares.[31,32] Horses that are actively racing or training and broodmares are likely to be supplemented with concentrates, which likely contribute to the high ulcer prevalence in these horses.

Clinical signs of ulcers are numerous and vague, and can include inappetence, poor body condition, weight loss, diarrhea, changes in behavior, and poor performance.[33] One of the most common clinical signs of equine gastric ulcer disease is colic, especially recurrent colic, although gastric ulcers can be seen on gastroscopy examination in horses without colic signs as well.[27] Other nonspecific signs include pain or discomfort when tightening the girth strap, as well as stereotypic or abnormal behavior, such as crib biting, head nodding, stall wall kicking, stall pawing, wood chewing, flehmen, and stall weaving.[33] In other studies, there was no association between crib biting/weaving and gastric ulceration.[34] The potential for EGUS to cause poor performance is of particular importance but, surprisingly, to date few studies have investigated the potential relationship between poor performance and the presence of EGUS.[35–37] In addition, clinical signs of ESGD do not necessarily correlate with presence or severity of gastric ulcers, although horses in one study that were presented with colic were more likely to have endoscopically confirmed gastric ulcers.[38]

The clinical signs of EGUS in foals with gastric outflow obstruction encompass those of gastroduodenal ulcer syndrome. Affected foals are often 2 to 6 months of age and typically show signs of lethargy, colic, an unthrifty appearance, frequent recumbency, bruxism, ptyalism, frothing or drooling of milk from the mouth, tongue lolling, diarrhea (present or recent), and frequent rolling into dorsal recumbency. Although clinical signs often do not correlate with a diagnosis of EGUS, they can be used to suggest the diagnosis and warrant gastroscopic examination.

DIAGNOSIS

The definitive diagnosis of EGUS is based on endoscopic visual evidence of gastric erosion, ulceration, or other lesions.[1] In addition, a presumptive diagnosis of EGUS can be made based on history, clinical signs, and response to treatment with a therapeutic trial. It is important to do a complete evaluation of the horse, including obtaining a thorough history, physical examination, and blood work, to rule out diseases that might lead to secondary gastric ulcers. Recently, a sucrose permeability test showed promise as a diagnostic aid in EGUS.[39] The sucrose permeability test requires testing urine for sucrose, which must be done in a laboratory using high-pressure liquid chromatography. In addition, a guaiac-based fecal occult blood test was used in one study and showed high specificity, low sensitivity, and high false-negative results for determining the location of ulceration (stomach or colon).[40] In a recent study, there was a high number of false-negative tests and no significant correlation was found between results of a new fecal blood test (Succeed FBT, Freedom Health LLC, Lexington, KY) and gastric ulcer scores in horses undergoing stall confinement and bolus feeding.[41] In foals, endoscopy and ultrasonography are the most important diagnostic tools for confirming mucosal ulcers and visually observing gastric and duodenal motility, respectively. Contrast radiography of the stomach following a barium swallow has also been used to confirm delayed gastric emptying.

Recently, an article presented an ulcer risk calculator for horse owners, highlighting key questions (**Table 1**).[42] Questions included how many meals the horse's concentrate provision is divided into per day; how much of the day the horse spends grazing or eating hay; how many days in a row the horse has been given NSAIDs in the past 3 months; and how many days per week the horse is in intense, high-speed work. Scores were calculated based on provided answers, with a score of 0 to 5 indicating low risk, a score of 6 to 15 indicating moderate risk, and a score of greater than 15 indicating a high risk for EGUS. The results have not been validated in other studies, but might help clients with understanding some of the risk factors.

THERAPY IN EQUINE GASTRIC ULCER SYNDROME

The goals of antiulcer therapy are to relieve pain, eliminate clinical signs, promote healing of ulcers, and prevent recurrence and secondary complications. Suppression of HCl and increasing stomach pH is the goal of EGUS treatment, regardless of where

Table 1
A gastric ulcer risk calculator

Gastric Ulcer Risk	Score					Score
	1	2	3	4	5	
1. How many meals is your horse's grain ration divided into per day?	3 or more	2	—	—	1	
2. How much of the day does your horse spend grazing or eating hay?	75%	50%	—	—	75%	
3. How many days in a row has your horse been on NSAIDs in the past 3 mo?	None	≤10 d	—	—	>10 d	
4. Over the past 3 mo, which of the following apply to your horse?	Spent 1 d away at show, clinic, or other	—				
	Took a trailer ride	—	—	—	—	
	Attended competition or clinic at unfamiliar location	—	—	—	—	
	Change in herd dynamics	—	—	—	—	
	Sustained injury or developed illness	—	—	—	—	
5. How many days per week is your horse in intense work?	None	1 or 2	—	—	≥ 3	
					Total	

Risk score: 0–5, low risk; 6–15, moderate risk; 16–25, high risk.
Adapted from Barakat C. What's your horse's ulcer risk. Equus 2016;454:68–77.

the lesions occur. Because of the high recurrence rate, effective acid control should be followed by altered management strategies or long-term treatment to prevent ulcer recurrence.

Environmental, Nutritional, and Dietary Management

Without alterations in management or initiation of preventive therapy, squamous ulcers quickly return if horses are maintained in training.[8] However, glandular ulcer recurrence has not been evaluated. Reducing exercise intensity, increasing pasture turnout, and amending dietary risk factors might help to decrease ulcer severity and the risk of recurrence in squamous ulcers, but it is unknown whether this will prevent recurrence of glandular ulcers. The following recommendations are primarily for squamous ulcers, but might also have a positive effect on glandular ulcers.

Modification of Exercise Intensity and Duration

Intense exercise, racing, and race training have been shown to contribute to worsening of squamous ulcers in horses, and pasture turnout or change in management might improve the condition.[35,37]

Pasture Turnout

Horses housed in pastures and constantly grazing appear less likely to develop squamous ulcers. Stall confinement generally has been associated with an increased risk of squamous ulcers and this type of ulcer might not improve in stall-confined horses even when horses are fed grass hay ad libitum. Although pasture turnout may be helpful in controlling squamous ulcers, the presence of certain other stressors and whether the horse continues to be fed high NSC (non-structural carbohydrates)-containing feed-stuffs may be greater determining factors.[19,43] In some situations changes in management, such as moving horses from stall to pasture housing, might be effective in reducing squamous ulcer scores in some horses.[44]

DIET

Pasture grazing, high-forage (dry matter [DM] intake, $\geq$1.5% body weight [BW]) and low-concentrate ($\leq$0.5% BW) diets, a diet low in NSC, feeding smaller and more frequent meals, and providing ad libitum forages might reduce the risk of squamous ulceration, as discussed below.

Eliminate Bolus Feeding and Increase Forage/Fiber Intake

One management practice that may help to decrease the risks of squamous ulcers is to feed a forage based diet ad libitum or at least ensure that forage is provided every few hours and before exercise (even in small amounts). Stabled horses should be fed 3 to 4 small grain meals (if required) per day, not to exceed 0.5 kg/100 kg BW every 6 hours.[15] Smaller grain meals decrease intragastric fermentation, reduce production of VFAs, and improve gastric emptying rate.

Providing alfalfa hay and good-quality grass hay as the forage and/or adding alfalfa chaff to any complementary feed may be advantageous, although the total ration needs to be balanced to account for the inclusion of alfalfa.[45,46] Straw should not be fed as the only or primary feed, because it was found to be at least 4.4 times more likely to increase squamous gastric ulcer severity scores.[47]

Although absolute requirements have not been determined for horses, current recommended levels of forage (grass and preserved forages) are ideally $\geq$1.5 kg DM/100 kg BW for all horses, including those with high energy requirements (in which case young, less mature, high-energy forages should be considered).[47] A target minimum, even for racehorses, is 1.25 kg DM/100 kg BW. Lower amounts may be required for those horses on a strict veterinary monitored weight loss program (but not <1 kg DM/100 kg BW), in which case appropriate measures need to be put into place to maximize the time spent chewing the restricted forage intake.[48,49] Examples of such measures include slow feeders and hay bags. Appropriate protein, vitamin, and mineral ration balancers are required to nutritionally balance the diet, especially if fortified concentrate feeds are not fed.

Reduce the Intake of Nonstructural Carbohydrate

Reduced-grain diets should be fed to decrease the risks of ulcers. Larger grain meals (700 g/100 kg BW) resulted in slower gastric emptying compared with a smaller (300 g/100 kg BW) grain meal.[50] Increased gastric retention time increases the fermentation by resident bacteria, resulting in higher VFA production and a greater potential for squamous injury. The intake of nonstarch polysaccharides, and particularly grains, should therefore be restricted through the use of lower NSC complementary feeds. Based on previous studies, feeding less than 0.5 kg grain (so-called sweet feed)/100 kg BW (NSC = 40%) should keep the stomach VFA concentration of acetic acid below a potentially injurious threshold (20 mmol/L) and minimize the effect on squamous ulcers.[15] Feeding less than 2g NSC/kg BW/d or less than 1g NSC/kg BW/meal has also been recommended.[50] This can be a challenge for trainers of high-intensity exercising horses, without an apparent (real or perceived) loss in performance, often resulting in their inclusion of various supplements in their horses' diets, as discussed later.

Antibiotics Versus Probiotics

Helicobacter pylori and other *Helicobacter* species have not been shown to cause squamous or glandular ulcers in horses, although *Helicobacter* DNA has been isolated from the squamous and glandular mucosa of horses.[51,52] Instead, other resident, acid-tolerant bacteria (*Escherichia coli*, *Lactobacillus*, and *Streptococcus*) are suspected to contribute to the worsening of squamous ulcers.[52] A large population of these bacteria was isolated from the gastric contents of horses fed various diets in one study.[53] In rats, which have a compound stomach similar to horses, bacteria (*E coli*) rapidly colonized acetic acid–induced glandular stomach ulcers and impaired glandular ulcer healing.[54] In that study, oral antibiotic treatment with streptomycin or penicillin suppressed bacterial colonization of the ulcer and markedly accelerated glandular ulcer healing compared with placebo-treated controls.[54] In addition, oral administration of lactulose resulted in increased *Lactobacillus* growth and colonization of the ulcer bed, which may facilitate glandular ulcer healing. These studies in rats only investigated healing of ulcers in the glandular mucosa. In a study evaluating horses with spontaneously occurring squamous ulcers, an antibiotic (trimethoprim-sulfadimidine) or a probiotic preparation containing *Lactobacillus agilis*, *Lactobacillus salivarius*, *Lactobacillus equi*, *Streptococcus equinus*, and *Streptococcus bovis* administered orally decreased ulcer number and severity compared with untreated controls.[53] These data suggest that resident stomach bacteria are important in maintenance and progression of squamous ulcers in horses. Treatment with antibiotic or probiotic preparations may facilitate squamous ulcer healing after 2 weeks of treatment, but a full effect was not seen until after 4 weeks of treatment. Antibiotic treatment may be indicated in horses with chronic nonresponsive squamous ulcers. However, antibiotic administration did not improve healing of glandular gastric ulceration in horses receiving omeprazole.[55] In any case, antibiotics should be used responsibly and only when acid-suppressive therapy alone is not effective.

PHARMACOLOGIC THERAPY

Once EGUS is diagnosed, therapy should be initiated to achieve the goals outlined earlier. Only approximately 4% to 6% of nonglandular ulcers heal spontaneously; to achieve significant healing, most horses need pharmacologic therapy, especially when they remain in athletic training.[8,56] There are many approaches to treating EGUS, but acid-suppressive therapy and establishing a permissive environment in the stomach to allow ulcer healing is the main approach. Many pharmacologic agents are available to treat gastric ulcers in humans, but few have been shown to be effective in the treatment and prevention of EGUS. Of these products, only omeprazole paste formulations (GastroGard paste and Ulcergard paste, Merial Limited, Duluth, GA) are registered by the US Food and Drug Administration (FDA) for treatment and prevention of recurrence of EGUS. Other therapies have been used with mixed success and their advantages, disadvantages, and evidence for use are presented later.

Although many drugs have been used to treat EGUS there are clear differences in efficacy of these agents in treating ulcers occurring in the nonglandular mucosa as opposed to the glandular mucosa. Nonglandular ulcers respond well to agents that increase gastric juice pH. Omeprazole treatment was more effective than ranitidine in a study of the treatment of racehorses with ESGD.[57] In contrast, the efficacy of pharmaceutical agents on EGGD has not been thoroughly studied; treatment of EGGD often follows the same principles as for ESGD, but a longer treatment period with omepra-zole might be required.[3] The physiologic aggressive and protective factors from each region of the equine stomach are shown in **Table 2**.[33]

Proton Pump Inhibitors

Omeprazole, a proton pump inhibitor, is the mainstay of treatment of EGUS in humans and horses. At present, omeprazole paste (GastroGard paste, Merial Limited, Duluth, GA) is registered in several countries for treatment and prevention of recurrence of EGUS.[8] However, other therapies have been used to treat EGUS, with mixed success. Doses of various pharmaceutical agents to treat EGUS are listed in **Table 3**.[33]

Omeprazole, a substituted benzimidazole, is a potent inhibitor of gastric acid secre-tion in humans, rats, dogs, and horses. Omeprazole decreases gastric acid secretion by blocking hydrogen-potassium-ATPase in the secretory membrane of parietal cells. This enzyme catalyzes the exchange of hydrogen ions for potassium ions in the final step of HCl production by parietal cells. Omeprazole, as an acid pump inhibitor, is 10 times more potent than ranitidine on an equimolar basis.[58] Omeprazole paste is one of the most extensively studied veterinary pharmaceutical agents.[8,59] Recently, the exclusive patent on omeprazole paste expired, and therefore several formulations, pharmacologic parameters, timing of administration, and dosing of omeprazole were reevaluated.[60,61] The results of those studied showed that a lower dose of omeprazole (1.0 mg/kg, by mouth, every 24 hours) might be effective if administered before exer-cise and following a brief fast. In that study, which evaluated 3 doses of omeprazole (1, 2, and 4 mg/kg), fewer glandular ulcers healed (36%), compared with squamous ul-cers (78%).[60] The results showed significant differences between the healing response of ESGD and EGGD after omeprazole therapy. These data support the notion that stomach acids are important risk factors in the cause of ESGD, whereas acids may play a lesser role in the pathogenesis of EGGD. In addition, the bioavail-ability of omeprazole is affected by the formulation, because omeprazole powder is acid labile and inactivated by stomach acid. Omeprazole formulations that are not pro-tected by enteric coating or mixed in an alkaline paste formulation are inactivated by stomach acid and have reduced bioavailability.[59,62]

Omeprazole is labeled for short-term administration (28 days) for the treatment of EGUS. Long-term administration of high doses of omeprazole caused hyperplasia of ECL cells and gastric carcinoid tumors in rats.[63] Gastric carcinoids seem to be species

Table 2		
Physiologic factors affecting ulcer development		
Aggressive Factors	**Protective Factors: Nonglandular Mucosa**	**Protective Factors: Glandular Mucosa**
HCl secretion	Epithelial restitution	Bicarbonate: mucus layer secretion
Organic acid production	Mucosal blood flow	Epithelial restitution
Pepsin conversion from pepsinogen		Mucosal blood flow
Duodenal reflux of bile acids		Prostaglandin E production

Adapted from Ward S, Sykes BW, Brown H, et al. A comparison of the prevalence of gastric ulcer-ation in feral and domesticated horses in the UK. Equine Vet Educ 2015;57(12):655–7; and Rabuffo TS, Hackett ES, Grenagar N, et al. Prevalence of gastric ulceration in horse with colic. J Equine Vet Sci 2009;29(6):540–6.

Table 3
Commonly used therapeutic agents for treatment and prevention of gastric ulcers in horses and foals

Drug	Dose	Dosing Interval	Route of Administration
Ranitidine	6.6 mg/kg	q 6–8 h	PO
Ranitidine	1.5 mg/kg	q 6 h	IV, IM
Omeprazole	4 mg/kg (treatment)	q 24 h	PO
Omeprazole	1–2 mg/kg (prevention)	q 24 h	PO
Omeprazole	0.5–1.0 mg/kg	q 24 h	IV
Esomeprazole	1.0 mg/kg	q 24 h	IV
Esomeprazole	1.0–2.0 mg/kg	q 24 h	PO
Pantoprazole	1.5 mg/kg	q 24 h	IV
Sucralfate	12–20 mg/kg	q 8 h	PO
Al or Mg hydroxide	0.5 mL/kg	q 4–6 h	PO
Misoprostol, Prostaglandin Analogues	1–4 µg	q 8 h	PO

Abbreviations: IM, intramuscular; IV, intravenous; PO, by mouth; q, every.
Adapted from Le Jeune SS, Nieto JE, Dechant JE, et al. Prevalence of gastric ulcers in Thoroughbred broodmares in pasture: a preliminary report. Vet J 2009;181:251–5.

specific and no significant side effects have been reported in horses treated for up to 90 days. Omeprazole has been shown to be safe in both foals and mature horses.[64]

However, omeprazole paste can only be administered orally. Administration of oral medications in horses with gastric reflux or dysphagia is contraindicated. A formulation of intravenous (IV) omeprazole was studied and showed significant increases in gastric pH, and squamous ulcers significantly improved after 5 days of treatment.[65] The compounded formulation of omeprazole is no longer available in the United States, but a human commercial IV formulation of omeprazole or ranitidine could be substituted.

Esomeprazole, the S-enantiomer of omeprazole, provides better gastric acid control and decreases interindividual variability in gastric juice pH in humans compared with omeprazole.[66] The improved efficacy of esomeprazole is likely caused by a lower plasma clearance and higher area under the curve for plasma concentration–time compared with omeprazole. Higher plasma concentrations result in greater drug availability to enter and inhibit parietal cell function in a dose-dependent manner, which leads to greater HCl suppression. Esomeprazole maintains an intragastric pH greater than 4 when given orally, once daily for 5 days in humans. It also has a faster onset of action compared with omeprazole and other racemic proton pump inhibitors. One study showed that IV administration of esomeprazole to horses for 14 days significantly increased gastric juice pH.[67] In addition, oral administration of esomeprazole (40 mg or 80 mg, orally, every 24 hours) controlled pH levels of gastric secretions in Thoroughbreds.[68] The results obtained corroborated the efficacy of esomeprazole magnesium in the control of gastric pH at both doses tested, with 100% of the mean pH being greater than 5. Moreover, no statistical difference was noted between the 2 doses tested.[68]

Pantoprazole, another proton pump inhibitor, has been evaluated in foals. Pantoprazole was administered intravenously (1.5 mg/kg) and enterally through a nasogastric tube (1.5 mg/kg, BW) to neonatal foals.[69] Gastric juice pH increased significantly after both IV and intragastric administration. Pantoprazole could be used intravenously in foals with pyloric outflow obstruction, especially because IV administration of ranitidine has shown inconsistent effects on increasing gastric juice pH. However, intragastric administration of pantoprazole resulted in a lower bioavailability compared with oral administration of omeprazole, so a higher dose should be used if administered orally in foals.[69]

Histamine Type 2 Receptor Blockers

Histamine type-2 receptor antagonists suppress HCl secretion by reversibly binding and competitively inhibiting the parietal cell H_2 receptors.[33] Ranitidine and cimetidine are two drugs of this type used in the horse. Ranitidine is available in tablet, syrup, suspension, and injectable forms. However, ranitidine requires thrice-daily oral administration and a longer treatment duration (45–60 days) compared with omeprazole (28 days) to achieve similar healing.[1,5] Ranitidine was less effective than omeprazole in healing gastric ulcers in racehorses.[57] In contrast, cimetidine does not seem to be effective in treatment of EGUS and is not recommended.

Famotidine is a potent histamine type-2 receptor antagonist used frequently in the treatment of EGUS. Famotidine (2.0 mg/kg BW) was approximately 3 times more potent at increasing gastric fluid pH compared with ranitidine (6.6 mg/kg BW).[70] Famotidine (2.0 mg/kg BW) increased mean gastric fluid pH (4.18), which was lower than the pH (5.34) achieved after ranitidine administration (6.6 mg/kg BW). In addition, gastric fluid pH increased to greater than 6 and for longer in each of the 5 horses receiving ranitidine, whereas only 3 of 5 horses receiving famotidine had a similar increase in gastric fluid pH and the duration was shorter.[71] Therefore, based on these data and pharmacologic data generated by Duran[71] (1999), the recommended oral dose of famotidine is 2.8 mg/kg, orally, every 12 hours and 0.3 mg/kg intravenously, every 12 hours. One horse treated with famotidine (6.0 mg/kg BW) at 3 times the therapeutic dose developed colic and was treated medically. Efficacy for treatment of gastric ulcers should be similar to that of ranitidine; however, there are no reported efficacy studies on the use of famotidine in treatment of EGUS.

Coating Agents

Sucralfate and bismuth subsalicylate are two compounds that bind to stomach ulcers and promote healing.[33] Sucralfate is an aluminum complex sulfated polysaccharide [α-D-glucopyranoside, β-D-fructofuranosyl, octakis-(hydrogen sulfate)], in combination with octasulfate and aluminum hydroxide. Its mechanism of action involves adherence to ulcerated mucosa, forming a proteinaceous bandage, and stimulating prostaglandin E_1 synthesis and mucus secretion. Sucralfate also inactivates pepsin and adsorbs bile acids. Recently, sucralfate (12 mg/kg every 8 hours, by mouth) was recommended to treat glandular ulcers.[3,4] The use of ranitidine and sucralfate at recommended doses has proved to be effective in treating phenylbutazone toxicosis in horses. Sucralfate alone may not be beneficial in the treatment of EGUS, but when used in conjunction with acid-suppressive therapy it might be effective in treatment of EGGD and right dorsal colitis (colonic ulcers).

Equine Mucosalfate (sucralfate malate paste, Brand of Orafate, Mueller Medical International LLC, Storrs, CT) was approved in 2013 by the FDA as a device to treat oral ulcerations and erosions, equine stomatitis, and periogingival inflammation.[72] The product is a polymerized, cross-linked 10% sucralfate paste. It also contains xanthan gum, calcium sulfate, purified water, calcium carbonate, methyl parabens, propyl parabens, malate, and sodium saccharin in a strawberry flavor. Water containing calcium chelated malic acid is added to sucralfate powder, thereby converting sucralfate granules into a polymerized paste. Mucosalfate forms a protective layer over the oral mucosa by adhering to the mucosal surface, which allows it to protect against further irritation and relieve pain. The paste may be used in the management of a variety of oral lesions in horses, including those caused by periodontal and gingival inflammation, tooth extractions, traumatic wounds, and wounds associated with oral surgery. The authors have used this product to successfully treat esophageal and colonic ulcers. It might also be effective, when administered with omeprazole, to treat EGGD, although data are lacking.

Bismuth subsalicylate, also a coating agent, inhibits the activation of pepsin and increases mucosal mucus and bicarbonate secretion.[33] One study showed that the addition of bismuth subsalicylate to antacids was effective in increasing gastric juice pH in horses for 2 hours after administration.[73] Bismuth subsalicylate might be converted to sodium subsalicylate in the gastrointestinal tract, which may cause gastric irritation. Salicylate, similar to aspirin, decreases prostaglandin secretion and may further compromise an already damaged mucosa; however, this has not been shown to occur in horses. Bismuth-containing compounds could possibly be effective in the treatment of EGGD, but data are lacking.

Porcine hydrolyzed collagen (HC; Hydro-P Premium, Sonac, A Darling Ingredient Company, Son, The Netherlands) was recently evaluated in stall-confined horses treated with omeprazole and undergoing intermittent feeding. The HC (45 g) was mixed with sweet feed twice daily for 56 days in a 2-period crossover study.[74] Mean gastric juice pH was higher in the HC-treated horses while the horses were on omeprazole treatment. In addition, HC-treated horses resulted in fewer ulcers at each gastroscopic examination and a significant effect on ulcer scores was seen on day 56 of treatment.

Antacids

Antacids (aluminum or magnesium hydroxide) alone are likely ineffective for the treatment of EGUS. They might ameliorate abdominal pain associated with EGUS or prevent gastric ulcer recurrence after successful treatment, but there are no data to support the use of antacids alone in treatment of EGUS.

Calcium carbonate is commonly used as an antacid in people. In in vitro studies, exposure of nonglandular mucosa to calcium carbonate resulted in recovery of tissue exposed to stomach acid. In addition, dietary studies feeding alfalfa hay, which contains a high concentration of calcium carbonate and protein, improved nonglandular gastric ulcer scores and increased gastric juice pH in stall-confined horses and horses that were exercising.[15]

Alfa-Lox Forage (Triple Crown Nutrition, Inc, Wayzata, MN), containing chopped alfalfa hay, mannan oligosaccharides, omega-3 fatty acids, and L-carnitine topdressed on grain (0.91 kg) and fed twice daily was evaluated in horses with ESGD.[75] When data were pooled, Alfa-Lox Forage did not have a treatment by day effect on squamous gastric ulcer scores or gastric juice pH during the study period.[75] Alfa-Lox Forage had no effect on gastric ulcer scores after omeprazole treatment or during feed deprivation compared with untreated controls. However, when forage had lower digestible energy and higher fiber content (during the first period of the study), Alfa-Lox Forage–fed horses had fewer ulcers and their body condition score were higher. Thus, Alfa-Lox Forage might provide gastric support when forage has marginal nutritional content. Note that the quantity of Alfa-Lox Forage fed may not have been adequate to affect gastric ulcer scores or gastric juice pH in horses in this study. Other nutritional benefits, such as higher glucose absorption in the horses after grain feeding, might improve overall nutrition as long as it is not contraindicated for individual horses.[76]

Synthetic Prostaglandins

The synthetic prostaglandin E2 analogue, misoprostol, has been recommended to treat EGUS.[3,4] Misoprostol is a methyl ester analogue of prostaglandin, and it showed a time-dependent increase in the basal gastric pH in horses. The gastric pH increased to greater than 3.5 at 3 to 5 hours after administration, with a concomitant reduction of 80% to 90% in the basal gastric free acid secretion over an 8-hour period.[77] Misoprostol also enhances mucosal protection by stimulating mucus and bicarbonate production, may aid in the treatment and prevention of gastric ulcers induced by NSAIDs, and might be effective in the treatment of EGGD caused by NSAIDs or inflammation.[78] In addition to increasing mucus and bicarbonate secretion, a recent report showed that misoprostol significantly inhibited inflammatory mediators (tumor necrosis factor-a, interleukin-1b, interleukin-6, and superoxide) produced ex vivo from equine leukocytes exposed to lipopolysaccharides.[78] This study showed that misoprostol has anti-inflammatory effects that might be effective in treating EGGD, because some lesions in the glandular mucosa are inflammatory.[79] Misoprostol may cause colic signs in horses, so use should be evaluated closely, and doses can be gradually increased over a few days to ensure that the drug is tolerated. Misoprostol should not be used in pregnant mares.

Somatostatin Analogue

A somatostatin analogue, octreotide acetate, has also been evaluated in horses. Octreotide (0.5–5 µg/kg) increased the gastric pH to greater than 7 for approximately 5 hours, with no adverse effects noted. The benefit of using a somatostatin analogue is the prevention of hypergastrinemia associated with long-term use of acid-suppressive drugs.[33] Hypergastrinemia has a positive trophic effect on gastric cells and may result in proliferation. Because somatostatin inhibits gastrin secretion, this hypertrophy is avoided; however, no cases of gastric hypertrophy have been reported in horses after long-term use of acid-suppressive drug therapy.

Motility Stimulants

Bethanechol is a synthetic muscarinic cholinergic agent that is not degraded by acetylcholinesterases. Bethanechol (0.25 mg/kg, IV) and erythromycin lactobionate (0.1 and 1 mg/kg, IV) increased solid-phase gastric emptying in horses.[80] No significant adverse effects were observed in healthy horses; however, other forms of erythromycin can cause fatal colitis in adult horses at antimicrobial doses.[33] The only side effect of bethanechol administration was increased salivation. Investigators have recommended a dose of 0.025 to 0.03 mg/kg subcutaneously every 3 to 4 hours, followed by oral maintenance therapy at 0.3 to 0.45 mg/kg 3 to 4 times daily. Prokinetics should not be used in horses with gastrointestinal obstructions, because gastroduodenal reflux may worsen after treatment in patients with proximal small intestinal obstructions.[33]

Antibiotics and Probiotics

Recently, trimethoprim-sulfadimidine (30 mg/kg for a 500-kg horse, by mouth) was evaluated in the healing of glandular gastric ulcers in a randomized, blinded, clinical trial.[55] Because H pylori is not likely to cause gastric ulcers in horses, the use of antibiotics should be limited to treatment of chronic nonhealing ulcers. A combination of omeprazole (4 mg/kg, every 24 hours), metronidazole (15 mg/kg, every 6 hours), and/or trimethoprim/sulfadiazine (25 mg/kg every 12 hours), with or without bismuth subsalicylate (3.8 mg/kg every 6 hours), could be used in these cases. An initial 14-day treatment period could be instituted, which should be followed by gastroscopy. Omeprazole therapy could be continued for the full 28 days if needed. Once the squamous mucosa is ulcerated, resident stomach bacteria might colonize the ulcer bed and delay healing. In one study, gram-positive cocci were observed in small ulcers in the squamous mucosa.[81] In addition, in the same study, acid-tolerant bacteria (*Lactobacillus* spp) were found adhered to the normal mucosa and could regulate microflora and protect the intact gastric mucosa from bacterial colonization by invasive species. There was a large population of these and other bacteria isolated from the gastric contents of horses fed various diets, and some of these bacteria could be synergistic and protective.[12,82,83] Antibiotic treatment may be indicated in horses with chronic nonresponsive gastric ulcers, but, more importantly, probiotic preparations containing *Lactobacillus* may be helpful to prevent colonization of the squamous mucosa and ulcers with more pathogenic bacteria; such probiotics may be an adjunct to pharmacologic treatment.[33] In contrast, the randomized controlled trial of trimethoprim-sulfadimidine showed that administering these antibiotics did not facilitate healing of glandular ulcers; therefore, antibiotic treatment might not be indicated for EGGD, although further research is required.[55]

Treatment and Prevention Recommendations

Table 4 shows the summary of treatment recommendations for ESGD.[3] **Table 5** shows the summary of treatment recommendations for EGGD. Two forms of omeprazole have been used for treatment of EGUS and approved by the FDA (enteric-coated and buffered formulations). Compounded omeprazole, formulated from bulk powders, has been used as a substitute for the FDA-approved and registered formulations. However, compounded pharmaceutical agents are not regulated and have varied widely in their efficacy in the treatment of gastric ulcers.[84] In addition, in the United States, use of compounded medications from bulk powders is currently illegal, according to the FDA, especially when there is an approved drug available.

For the treatment and prevention of EGUS in foals, clinicians should follow similar principles as for adult horses. However, prophylactic treatment of hospitalized neonatal foals could increase the risk of diarrhea.[85] A multicenter retrospective study including 1710 foals ($\leq$10 days of age) showed that the use of antiulcer medications, including sucralfate, increased the odds of in-hospital diarrhea by 2.0, relative to the use of no antiulcer medications. However, there was no significant association of antiulcer medication administration with *Clostridium difficile*–associated diarrhea. In addition, results suggested that the prevalence of gastric ulceration was not decreased

Table 4	
Treatment recommendations for equine squamous gastric disease	
Primary Recommendation	**Secondary Recommendation**
Omeprazole	Omeprazole
Buffered formulations: 4 mg/kg PO, q 24 h; or	Buffered formulation: 2 mg/kg PO q 24 h
Enteric coated granule formulations: 1 mg/kg	Or
PO q 24 h; or	Ranitidine: 6.6 mg/kg PO q 8 h
Plain formulations: 4 mg/kg PO q 24 h	
Treatment duration 3 wk	
Control gastroscopy before the discontinuation of treatment	

Table 5
Treatment recommendation for equine glandular gastric disease

Primary Recommendation	Secondary Recommendation
Omeprazole Buffered formulations: 4 mg/kg PO q 24 h; or Enteric coated granule formulations: 1 mg/ kg PO q 24 h; or Plain formulations: 4 mg/kg PO q 24 h	Omeprazole Buffered formulations: 2 mg/kg PO q 24 h
Plus	Plus
Sucralfate 12 mg/kg PO q 12 h	Sucralfate: 12 mg/kg PO q 12 h Or Specific nutraceutical with published efficacy

Treatment duration: 4 wk (minimum of 8 wk before additional adjunctives are considered)
Control gastroscopy before the discontinuation of therapy

with the use of antiulcer drugs; however, because this was a retrospective study, the findings warrant study with prospective, randomized controlled trials. The use of anti-ulcer medications in hospitalized neonatal foals should be carefully evaluated on an individual basis, because gastric ulcers in neonatal foals may not be caused by HCl, although this requires additional study.

SUPPLEMENTS AND FEED ADDITIVES

Recently, there has been interest in the use of herbs, botanic products (nutraceuticals), oils, and trace minerals to maintain stomach health in horses with EGUS. The reasons for evaluation of these feed supplements include:

- The high expense of pharmacologic agents
- Daily handling and oral administration of paste or tablet formulations
- Pharmaceutical agents require a prescription
- Gastric ulcer recurrence is common once treatment is discontinued
- Long-term treatment with omeprazole results in high gastric juice pH and might negatively affect digestion in the stomach or small intestine
- Use of medications in performance and show horses is now forbidden or under tight control

Table 6 shows a summary of natural products that have recently been studied for the treatment of equine gastric ulcers.

Sea Buckthorn Berries and Pulp

There is increasing interest in the use of herbs and berries to maintain stomach health. Berries and pulp from the sea buckthorn plant (*Hippophae rhamnoides*) have been used successfully to treat gastric and duodenal ulcers in humans and rats. These plants have high concentrations of vitamins, trace minerals, amino acids, antioxidants, and other bioactive substances. Recent studies of oral supplements containing sea buckthorn berries or the berries and other agents such as probiotics suggest that they have a protective and possibly therapeutic effect.[86] This studied preparation of sea buckthorn berries prevented glandular ulcers from increasing in severity compared with control horses; however, nonglandular gastric ulcer scores were not affected.[79]

Table 6
Summary of natural products that have recently been studied for the treatment of equine gastric (glandular and/or nonglandular) ulcer syndrome

Name of Product	Study, Date of Research
Sea buckthorn (*Hippophae rhamnoides*)	Huff et al,[86] 2009
Egusin	Woodward et al,[44] 2014
Apolectol, *Saccharomyces cerevisiae*, magnesium hydroxide	Sykes et al,[89] 2014
Pectin-lecithin	Sanz et al,[88] 2014
SmartGut Ultra	Andrews et al,[90] 2015
GastroTech	Conover et al,[91] 2015
Alfa-Lox Forage	Andrews et al,[75] 2016; Garza et al,[76] 2016
HC	Keowen et al,[74] 2016

Pectin and Lecithin

Pectin is found in numerous fruits, tubers, and stem plants and is rendered into a gel when exposed to an acidic environment. Pectin may bind to bile acids and prevent them from having deleterious effects on the gastric mucosa. Lecithin is a phospholipid that reduces surface tension at the air-water interface. Supplements containing pectin and lecithin alone and in combination with antacids improved gastric ulcer scores in horses after 5 weeks of treatment.[87] However, in another study, a pectin-lecithin complex–containing supplement did not improve nonglandular ulcer scores in treated mares compared with control horses.[88] In a more recent study, horses treated with a supplement containing pectin and lecithin and antacids (Egusin, Centaur Animal Health, Olathe, KS) showed lower nonglandular ulcer scores in stall-confined horses after feed stress compared with control horses after 35 days of feeding.[44] In addition, a supplement containing Apolectol, live yeast (*Saccharomyces cerevisiae* [CNM I-1077]) and magnesium hydroxide showed improvement in glandular ulcers in Australian Thoroughbred racehorses, but did not improve squamous ulcer scores.[89]

Multiple-Component Supplements

SmartGut Ultra (SmartPak Equine, Plymouth, MA) pellets, a commercially available supplement, contain a proprietary blend of sea buckthorn, glutamine, aloe vera, pectin, and lecithin, as well as other herbs, amino acids, soluble fibers and probiotics, polysaccharides, amino acids, natural antioxidants, and probiotics. In a study, Smart-Gut Ultra supplement added to the grain of stall-confined horses prevented the worsening of gastric ulcer numbers, 2 weeks after omeprazole treatment, without altering the gastric juice pH.[90] SmartGut Ultra is not a pharmaceutical agent and is not intended to be used to treat gastric ulcers in horses; however, it can be used to improve overall stomach health after successful treatment of nonglandular gastric ulcers.

Conover and colleagues[91] (2015) reported improvement in gastric ulcer scores using a supplement containing a proprietary blend of natural ingredients (GastroTech, Southern States Feeds, Richmond, VA) for 44 days (14 days of adaptation and 30 days of treatment) in the feed of horses. The supplement was fed to horses at 2 different sites and differences in management factors at the 2 sites may have affected the results of the study. More horses at location A had access to pasture turnout compared with location B. Stall confinement has been shown to increase the incidence of lesions, whereas pasture turnout has been associated with fewer ulcers, and therefore these management practices may have confounded the results.

Dietary Oils

Oils have been added to horse diets for several years and they might have benefits in maintaining gastric health. Dietary oils and fats delay gastric emptying time in humans. However, in contrast, gastric emptying rates are similar in horses fed high-carbohydrate diets, compared with those fed diets high in fat. Horses fed corn oil (0.3–0.5 mL/kg BW/d; 150–250 mL/d for a 500-kg horse) showed decreased gastric acid output and increased prostaglandin E_2 production, which might be beneficial for the treatment and prevention of EGGD.[92] Gastric ulcer scores were not provided in that study, but corn oil might contribute to glandular stomach health. In contrast, in another study in which corn oil, refined rice bran oil, and crude rice bran oil (240 mL, once daily, mixed in grain) were fed to horses there was no significant difference in nonglandular gastric ulcer scores between treatment groups.[93] There were very few glandular ulcers in that study, so the effect on such ulcers could not be evaluated. The balance between omega-3 and omega-6 fatty acids may be important in inflammatory diseases of the gastrointestinal tract, but the antiinflammatory properties, influence on mucosal circulation, cytoprotective effects, and effects on gastric ulcer scores remain unknown. Furthermore, nutritional changes, such as a reduction of starch and an increase of digestible fiber, are key factors in preventing EGUS.

Chelated Minerals (Zinc, Manganese, and so Forth)

In addition to botanicals and coating agents, chelated minerals containing zinc have been evaluated in horses with squamous ulcers. Zinc has been recognized as an important trace mineral for healing epithelial tissue in multiple species, and is essential for the immune system, including providing antioxidant protection against free radicals.[94,95] A recent study feeding a mineral/vitamin supplement containing complexed mineral sources (ZINPRO [zinc methionine], CuPLEX [copper lysine], MANPRO [manganese methionine], and COPRO [cobalt glucoheptonate]) resulted in lower squamous ulcer scores in horses after omeprazole treatment and during an alternating feed-deprivation model compared with the control supplement containing inorganic trace minerals.[96] This difference was observed in period 2, when a good nutritional plane was provided. Although the mechanism is yet to be clearly defined, other studies have shown a gastroprotective action of zinc through its involvement with gastric mucosa integrity.[97–100] Zinc evaluated in a cell culture model seems to promote signaling for epithelial repair. In work with rat models, zinc compounds have been shown to be effective for healing ulcerated glandular gastric mucosa.[97]

REFERENCES

1. Andrews FM, Bernard W, Byars D, et al. Recommendation for the diagnosis and treatment of equine gastric ulcer syndrome (EGUS). Equine Vet Educ 1999;11: 262–72.
2. Sykes BW, Jokisalo JM. Rethinking equine gastric ulcer syndrome: part 1–terminology, clinical signs and diagnosis. Equine Vet Educ 2014;26(10):543–7.
3. Sykes BW, Hewetson M, Hepburn RJ, et al. European College of Equine Internal Medicine Consensus Statement- equine gastric ulcer syndrome in adult horse. J Vet Intern Med 2015;29:1288–99.
4. Sykes B, Jokisalo JM. Rethinking equine gastric ulcer syndrome: part 3–equine glandular gastric ulcer syndrome (EGGUS). Equine Vet Educ 2015;27(7):372–5.

5. Sykes BW, Jokisalo JM. Rethinking equine gastric ulcer syndrome: part 2– equine squamous gastric ulcer syndrome (ESGUS). Equine Vet Educ 2015; 27(5):264–8.

6. Sandin A, Skidell J, Haggstrom J, et al. Post-mortem findings of gastric ulcers in Swedish horses up to 1 year of age: a retrospective study 1924–1996. Acta Vet Scand 1999;40:109.

7. Merritt AM. Appeal for proper usage of the term "EGUS": equine gastric ulcer syndrome. Equine Vet J 2009;41:616.

8. Andrews FM, Sifferman RL, Bernard W, et al. Efficacy of omeprazole paste in the treatment and prevention of gastric ulcers in horses. Equine Vet J Suppl 1999; 29:81–6.

9. Malfertheiner P, Chan FFKL, McColl KEL, et al. Peptic-ulcer disease. Lancet 2009;374:1449–61.

10. Ethell M, Hodgson DR, Hills BA. Evidence of surfactant contributing to the gastric mucosa barrier of the horse. Equine Vet J 2000;32:470–4.

11. Bullimore SR, Corfield AP, Hicks SJ, et al. Surface mucus in the non-glandular region of the equine stomach. Res Vet Sci 2001;70:149–55.

12. Al Jassim RAM, Andrews FM. The bacterial community of the horse gastrointestinal tract and its relation to fermentative acidosis, laminitis, colic, and stomach ulcers. Vet Clin N Am Equine 2009;25:199–215.

13. Nadeau JA, Andrews FM, Patton CS, et al. Effects of hydrochloric, acetic, butyric, and propionic acids, on pathogenesis of ulcers in the non-glandular portion of the stomach of horses. Am J Vet Res 2003;64(4):404–12.

14. Nadeau JA, Andrews FM, Patton CS, et al. Effects of hydrochloric, valeric, and other volatile fatty acids on pathogenesis of ulcers in the nonglandular portion of the stomach of horses. Am J Vet Res 2003;64:413–7.

15. Andrews FM, Buchanan BR, Smith SH, et al. In vitro effects of hydrochloric acid and various concentrations of acetic, propionic, butyric, or valeric acids on bioelectric properties of equine gastric squamous mucosa. Am J Vet Res 2006;67(11):1873–82.

16. Andrews FM, Buchanan BR, Elliott SB, et al. In vitro effects of hydrochloric acid and lactic acid on bioelectric properties of equine gastric squamous mucosa. Equine Vet J 2008;40:301–5.

17. Sandin A. Studies of gastrin and gastrin secretion in the horse [Doctoral thesis]. Uppsala(Sweden): Swedish University of Agricultural Sciences; 1999. p. 69.

18. Argenzio RA, Eisemann J. Mechanisms of acid injury in porcine gastroesophageal mucosa. Am J Vet Res 1996;57:564–73.

19. Malmkvist J, Poulsen JM, Luthersson N, et al. Behavior and stress responses in horses with gastric ulceration. Appl Anim Behav Sci 2012;142:160–7.

20. Moyaret H, Pasmans F, Decostere A, et al. *Helicobacter equorum*: prevalence and significance for horses and humans. FEMS Immunol Med Microbiol 2009; 57:14–6.

21. Bezdekova B, Futas J. *Helicobacter* species and gastric ulceration in horses: a clinical study. Vet Med-CZECH 2009;54(12):577–82.

22. Orsini JA, Hackett ES, Grenager N. The effect of exercise on equine gastric ulcer syndrome in the thoroughbred and standardbred athlete. J Equine Vet Sci 2009;29(3):167–71.

23. Bertone JJ. Prevalence of gastric ulcers in elite heavy use western performance horses. In: Proceedings 48th Annual AAEP Convention, vol. 48. Orlando (FL), 2002. p. 256–9.

24. Vatistas NJ, Synder JR, Carlson GP, et al. Epidemiology study of gastric ulceration in the Thoroughbred race horse; 202 cases. In: Proceeding Ann. Conv. Amer. Assoc. Equine Pract. Vancouver (Canada), 1994. p. 125–6.

25. Habershon-Butcher JL, Hallowell GD, Bowen IM, et al. Prevalence and risk factors for ulceration of the gastric glandular mucosa in thoroughbred racehorses in training in the UK and Australia [abstract]. J Vet Intern Med 2012;26:731.

26. Ward S, Sykes BW, Brown H, et al. A comparison of the prevalence of gastric ulceration in feral and domesticated horses in the UK. Equine Vet Educ 2015; 57(12):655–7.

27. Rabuffo TS, Hackett ES, Grenagar N, et al. Prevalence of gastric ulceration in horse with colic. J Equine Vet Sci 2009;29(6):540–6.

28. Wilson JH. Gastric and duodenal ulcers in foals: a retrospective study. In: Proceedings of the 2nd Equine Colic Res Symp, vol. 2. 1986. p. 126–8.

29. Rabuffo TS, Orsini JA, Sullivan E, et al. Association between age or sex and prevalence of gastric ulceration in Standard bred racehorses in training. Am J Vet Med 2002;221:1156–9.

30. Reese R, Andrews FM. Nutrition and dietary management of equine gastric ulcer syndrome. Vet Clin Equine 2009;25:79–92.

31. Bell RJW, Kingston JK, Mogg TD, et al. The prevalence of gastric ulceration in racehorses in New Zealand. N Z Vet J 2007;55:13–8.

32. Le Jeune SS, Nieto JE, Dechant JE, et al. Prevalence of gastric ulcers in thoroughbred broodmares in pasture: a preliminary report,. Vet J 2009;181:251–5.

33. Buchanan BR, Andrews FM. Treatment and prevention of equine gastric ulcer syndrome. Vet Clin Equine 2003;19:575–97.

34. Wickens C, McCall CA, Bursian S, et al. Assessment of gastric ulceration and gastrin response in horses with history of crib-biting. J Equine Vet Sci 2013; 33:739–45.

35. Vatistas NJ, Snyder JR, Carlson G, et al. Cross-sectional study of gastric ulcers of the squamous mucosa in thoroughbred racehorses. Equine Vet J 1999; 29(Suppl):40–4.

36. Franklin SH, Brazil TJ, Allen KJ. Poor performance associated with equine gastric ulceration syndrome in four thoroughbred racehorses. Equine Vet Educ 2008;20:119–24.

37. Nieto JE, Synder JR, Vatistas NJ, et al. Effect of gastric ulceration on physiologic responses to exercise in horses. Am J Vet Res 2009;70:787–95.

38. Murray MJ, Grodinsky CA, Anderson CW, et al. Gastric ulcers in horses: a comparison of endoscopic findings in horses with and without clinical signs. Equine Vet J 1989;(Suppl 7):68–72.

39. Hewetson M, Sykes BW, Hallowell G, et al. Diagnostic accuracy of blood sucrose as a screening test for diagnosis of gastric ulceration in adult horses. Equine Vet J 2015;47(Suppl 48):2–28.

40. Pellegrini FL. Results of a large-scale necroscopic study of equine colonic ulcers. J Equine Vet Sci 2005;25(3):113–7.

41. Andrews FM, Camacho-Luna P, Loftin PG, et al. Effect of a pelleted supplement fed during and after omeprazole treatment on non-glandular gastric ulcer scores and gastric juice pH in horses. Equine Vet Educ 2015;28(4):196–202.

42. Barakat C. What's your horse's ulcer risk. Equus 2016;454:68–77.

43. Luthersson N, Hou Nielsen K, Harris P, et al. Risk factors associated with equine gastric ulceration syndrome in 201 horses in Denmark. Equine Vet J 2009;41: 625–30.

44. Woodward MC, Huff NK, Garza F Jr, et al. Effect of pectin, lecithin, and antacid feed supplements (Egusin) on gastric ulcer scores, gastric fluid pH and blood gas values in horses. BMC Vet Res 2014;10(Suppl 1):54–62.
45. Nadeau JA, Andrews FM, Mathew AG, et al. Evaluation of diet as a cause of gastric ulcers in horses. Am J Vet Res 2000;61(7):784–90.
46. Lybbert T, Gibbs P, Cohen N, et al. Feeding alfalfa hay to exercising horses reduces the severity of gastric squamous mucosal ulceration. In: Proceedings Am Assoc Equine Pract, vol. 53. 2007. p. 525–6.
47. Harris PA, Coenen M, Geor RJ. Controversial areas in equine nutrition and feeding management: the editors' views. In: Geor RJ, Harris PA, Coenen M, editors. Equine applied and clinical nutrition: health, welfare and performance. Waltham (MA): Elsevier Health Sciences; 2013. p. 455–68.
48. Bruynsteen L, Janssens GPJ, Harris PA, et al. Changes in oxidative stress in response to different levels of energy restriction in obese ponies. Br J Nutr 2014;112:1402–11.
49. Ellis AD, Redgate S, Zinchenko S, et al. The effect of presenting forage in multilayered hay nets and at multiple sites on night time budgets of stabled horses. Appl Anim Behav Sci 2015;165:88–94.
50. Metayer N, Lhote M, Bahr A, et al. Meal size and starch content affect gastric emptying in horses. Equine Vet J 2004;36:436–40.
51. Scott DR, Marcus EA, Shirazi-Beechey SSP. Evidence of Helicobacter infection in the horse. In: Proceedings, American Society of Microbiologists. Washington, DC, June 20–24, 2001. p. 35–37.
52. Contreras M, Morales A, Garcıa-Amado MA, et al. Detection of *Helicobacter*-like DNA in the gastric mucosa of thoroughbred horses. Lett Appl Microbiol 2007; 45:553–7.
53. Rafat Al Jassim, McGowan T, Andrews FM, et al. Role of bacteria and lactic acid in the pathogenesis of gastric ulceration. In: Rural industries research and development corporation final report. Brisbane (Queensland): 2008. p. 1–26.
54. Elliott SN, Buret A, McKnight W, et al. Bacteria rapid colonize and modulate healing of gastric ulcer in rats. Am J Phys 1998;275:425–32.
55. Sykes BW, Sykes MK, Hallowell GD. Administration of trimethoprim-sulphadimidine does not improve healing of glandular gastric ulceration in horses receiving omeprazole: a randomized, blinded, clinical study. BMC Vet Res 2014;10:180.
56. Sykes BW, Sykes KM, Hallowell GD. A comparison between pre-and post-exercise administration of omeprazole in the treatment of equine gastric ulcer syndrome: a blinded, randomized, clinical trial,. Equine Vet J 2014;46:422–6.
57. Lester GD, Robertson I, Secombe C. Risk factor for gastric ulceration in thoroughbred racehorses, Rural industries research and development corporation, Australian Government, publication number. 2008. 08/061.
58. Walt RP, Gomes WD, Wood EC, et al. Effect of daily oral omeprazole on 24 hour intragastric acidity. Br Med J (Clin Res Ed) 1983;287:12–20.
59. Daurio CP, Holste JE, Andrews FM, et al. Effect of omeprazole paste on gastric acid secretion in horses. Equine Vet J Suppl 1999;29:59.
60. Sykes BW, Sykes KM, Hallowell GD. A comparison of three doses of omeprazole in the treatment of equine gastric ulcer syndrome: A blinded, randomized, dose-response clinical trial,. Equine Vet J 2015;47:285–90.
61. Sykes BW, Sykes KM, Hallowell GD. A comparison of two doses of omeprazole in the treatment of equine gastric ulcer syndrome: a blinded, randomized, clinical trial. Equine Vet J 2014;46:416–21.

62. Andrews FM, Doherty TJ, Blackford JT, et al. Effect of orally administered enteric-coated omeprazole on gastric acid secretion in horses. Am J Vet Res 1999;60(8):929–31.
63. Tielemans Y, Hakason R, Sundler F, et al. Proliferation of enterochromaffin like cells in omeprazole-treated hypergastrinemic rats. Gastroenterology 1989;96:723–9.
64. Plue RE, Wall HG, Daurio C, et al. Safety of omeprazole paste in foals and mature horses. Equine Vet J 1999;31(Suppl 29):63–6.
65. Andrews FM, Frank N, Sommardahl CS, et al. Effects of intravenously administrated omeprazole on gastric juice pH and gastric ulcer scores in adult horses. J Vet Intern Med 2006;20:1202–6.
66. Scott LJ, Mallarkey G, Sharpe M. Esomeprazole. A review of its use in the management of acid-related disorders. Drugs 2002;62:1503–38.
67. Videla R, Sommardahl CS, Elliott SB, et al. Effects of intravenously administration esomeprazole sodium on gastric juice pH in adult female horses. J Vet Intern Med 2011;25:558–62.
68. Pereira MC, Levy FL, Valadão CAA, et al. Preliminary study of the gastric acidity in thoroughbred horses at rest after enteral administration of esomeprazole magnesium (Nexium). J Equine Vet Sci 2009;29:791–4.
69. Ryan CA, Sanchez LC, Giguere S, et al. Pharmacokinetics and pharmacodynamics of pantoprazole in clinically normal neonatal foals. Equine Vet J 2005;4:336–41.
70. Murray MJ. Drugs acting on the gastrointestinal system. In: Bertone J, Horspool LJI, editors. Equine pharmacology. London: WB Saunders; 2004. p. 85–120.
71. Duran SH. Famotidine. Compend Continuing Education Practicing Veterinarian 1999;21:424–5.
72. Equine Mucosalfate™ Prescribing information [package insert]. 2013.
73. Clark CK, Merritt AM, Burrow JA, et al. Effect of aluminum hydroxide/magnesium hydroxide antacid and bismuth subsalicylate on gastric pH in horses. J Am Vet Med Assoc 1996;208:1687–91.
74. Keowen ML, Camacho-Luna P, Micheau L, et al. Effects of collagen hydrolysates on equine gastric ulcer scores and gastric juice pH. J Vet Intern Med 2016;68:E44. Early View.
75. Andrews F, Camacho-Luna P, Bailey K, et al. Effects of a supplement (Alfa-Lox Forage) on equine gastric ulcer scores and gastric juice pH. J Vet Intern Med 2016;99:E24. Early View.
76. Garza F Jr, Camacho-Luna P, Bailey K, et al. Effects of Alfa-Lox Forage on blood glucose and insulin activity after grain feeding in horses. J Vet Intern Med 2016;108:E52. Early View.
77. Sangiah S, MacAllister CC, Amouzadeh HR. Effects of misoprostol and omeprazole on basal gastric pH and free acid content in horses. Res Vet Sci 1989;47(3):350–4.
78. Medlin E, Jones S. Investigation of misoprostol as a novel anti-inflammatory in equine leukocytes. ACVIM Forum, June 7-10, 2016, Denver, CO [abstract]. J Vet Intern Med 2016;30:1520.
79. Murray MJ. Pathophysiology of peptic disorders in foals and horses: a review. Equine Vet J Suppl 1999;29:14–8.
80. Ringger NC, Lester GD, Neuwirth L, et al. Effect of bethanechol or erythromycin on gastric emptying in horses. Am J Vet Res 1996;57(12):1771–5.

81. Yuki N, Shimazaki T, Kushiro A, et al. Colonization of the stratified squamous epithelium of the nonsecreting area of horse stomach by lactobacilli. Appl Environ Microbiol 2000;66:5030–4.

82. Al Jassim RAM, Scott PT, Krause D, et al. Cellulolytic and lactic acid bacteria in the gastro–intestinal tract of the horse. Recent Adv Anim Nutrit Aust 2005;15: 155–63.

83. Al Jassim RAM, Scott PT, Trebbin AL, et al. The genetic diversity of lactic acid producing bacteria in the equine gastrointestinal tract. FEMS Microbiol Lett 2005;248:75–81.

84. Merritt AM, Sanchez LC, Burrow JA, et al. Effect of GastroGard and three compounded oral omeprazole preparations on 24 h intragastric pH in gastrically cannulated mature horses. Equine Vet J 2003;35:691–5.

85. Furr M, Cohen ND, Axon JE, et al. Treatment with histamine-type 2 receptor antagonists and omeprazole increase the risk of diarrhoea in neonatal foals treated in intensive care units. Equine Vet J 2012;44(Suppl 41):80–6.

86. Huff NK, Auer AD, Garza F Jr, et al. Effect of sea buckthorn berries and pulp in a liquid emulsion on gastric ulcers scores and gastric juice pH in horses. J Vet Intern Med 2012;26:1186–91.

87. Venner M, Lauffs S, Deegen E. Treatment of gastric lesions in horses with pectin-lecithin complex. Equine Vet J Suppl 1999;(Suppl 31):91–6.

88. Sanz MG, Viljoen A, Saulez MN, et al. Efficacy of pectin- lecithin complex for treatment and prevention of gastric ulcers in horses. Vet Rec 2014;175:6.

89. Sykes BW, Sykes KM, Hallowell GD. Efficacy of a combination of Apolectol, live yeast (*Saccharomyces cerevisiae* [CNCM I-1077]), and magnesium hydroxide in the management of equine gastric ulcer syndrome in thoroughbred racehorse: a blinded, randomized, placebo-controlled clinical trial. J Equine Vet Sci 2014;34:1274–8.

90. Andrews FM, Camacho-Luna P, Loftin PM, et al. Effect of a commercial supplement on nonglandular gastric ulcer scores and pH. Equine Vet Educ 2015;28(4): 196–202.

91. Conover AL, Shultz AM, Wagner AL. Effects of GastroTech on equine gastric ulcer syndrome (EGUS). J Equine Vet Sci 2015;35:418–36.

92. Cargile JL, Burrow JA, Kim I, et al. Effect of dietary corn oil supplementation on equine gastric fluid acid, sodium, and prostaglandin E2 content before and during pentagastrin infusion. J Vet Intern Med 2004;18:545–9.

93. Frank N, Andrews FM, Elliott SB, et al. Effects of dietary oils on the development of gastric ulcers in mares. Am J Vet Res 2005;66:2006–11.

94. Sturniolo GC, Di Leo V, Barollo M, et al. The many functions of zinc in the inflammatory conditions of the gastrointestinal tract. J Trace Elem Exp Med 2000;13: 33–9.

95. McDowell LR. Zinc, physiological functions. In: Minerals in animal and human nutrition. 2nd edition. Amsterdam (The Netherlands): Elsevier Science BV; 2003. p. 362–7.

96. Loftin P, Woodward M, Bidot W, et al. Evaluating replacement of supplemental inorganic minerals with Zinpro performance minerals on prevention of gastric ulcers in horses. J Vet Intern Med 2012;26:737–8.

97. Watanabe T, Arakawa T, Fukuda T, et al. Zinc deficiency delays gastric ulcer healing in rats. Dig Dis Sci 1995;40:1340–4.

98. Sharma J, Singla AK, Dhawan S. Zinc-naproxen complex: synthesis, physico-chemical and biological evaluation. Int J Pharm 2003;260:217–27.

99. Opoka W, Adamek D, Plonka M, et al. Importance of luminal and mucosal zinc in the mechanism of experimental gastric ulcer healing. J Physiol Pharmacol 2010; 61:581–91.

100. Sharir H, Zinger A, Nevo A, et al. Zinc released from injured cells is acting via the Zn2+ sensing receptor, ZnR, to trigger signaling leading to epithelial repair. J Biol Chem 2010;285:26097–105.

Equine Cardiovascular Therapeutics

 CrossMark

Meg M. Sleeper, VMD

KEYWORDS

- Congestive heart failure • Valve disease • Dysrhythmia • Atrial fibrillation
- Antiarrhythmic

KEY POINTS

- The most common acquired heart disease in horses include acquired valve disease (mitral and aortic are most common) and atrial fibrillation.
- Appropriate medical management and prognosis requires a complete evaluation, including electrocardiogram (ECG), echocardiogram, and in some cases Holter or exercising ECG.
- In clinical animals, therapy can be initiated before further diagnostics.

 Video content accompanies this article at http://www.vetequine.theclinics.com.

INTRODUCTION

Signs associated with primary heart disease are due to either inadequate cardiac output (signs include exercise intolerance, weakness, and fainting) or elevated cardiac filling pressure (venous engorgement, jugular pulsations [Video 1]). Ultimately signs of congestive heart failure (CHF) with fluid retention may develop (subcutaneous edema [**Fig. 1**], pulmonary edema). Generally, because of sympathetic activation, most horses with heart failure have an increased resting heart rate. Although long-term prognosis for equine heart failure is poor unless the primary defect can be corrected, heart disease in horses is being treated more commonly than previously. Many therapies are empirical and based on data from other species; however, more information is becoming available regarding their efficacy in the horse. Nevertheless, it is important to remember that most agents used for therapy for heart disease are not specifically approved for use in horses. Those studies that are available have often evaluated only a small number of horses, making it impossible to predict idiosyncratic adverse effects. Moreover, many studies are conducted on healthy horses making extrapolation

Cardiology, Department of Small Animal Clinical Sciences, College of Veterinary Medicine, University of Florida, 2015 Southwest 16th Avenue, PO Box 100126, Gainesville, FL 32610-0126, USA
E-mail address: margaretmsleeper@ufl.edu

Vet Clin Equine 33 (2017) 163–179
http://dx.doi.org/10.1016/j.cveq.2016.11.005
0749-0739/17/© 2016 Elsevier Inc. All rights reserved.

vetequine.theclinics.com

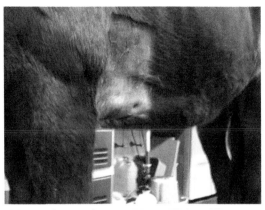

Fig. 1. A horse with ventral subcutaneous edema caused by CHF. Note the impression in the plaque of edema caused by a finger indentation. This phenomenon has led to the term *pitting edema*. Subcutaneous edema in the horse often accumulates ventrally, as in this case, in the lower limbs and around the sheath in males.

to horses with heart disease tenuous at best. This article focuses on the current recommendations for the treatment of acute and chronic CHF and the acute and chronic medical management of cardiac arrhythmias in horses.

CONGESTIVE HEART FAILURE
Patient Overview

CHF in horses occurs most commonly secondary to acquired valve disease. However, heart failure in horses can occur because of congenital heart disease, such as a large ventricular septal defect, or any acquired disorder, such as myocardial diseases.[1] See **Table 1** for a list of clinical signs consistent with CHF in the horse. Regardless of the underlying cause of CHF, the goals of treatment are to improve cardiac output, tissue perfusion, and oxygenation and to promote diuresis of excessive body fluid thereby improving edema. If available, referral to a specialist is optimal; however, early initiation of medical management is often critical for successful case outcomes and referral is not always an option. Cardiac output is determined by preload, afterload, myocardial contractility (inotropy), and heart rate.

Table 1		
Common clinical signs of heart disease in the horse		
Heart Disease	**Cardiac Arrhythmia**	**CHF**
• Heart murmur	• Heart arrhythmia	• Tachycardia
• Heart arrhythmia	• Exercise intolerance	• Exercise intolerance
• Asymptomatic	• Weakness	• Weakness
• Weight loss	• Collapse	• Systemic venous congestion
• Poor performance	• Syncope	• Jugular pulsations
• Exercise intolerance	• CHF	• Subcutaneous edema (pitting edema)
• Abnormal pulses		• Cough
• Weakness		• Tachypnea
• CHF		
• Death		

Pharmacologic Treatment Options of Congestive Heart Failure

In other species, treatment is often divided into acute versus chronic treatment strategies. Although this division remains useful to consider in the horse, whereby some drugs are rapidly available as injectable agents and others are oral and more suited to chronic use, horses in CHF are not treated with oxygen therapy as often as are dogs and cats, except at referral centers and hospitals. Therefore, this discussion focuses on the mechanism of action of medications rather than the acute versus chronic phase of treatment.

Preload Reducers

Preload reduction is one of the mainstays in the treatment of heart failure. Furosemide is the most commonly used medication to achieve this goal. Furosemide acts in the ascending loop of Henle, leading to increased excretion of water and electrolytes, including sodium, chloride, potassium, calcium, magnesium, phosphate, bicarbonate, as well as acid. Furosemide (**Table 2**) should be administered intravenously (IV) or intramuscularly (IM) at a dose of 1 to 2 mg/kg every 6 to 12 hours to control volume overload (ie, pulmonary edema, subcutaneous edema, and so forth) in the acute stages. Subsequent dosing for chronic therapy can be titrated to the patient's individual response and optimally administered less frequently and at lower doses to prevent chronic electrolyte depletion. IV-administered furosemide (1 mg/kg) results in a peak

Table 2	
Common drugs to treat cardiovascular disease in the horse	
Common Drugs to Treat Equine Arrhythmias	
Drug	**Dose**
Quinidine	Oral: 22 mg/kg quinidine sulfate by NGT every 2 h, up to total dose of 88 mg/kg (see text) IV: quinidine gluconate in 1.1–2.2 mg/kg q 10 min up to total dose of 9–11 mg/kg
Procainamide	Oral: 25–35 mg/kg every 8 h IV: 1 mg/kg/min up to a total dose of 20 mg/kg has been given
Magnesium	IV: 1 g/min/450 kg horse (2.2 mg/kg/min) to effect up to a maximum of 25 g/450 kg horse
Lidocaine	IV: 0.1–0.5 mg/kg slowly q 5 min, up to a total dose of 1.5 mg/kg; recommended CRI dose for postoperative ileus: 1.3 mg/kg IV followed by 0.05 mg/kg
Propranolol	IV: 0.02–0.22 mg/kg q 12 h (administer over 1 min)
Common Drugs to Treat Equine CHF	
Furosemide	IV or IM: 0.25–2.0 mg/kg as needed to control pulmonary edema; CRI: 0.12 mg/kg/h following an IV 0.12 mg/kg loading dose
Benazepril	Oral: 0.5 mg/kg once daily
Quinapril	Oral: 0.5 mg/kg once daily
Digoxin	Oral: 11–35 µg/kg q 12 h (use lower dose with tablets and higher dose with elixir)
Hydralazine	Oral: 0.5–1.5 mg/kg q 12 h IV: 0.5 mg/kg q 12 h

Abbreviations: CRI, constant rate infusion; IM, intramuscular; IV, intravenous; NGT, nasogastric tube.

diuretic effect 15 to 30 minutes after injection. After this peak effect there is rapid elimination of the drug. IM administration resulted in more prolonged diuretic effect in horses as compared with IV administration, with excretion of about 50% more urine.[2] Aggressive therapy with furosemide can lead to significant metabolic disturbances, including hypokalemia or metabolic alkalosis; these patients should be monitored closely with measurement of packed-cell volume and total protein and electrolyte concentrations.

Constant rate infusion (CRI) of furosemide has been suggested to be superior to bolus administration in human[3] and canine patients.[4] Results from one study comparing furosemide CRI (0.12 mg/kg/h, after a single loading dose of 0.12 mg/kg) with IV dosing of 1 mg/kg furosemide every 8 hours in horses suggest the CRI administration method may be a better approach in cases that require profound diuresis.[5] However, the advantages compared with bolus administration are minimal, so that if CRI administration is not possible, intermittent bolus administration is still a good option. Most equine patients with heart failure respond well to IV boluses of furosemide followed by IM administration for chronic administration.

Once an animal has developed CHF, it is rare that medications can ever be discontinued. Furosemide therapy is expected to continue for the remainder of the life of the horse with CHF. Exceptions to this rule would be those cases in which cardiac function improves (eg, CHF secondary to a rapid tachyarrhythmia or myocarditis, which responds to medical management). However, for most cases, long-term therapy with furosemide is necessary (0.25–2.0 mg/kg every 8–24 hours IM or IV). Unfortunately, furosemide is not effective after oral administration in normal horses[6]; the drug is not recommended for administration by this route.

Afterload Reducers

Afterload reduction is an important component of CHF therapy in other species; although there are little data to evaluate afterload reducers in horses with CHF, it is reasonable to hypothesize that they are helpful. Arteriodilators increase forward stroke volume and cardiac output; these result in a reduction in regurgitant fraction. Angiotensin-converting enzyme inhibitors (ACEIs) are the most commonly used afterload reducers in veterinary cardiology. These ACEIs act by inhibiting the conversion of angiotensin I to angiotensin II, thereby reducing angiotensin II production. Angiotensin II is a potent vasoconstrictor, which increases systemic blood pressure, myocardial work, and myocardial oxygen demand. Enalapril is a common ACEI. Enalaprilat, the active metabolite of enalapril, has been shown to cause arterial dilation in anesthetized horses[7]; however, 2 other studies suggested the oral drug is not effective in horses.[8,9]

Several reports suggest alternative ACEIs are likely more effective in horses. One case report described subjective improvement with the use of ramipril in a horse with CHF.[10] Also, ramipril reduced the hypertensive response to angiotensin I and reduced arterial pressure in healthy horses when administered orally.[11,12] Twenty horses with mitral valve disease were treated with quinapril, and catheterization studies showed improved stroke volume and cardiac output.[13] Pretreatment with quinapril also improved the prognosis for cardioversion of horses with atrial fibrillation (AF).[14] A more recent study demonstrated that quinapril was absorbed orally and converted to the active metabolite, quinaprilat, in normal horses. Moreover, it reduced plasma ACE activity.[15] However, quinapril had low oral bioavailability, and a dose of 240 mg per horse of quinapril was necessary to inhibit plasma ACE activity for 24 hours.[15] A study comparing ACE inhibition of 4 ACEIs in healthy horses (benazepril, ramipril, quinapril, and perindopril) noted marked differences in ACE inhibition, although all caused a similar decrease in indirect blood pressure. Administration of benazepril at 0.5 mg/kg was the only one resulting in significant serum ACE inhibition.[16] However, the dose of quinapril used in this study was actually lower than the dose used by Davis and colleagues,[15] which did demonstrate ACE inhibition with quinapril.[15] Therefore, from the current literature, benazepril or quinapril at 0.5 mg/kg once daily, by mouth, seems to be a reasonable option in the horse.

Hydralazine is primarily an arterial vasodilator, with minimal venous effects. It is available in an injectable formulation and can, therefore, be administered in the acute stage of heart failure. Results from one study suggest the drug may have a direct, positive inotropic effect independent of afterload reduction. It was shown to decrease peripheral vascular resistance and pulmonary arterial pressure when administered at a dose of 0.5 mg/kg IV to horses.[17] It resulted in both cardiac output and heart rate increases, without changing mean arterial and central venous blood pressures.[17] For long-term therapy, a dosage of 0.5 to 1.5 mg/kg by mouth every 12 hours has been suggested; but the efficacy of the oral administration route has not been evaluated.[18]

Diltiazem is a calcium channel blocker. It is commonly used for the management of supraventricular arrhythmias in dogs. In humans, it has been used for rhythm control and has also been shown to reduce systemic blood pressure.[19] Studies have shown the response to diltiazem to be highly variable in horses, and its efficacy after oral administration is uncertain.[20,21] Until further study, the use of diltiazem in horses requires careful monitoring of hemodynamic parameters; it should only be used with extreme caution in horses with CHF. The cardiovascular effects of other arteriodilators, such as the angiotensin receptor blockers, nitrovasodilators, and promazine, have not been evaluated in horses to date.

Inotropic Agents

Sympathomimetic agents are commonly used for equine patients with myocardial failure in which systolic dysfunction is present, but these agents are short acting and must be administered by CRI. Sympathomimetic administration in the horse serves to increase cardiac inotropy (contractility) during the acute management of CHF. Dobutamine (1–10 μg/kg/min IV) is a synthetic catecholamine with primarily β1 agonism. It is the least arrhythmogenic catecholamine and is the most frequently used sympathomimetic in horses. Dobutamine acts on cardiac ß-adrenergic receptors to increase contractility resulting in increased cardiac output and arterial pressure with minimal effect on peripheral vascular resistance in horses.[22] Dobutamine does not significantly affect heart rate in horses.[22]

Dopamine, in contrast, acts on variable receptors depending on the dose of administration. Although it has been shown to increase cardiac output in healthy, halothane-anesthetized horses,[23,24] and during infusion of endotoxin in anesthetized horses,[25] it has the potential to cause vasoconstriction and increase cardiac afterload. Therefore, dobutamine is preferred over dopamine in horses with heart failure.[22,26] Similarly, catecholamines with mixed adrenergic activity, such as norepinephrine, are generally avoided because of the potential for vasoconstriction causing an increase in cardiac afterload as well as arrhythmogenesis.

Phosphodiesterase III inhibitors (PDEIII-Is) have become a key component of heart failure management in small animal cardiology.[27] These drugs are called inodilators because they result in both an increase in cardiac contractility and vasodilation. Pimobendan is a PDEIII-I, which sensitizes the cardiomyocyte mechanical apparatus to calcium, thereby increasing contractility. Although pharmacokinetic studies with pimobendan have not been performed in the horse to date, it has positive inotropic and chronotropic effects in healthy adult horses when administered IV.[28] Milrinone, an injectable PDEIII-I agent, has been shown to produce beneficial hemodynamic effects in halothane-anesthetized horses.[29] Milrinone is used in human patients for short-term treatment of severe myocardial failure, but it is also likely to be cost prohibitive in equine patients.

Digoxin has historically been considered a positive inotropic agent; however, this effect is nearly negligible, particularly compared with the drugs described earlier. However, because pimobendan is often cost prohibitive in horses, it is likely that digoxin will continue to be used for this purpose in horses. Digoxin results in increased intracellular calcium concentrations by blocking the myocardial sodium ion (Na+)/potassium ion pump leading to increased intracellular Na+, which is then exchanged for calcium ions. In addition to this increase in contractility, digoxin increases parasympathetic activity, thereby slowing atrioventricular (AV) nodal conduction (see section on treating cardiac arrhythmias). The recommended dosage is 11 μg/kg, by mouth, every 12 hours.[30,31] IV administration of digoxin is not recommended in horses because rapid digitalization significantly increases the risk of toxicity. Because there is wide variability in an individual horse's response to digoxin, therapeutic drug monitoring (TDM) is recommended. When performing TDM after oral administration, the desired plasma concentrations of digoxin are between 0.5 and 2.0 ng/mL approximately 2 hours after administration.[30]

When TDM is not available, signs of toxicity should be monitored for closely, including electrocardiographic (ECG) changes, lethargy, anorexia, and/or constipation.[22] The ECG changes consistent with digoxin toxicity include bradycardia, PR interval prolongation, shortened QT interval, ST segment depression, and T-wave configuration changes (eg, flattened, change to inverted or biphasic appearance). Hypokalemia, hypoproteinemia, renal dysfunction, and dehydration each predispose to digoxin toxicity.[22] Acute digoxin toxicity can be treated by discontinuation of the digoxin and promoting diuresis with IV fluids.[22] Commercially available digoxin antibodies can be used; however, they are cost prohibitive for use in large animals in most cases. In horses with reduced renal function, digoxin should be administered with a high degree of caution; digoxin is contraindicated in horses with suspected or confirmed ionophore (eg, monensin) or cardiac glycoside (eg, oleander) toxicosis.

Although arrhythmia management is discussed in a separate section of this article, it is important to remember that significant bradycardia (<20 beats per minute [bpm]) or tachycardia (>80 bpm) will negatively impact cardiac output. Therefore, optimizing the heart rate is another important part of therapy for patients with CHF.

Evaluation of Outcome and Long-Term Recommendations

Unfortunately, the long-term prognosis for most horses with CHF is poor unless an underlying cause is present that can be addressed. For example, tachycardia-induced heart failure can often be treated, as can many cases of myocarditis or selenium-deficiency–induced myocardial dysfunction. In addition, because furosemide must be administered by injection, for many owners, the long-term management of horses with CHF is not feasible. For those who are able to make this commitment, regular monitoring of renal function and serum electrolyte status is important.

MEDICAL MANAGEMENT OF CARDIAC ARRHYTHMIAS
Patient Evaluation Overview

Occasionally horses with arrhythmias will be subclinical; the rhythm disturbance will be detected during routine cardiac auscultation, which is often the case with lone

AF. More frequently, clinical signs will prompt veterinary consultation. See **Table 1** for a list of common clinical signs associated with cardiac arrhythmias in horses. With the exception of AF, it can be very difficult to diagnose the type of arrhythmia on auscultation alone; an ECG is essential to define the arrhythmia and the optimal therapeutic options. Further workup (for example, an echocardiogram and/or exercising ECG) may also be warranted.

The possibility of underlying disease processes should always be considered in patients with arrhythmias. Echocardiography is important in these cases to evaluate for potential structural heart disease. Myocarditis often results in ventricular, or sometimes supraventricular, arrhythmias. Sometimes the arrhythmias secondary to myocarditis will respond to corticosteroid therapy administered to treat the underlying myocarditis. Therapy with antiarrhythmic drugs is only recommended if the rhythm disturbance is causing clinical signs or if a rapid ventricular tachycardia is present, because these medications can be proarrhythmic. Serum electrolytes and acid base status should also be evaluated as potential contributing factors to arrhythmias.

Pharmacologic Treatment Options

Supraventricular arrhythmias
Atrial fibrillation AF is by far the most common arrhythmia in horses, after second-degree AV block; it is the most common cardiovascular cause of poor performance in the equine athlete.[31,32] Large atrial size is a predisposing factor for the development of AF, which explains why horses as a species are structurally predisposed. AF often occurs in horses with no evidence of underlying cardiac disease, and this form is termed *lone AF*.[32,33] However, even in lone AF cases the longer the arrhythmia is present, the more likely electrical remodeling will occur. This chronic remodeling results in a reduced likelihood of successful conversion to sinus rhythm.[34] Therefore, the longer a horse has had AF, the more difficult it is to convert the horse to sinus rhythm and the more likely recurrence is. Similarly, in horses with AF and underlying heart disease, conversion to sinus rhythm is difficult and recurrence of AF is more likely.[34] Therefore, it is important to perform a complete cardiac examination, including echocardiography, before attempting conversion.

Traditionally, oral quinidine sulfate has been the treatment of choice for horses with AF; it remains the most common therapy today. Quinidine is a class IA sodium channel blocker (see **Table 2**). In horses with recent-onset AF (<2 months), AF may be treated effectively with IV administration of quinidine, in the form of quinidine gluconate.[33] Quinidine gluconate is administered IV in 1.1 to 2.2 mg/kg boluses every 10 minutes, up to a total dose of 8.8 to 11 mg/kg, or until conversion or signs of toxicity develop.[18] If IV quinidine therapy is unsuccessful, or if AF has been present for longer than 2 months, oral quinidine (quinidine sulfate) should be used. The dosing regimen consists of 22 mg/kg administered through a nasogastric tube every 2 hours, up to a total dose of 88 mg/kg, or until conversion occurs or signs of toxicity develop.[35,36] It is important that the horse is observed closely for 2 hours following treatment with oral quinidine (time of peak blood concentration). Idiosyncratic or adverse reactions to quinidine, such as nasal edema, urticaria, laminitis colic, diarrhea, or ataxia, can develop. If no reactions are noted, then a surface ECG should be recorded and the QRS interval should be measured. Use of a telemetry device allows for continuous monitoring of the ECG during quinidine therapy. If the QRS interval is not prolonged by more than 25%, then a second dose of quinidine can be administered. Similarly, subsequent doses can be administered using the same criteria. TDM can also be performed on plasma quinidine concentrations. If plasma quinidine concentrations cannot be obtained promptly, a total dosage of 88 mg/kg should not be exceeded.

If neither conversion nor signs of toxicity occur after this total dose of 88 mg/kg, then quinidine therapy can be continued at a dosing rate of 22 mg/kg with reduced frequency (every 6 hours), through nasogastric tube administration.[35] TDM of plasma or serum quinidine concentrations is very helpful to avoid toxicity, and it is particularly important in horses that are treated beyond the first day. The therapeutic serum or plasma concentration range for quinidine is 2 to 5 μg/mL. When concentrations exceed 5 μg/mL, toxic signs are common and conversion to sinus rhythm is unlikely to occur.[35] Quinidine administration is contraindicated in horses with AF that is associated with heart failure, again emphasizing the importance of echocardiography before treatment. These horses with heart failure should be treated as described earlier for CHF. The reported success rate of quinidine therapy in conversion of AF to normal sinus rhythm in horses without underlying heart disease ranges from 62% to 92%.[32,35,36,40]

Therapy with quinidine can result in potentially serious consequences. Adverse effects include depression, diarrhea, colic, laminitis upper respiratory tract edema, urticaria, hypotension, ataxia, and even sudden death.[22,35] Horses undergoing treatment should be kept in quiet surroundings, with telemetry for continuous ECG monitoring or frequent, intermittent ECG monitoring at a minimum. It is important to monitor the ECG during treatment for changes consistent with quinidine toxicity. These changes include QRS prolongation as well as the development of new cardiac arrhythmias. Rapid supraventricular or ventricular arrhythmias (>100 bpm) can develop, which should prompt discontinuation of the drug. In humans, high serum quinidine concentrations have abortogenic and teratogenic effects; but this effect has not been described in the horse, including in one reported pregnant mare treated with quinidine for AF.[37]

Accelerated AV conduction occurs in a significant proportion of horses treated with quinidine because of its vagolytic effect, resulting in tachycardia.[35] In order to reduce the risks of developing significant tachycardia, treatment with digoxin has been recommended before initiating quinidine therapy in horses with increased heart rates. In addition, many clinicians initiate treatment with digoxin if conversion to sinus rhythm has not occurred after 2 days of quinidine therapy.[22] However, the concurrent administration of these two drugs increases free-plasma drug concentrations of both, thereby increasing risks of toxicity; therefore, TDM of plasma concentrations is indicated.[38] Quinidine-induced supraventricular arrhythmias that are greater than 100 bpm can be treated with digoxin (0.0022 mg/kg IV or 0.011 mg/kg by mouth).

Supraventricular tachycardia during quinidine administration can also be addressed using a β-adrenergic blocker, such as propranolol (0.02–0.22 mg/kg IV).[18] Efficacy of propranolol depends on the degree of sympathetic tone present. Injectable propranolol should be used because the bioavailability of oral propranolol is very low.[39] Ventricular arrhythmias can also develop following quinidine administration; these are best treated with magnesium sulfate (treatment of choice for torsades de pointes), lidocaine, or propranolol. These therapeutics and others are further discussed under ventricular antiarrhythmic therapy.

Ancillary therapies, such as mineral oil or activated charcoal, may help to limit further quinidine absorption. Fluid therapy is also recommended to treat quinidine-induced hypotension and for cardiovascular support. IV sodium bicarbonate (1 mEq/kg) increases protein binding of free quinidine, thereby decreasing the circulating plasma concentrations of free or active drug. In cases of severe hypotension, phenylephrine (1 μg/kg/min, up to a total dose of 0.01–0.02 mg/kg IV) can be administered; blood pressure should be monitored.[35]

Alternative Atrial Fibrillation Medical Therapies

Alternatives to quinidine for AF conversion continue to be evaluated because of the risks associated with quinidine administration and the fact that it is not effective in all horses.

Procainamide is a class Ia antiarrhythmic, similar to quinidine.[22] The direct hemodynamic effects of procainamide are the same as quinidine, but they are less pronounced.[22] The recommended dose of procainamide in the horse is 1 mg/kg/min IV, up to a total dose of 20 mg/kg. The recommended oral dose is 25 to 35 mg/kg, administered every 8 hours.[18]

Amiodarone is a class III antiarrhythmic, which has been evaluated in the treatment of AF in horses. Oral amiodarone therapy likely has too many limitations, including variable bioavailability, to be useful in the horse.[41] However, in normal ponies a single IV dose was well tolerated and no side effects were noted.[42] In 2 clinical reports, approximately half the treated horses (7 of 12) were successfully converted to sinus rhythm and side effects were usually mild and transient, although 3 of 6 horses in one of the studies that did not convert also developed diarrhea that lasted 10 to 14 days.[41,43] Hind limb weakness with weight shifting was also noted but was transient and resolved after the drug was discontinued.[41] From the small amount of data currently available, amiodarone may be an effective antiarrhythmic for use in the horse; however, caution should be exercised in using the drug as a prolonged infusion, where side effects are more likely to occur.

Flecainide is a class IC sodium channel blocker, used for treating both supraventricular and ventricular arrhythmias in humans. Ohmura and colleagues[44] found that flecainide given at a dose of 0.2 mg/kg/min IV, up to a total dose of 2 mg/kg, successfully converted experimental and acute AF in horses. Flecainide seems to be absorbed orally,[47] and a case report described the successful conversion of AF using 5 doses of oral flecainide; however, the horse exhibited colic during the conversion.[48] Despite its reported success with acute AF, flecainide has not been particularly useful in converting horses with chronic AF.[45] In addition, the drug was shown to temporarily prolong ventricular repolarization, which is considered a proarrhythmic effect.[49] A proarrhythmic effect was also noted in a case report of a horse with supraventricular tachycardia that developed a presumed fatal arrhythmia following treatment with flecainide.[46] Taken together, these reports suggest that, although flecainide might be effective in acute cases of equine AF, it is unlikely to be useful in cases of chronic AF and may cause significant adverse effects.

Sotalol, a class III antiarrhythmic drug with additional ß-adrenergic blocking effects, and propafenone, a class IC antiarrhythmic, have also been investigated in the treatment of AF in horses; however, neither seems particularly effective in this regard.[50]

Surgical Treatment Options

Electrical cardioversion is routinely used in humans for restoration of sinus rhythm in cases of AF.[51] Transvenous electrical cardioversion (TVEC) has proven to be effective for equine lone AF as well.[52,53] The TVEC procedure seems successful for the short-[54] and long-term[55] successful treatment of horses with AF. It is particularly useful for horses that develop idiosyncratic reactions or toxicity before conversion with quinidine therapy. The TVEC procedure requires specialized equipment and training that is not widely available, and it requires general anesthesia. Therefore, medical management will continue to be widely used for equine patients with AF. At this time, quinidine or electrical cardioversion remain the best choices for treatment of horses with lone AF.

Supraventricular Arrhythmias Other than Atrial Fibrillation

Supraventricular arrhythmias other than AF, including supraventricular tachycardia and frequent atrial premature contractions (APCs), can also cause clinical signs in the horse, although they are less common than AF. Occasional or intermittent APCs rarely result in clinical signs or require specific therapy. Atrial tachycardia rarely results in increased resting heart rates in horses that are otherwise healthy, because the normally high resting vagal tone in horses leads to physiologic AV block and prevents the ventricular rate from increasing. However, with any cause of vagal inhibition, including exercise and sympathetic stimulation, significant tachycardia can develop in such horses.

The medical management of supraventricular tachycardia, when causing sustained and marked tachycardia, could include most of the drugs listed in the earlier section on AF (eg, propranolol, procainamide). Digoxin can be used to slow AV nodal conduction and the ventricular response rate. Alternatively, conversion of atrial tachycardia can be attempted with electrical cardioversion.

Ventricular arrhythmias

Because most ventricular antiarrhythmic agents can be proarrhythmic, therapy is generally only recommended in symptomatic or clinical cases. If ectopy is severe enough to cause signs of low cardiac output, which generally occurs when the heart rate is greater than 100 bpm in adult horses, then treatment is recommended. Moreover, if tachycardia is persistent, secondary heart failure is a likely sequel if left untreated.[18] Other risk factors suggesting there is benefit to suppress ventricular ectopy have been extrapolated from human studies. These risk factors include multiform complexes and R on T phenomenon. Lidocaine, magnesium sulfate, quinidine gluconate, propranolol, procainamide, phenytoin, amiodarone, and propafenone have been advocated for the treatment of ventricular tachycardia in horses.[56]

Lidocaine is a class IB sodium channel blocker. Unlike most other sodium channel blockers, lidocaine is not effective in treating supraventricular arrhythmias.[22] The recommended dosing regimen for lidocaine conversion of ventricular dysrhythmias is 0.1 to 0.5 mg/kg IV, as a slow injection every 5 minutes, up to a total dose of 1.3 to 1.5 mg/kg (see **Table 2**).[31] Lidocaine infusions of 0.05 mg/kg/min (as a CRI) can then be instituted immediately after the slow boluses for persistent or recurrent ventricular tachycardia or to prevent recurrence in horses with myocardial disease until the disease process resolves (eg, oleander toxicity). The most significant side effects of lidocaine are neurologic and occur secondary to central nervous system stimulation. These side effects include excitement, ataxia, muscle fasciculations, weakness, and seizures. If any of these are noted, the lidocaine should be discontinued. If seizure activity is noted, diazepam (0.05–0.4 mg/kg IV) can be effective. Lidocaine is fast acting but has a short duration of action and minimal cardiovascular depressant effects.[57] The equine nervous system, however, is more sensitive to the effects of lidocaine than is the cardiovascular system.[58] The target or therapeutic plasma concentration of lidocaine in the treatment of ventricular arrhythmias is 1 to 2 μg/mL, with toxic effects occurring in the 1.9 to 4.5-μg/mL range.[59] Coadministration of highly protein-bound drugs increases the risk of lidocaine toxicity because of displacement of lidocaine from protein, thereby increasing the plasma concentration of free drug.[59,60]

Phenytoin sodium has similar actions to lidocaine and is generally considered to be the drug of choice for ventricular arrhythmias caused by digoxin toxicity.[61,62] The drug has also been effective at abolishing ventricular ectopy in horses that did not respond to lidocaine or procainamide.[63] The recommended protocol is 20 mg/kg by mouth every 12 hours for 2 days and then reduced to 10 to 15 mg/kg by mouth every 12 hours.[63] IV administration may be irritating to surrounding tissue because of its alkalinity.[63] If possible, TDM is recommended, with the effective plasma concentrations between 5 and 10 µg/mL.[63] Signs of sedation, periods of recumbency, or muscle fasciculations suggest an excessively high plasma concentration; the dose should be reduced.

Magnesium sulfate is a physiologic calcium channel blocker that enhances repolarization homogeneity and, thereby, suppresses ventricular arrhythmias.[64] Magnesium sulfate is slower acting than lidocaine as an antiarrhythmic agent. It has no significant cardiovascular effects, which is a potential advantage when only ventricular antiarrhythmic effects are sought. In humans, it is specifically recommended as the first-line therapy for polymorphous ventricular tachycardia with prolonged QT interval (a specific type of ventricular tachycardia, termed *torsade de pointes*).[64,65] It is recommended to be administered at a dosage of 1 g/min/500-kg horse (ie, 2.2 mg/kg/min) to effect, up to a maximum of 25 g for a 500-kg horse.[31] Magnesium solutions containing calcium should not be used for this purpose.

Quinidine gluconate (1.1–2.2 mg/kg IV boluses every 10 minutes up to a total of 8.8–11.0 mg/kg) can also be used to treat ventricular tachycardia.[31] As noted previously in the section on AF, quinidine has many potential undesirable side effects; therefore, hemodynamic and clinical monitoring is important. Quinidine should be avoided in horses with systolic dysfunction. When it must be used in animals with hypotension, concurrent IV administration of a balanced electrolyte solution at the rate of 3 to 4 mL/kg/h has been recommended.[31] Oral quinidine was used successfully to treat a quarter horse with ventricular tachycardia.[66]

As stated earlier, procainamide has similar actions to quinidine with fewer cardiovascular side effects, such as hypotension. Recommended dosing regimens for procainamide in horses include 1 mg/kg/min, IV, up to a total dose of 20 mg/kg. A suggested oral dosage is 25 to 35 mg/kg administered every 8 hours.[31]

Propafenone is a class I antiarrhythmic with mild β-adrenoceptor antagonistic properties as well as mild class III and class IV activity.[67] It is useful for both supraventricular and ventricular arrhythmias in humans. A pharmacokinetic study in horses demonstrated that propafenone has rapid distribution after IV administration; however, there is large interindividual variability, and plasma concentrations quickly decreased to less than the concentrations considered therapeutic in other species.[67] Proposed dosing regimens include 0.5 to 1.0 mg/kg IV administered slowly, in 5% dextrose. A suggested oral dosage includes 2 mg/kg administered every 8 hours; however, propafenone has not been evaluated by the oral route in either healthy horses or in horses with heart disease.

Amiodarone is an alternative antiarrhythmic with primarily class III effects. It was successfully used to treat a horse with refractory ventricular tachycardia after therapy with magnesium, lidocaine and propafenone was unsuccessful in converting the arrhythmia (CRI administration with 5 mg/kg/h for 1 hour, followed by 0.83 mg/kg/h for 24 hours).[68] Because there is not much experience using this drug in the horse, it is probably best reserved for use in refractory VT cases.

Propranolol is a nonselective β-adrenoceptor antagonist. It can be particularly effective in arrhythmias whereby sympathetic overdrive is a factor. Dose rates range from 0.02 to 0.22 mg/kg IV.[69] Therapeutic concentrations of propranolol reduce myocardial contractility; therefore, it should be used with caution in patients with structural heart disease and should be avoided when heart failure is present. Because it is a nonselective adrenoceptor β antagonist, it should be avoided in horses with lower airway disease. The oral form of propranolol has not been effective in the horse.[22]

Ventricular fibrillation is a far more serious dysrhythmia than even ventricular tachy-cardia. The pharmacologic treatment of ventricular fibrillation is rarely successful in horses. Defibrillation is the treatment of choice in conversion of ventricular fibrillation. Drugs that have been suggested for ventricular fibrillation include lidocaine and brety-lium (0.5–5 mg/kg, IV).[18]

Bradyarrhythmias

Bradyarrhythmias include sinus bradycardia, high-grade second-degree AV block, and third-degree AV block. These bradyarrhythmias require treatment if the heart rate is slow enough to negatively impact cardiac output (usually <24 bpm). The anti-cholinergic drugs atropine (0.01–0.02 mg/kg IV) and glycopyrrolate (5–10 μg/kg IV) can increase heart rate if elevated vagal tone is a factor (most often during anesthesia). Possible side effects include decreased gastrointestinal motility and secretions (potentially leading to colic), increased respiratory dead space, and mydriasis.[22] Atro-pine should not be used more than once, and even then it can lead to significant ileus in horses. In patients with symptomatic bradyarrhythmias, a positive response following anticholinergic administration (ie, increased heart rate) suggests the drug may be effective for therapeutic purposes. However, ventricular escape rhythms (as in third-degree AV block) rarely respond to medical therapy; the risk of reducing gastrointestinal motility is significant with chronic use. Instead of anticholinergics, or in addition, theophylline and aminophylline can also be used to try to increase the heart rate. These drugs are more often used for airway disease but usually stimulate an increase in heart rate.[70] Side effects include excitement, cardiac arrhythmias, and tachycardia.[22] Aminophylline is recommended at 2 to 7 mg/kg IV every 6 to 12 hours or 5 mg/kg orally. Theophylline can be administered at 5 to 15 mg/kg by mouth every 12 to 24 hours (sustained-release product).[70] TDM can be performed for theophylline, with the therapeutic goal being 5 to 12 μg/mL. Toxicity occurs at theophylline concentrations greater than 15 μg/mL.

When anesthesia-associated bradyarrhythmias do not respond to anticholinergics, sympathomimetics may be required to increase the heart rate. As stated earlier, dobutamine is the least arrhythmogenic of the sympathomimetic drugs. Isoproterenol is another sympathomimetic drug used to address bradycardia in other species. It effectively increased heart rate at 1.0 μg/kg/min in normal horses but also has β_2 adrenergic activity and causes peripheral vasodilation.[71]

It is important to consider possible causes of the bradycardia. For example, hyper-kalemia can cause severe bradycardia; addressing it with insulin and dextrose or calcium gluconate often results in an improved heart rate. Alternatively, echocardiog-raphy, to look for a structural cause of complete heart block, could reveal evidence for immune-mediated myocarditis, along with increased cardiac troponin-I. Corticoste-roid therapy may lead to resolution of complete heart block in these cases.

Treatment Resistance and Surgical Treatment Options

If the bradycardia is not transient, as in anesthetized patients, and an underlying cause cannot be identified and addressed, long-term medical management for symptomatic bradycardia is rarely successful in the horse. Drug efficacy is limited and side effects are common. A permanent pacemaker results in long-term control of bradycardia, and the procedure has been successfully performed in horses[72–75]; but risks associated with pacemaker failure, although very low, make it difficult to recommend using the animal for performance.

In part, the reason so many different medical options are available for the various arrhythmias that occur in horses is that some individuals simply do not respond to the drug of first choice and alternative approaches are necessary. In these intractable cases, repeated evaluation of electrolyte status and the possibility of underlying structural heart disease is warranted.

Evaluation of Outcome and Long-Term Recommendations

The prognosis for individual equine cases with cardiac arrhythmias is highly variable and depends on the rhythm, underlying structural heart disease, and response to therapy. Although some cases may ultimately not need chronic medical therapy following conversion and have a good prognosis (eg, AF, or ventricular tachycardia associated with oleander toxicity that resolves), some arrhythmias, such as persistent ventricular ectopy, put patients at risk of a future, potentially fatal arrhythmia, even if apparently managed with antiarrhythmic therapy. Recommendations regarding future care and use of the horse require an understanding of the potential risk for the horse as well as the owner/rider.

SUPPLEMENTARY DATA

Supplementary data related to this article can be found online at http://dx.doi.org/10. 1016/j.cveq.2016.11.005.

REFERENCES

1. Nout YS, Hinchcliff KW, Bonagura JD, et al. Cardiac amyloidosis in a horse. J Vet Intern Med 2003;17:588–92.
2. Tobin T, Roberts BL, Swerczek TW, et al. The pharmacology of furosemide in the horse. III. Dose and time response relationships, effects of repeated dosing, and performance effects. Journal of Equine Med Surg 1978;2:216–26.
3. Lahav M, Regev A, Ra'anani P, et al. Intermittent administration of furosemide vs continuous infusion preceded by a loading dose for congestive heart failure. Chest 1992;102:725–31.
4. Adin DB, Taylor AW, Hill RC, et al. Intermittent bolus injection versus continuous infusion of furosemide in normal adult greyhound dogs. J Vet Intern Med 2003;17: 632–6.
5. Johansson AM, Gardner SY, Levine JF, et al. Furosemide continuous rate infusion in the horse: evaluation of enhanced efficacy and reduced side effects. J Vet Intern Med 2003;17:887–95.
6. Johansson AM, Gardner SY, Levine JF, et al. Pharmacokinetics and pharmacodynamics of furosemide after oral administration to horses. J Vet Intern Med 2004; 18:739–43.
7. Muir WW 3rd, Sams RA, Hubbell JA, et al. Effects of enalaprilat on cardiorespiratory, hemodynamic, and hematologic variables in exercising horses. Am J Vet Res 2001;62:1008–13.
8. Gardner SY, Atkins CE, Sams RA, et al. Characterization of the pharmacokinetic and pharmacodynamic properties of the angiotensin-converting enzyme inhibitor, enalapril, in horses. J Vet Intern Med 2004;18:231–7.
9. Sleeper MM, McDonnell SM, Ely JJ, et al. Chronic oral therapy with enalapril in normal ponies. J Vet Cardiol 2008;10:111–5.
10. Guglielmini C, Giuliani A, Testoni S, et al. Use of an ACE inhibitor (ramipril) in a horse with congestive heart failure. Equine Vet Educ 2002;14:297–306.
11. De Luna R, Oliva G, Ambrosio R, et al. Angiotensin-converting enzyme (ACE) inhibitors in horses: evaluation of the renin angiotensin-aldosterone system after administration of ramipril (preliminary studies). Acta Med Vet 1995;41:41–50.

12. Luciani A, Civitella C, Santori D, et al. Haemodynamic effects in healthy horses treated with an ACE-inhibitor (ramipril). Vet Res Comm 2007;31:S297–9.
13. Gehlen H, Vieht JC, Stadler P. Effects of the ACE inhibitor quinapril on echocardiographic variables in horses with mitral valve insufficiency. J Vet Med A Physiol Pathol Clin Med 2003;50:460–5.
14. Goltz A, Gehlen H, Rohn K, et al. Therapy of atrial fibrillation with class-1A and class-1C antiarrhythmic agents and ACE inhibitors. Pferdeheilkunde 2009;25:220–7.
15. Davis JL, Kruger K, Lafevers DH, et al. Effects of quinapril on angiotensin converting enzyme and plasma renin activity as well as pharmacokinetic parameters of quinapril and its active metabolite, quinaprilat, after intravenous and oral administration to mature horses. Equine Vet J 2014;46:729–33.
16. Afonso T, Guguere S, Rapoport G, et al. Pharmacodynamic evaluation of 4 angiotensin-converting enzyme inhibitors in healthy adult horses. J Vet Intern Med 2013;27:1185–92.
17. Bertone JJ. Cardiovascular effects of hydralazine HCl administration in horses. Am J Vet Res 1988;49:618–21.
18. Mogg TD. Equine cardiac disease. Clinical pharmacology and therapeutics. Vet Clin North Am Equine Pract 1999;15:523–34.
19. Opie LH. Calcium channel blockers (calcium antagonists). In: Opie LH, Gersh BG, editors. Drugs for the heart. 7th edition. Philadelphia: Saunders Elsevier; 2009. p. 59–87.
20. Schwarzwald CC, Bonagura JD, Luis-Fuentes V. Effects of diltiazem on hemodynamic variables and ventricular function in healthy horses. J Vet Intern Med 2005;19:703–11.
21. Schwarzwald CC, Hamlin RL, Bonagura JD, et al. Atrial, SA nodal, and AV nodal electrophysiology in standing horses: normal findings and electrophysiologic effects of quinidine and diltiazem. J Vet Intern Med 2007;21:166–75.
22. Muir WW 3rd, Mcguirk S. Cardiovascular drugs. Their pharmacology and use in horses. Vet Clin North Am Equine Pract 1987;3:37–57.
23. Trim CM, Moore JN, White NA. Cardiopulmonary effects of dopamine hydrochloride in anaesthetized horses. Equine Vet J 1985;17:41–4.
24. Swanson CR, Muir WW, Bednarski RM, et al. Hemodynamic responses in halothane-anesthetized horses given infusions of dopamine or dobutamine. Am J Vet Res 1985;46:365–70.
25. Trim CM, Moore JN, Hardee MM, et al. Effects of an infusion of dopamine on the cardiopulmonary effects of Escherichia coli endotoxin in anesthetized horses. Res Vet Sci 1991;50:54–63.
26. Geor RJ. Acute renal failure in horses. Vet Clin North Am Equine Pract 2007;23:577–91.
27. Gordon SG, Miller MW, Saunders AB. Pimobendan in heart failure therapy–a silver bullet? J Am Anim Hosp 2006;42:90–3.
28. Afonso T, Giguere S, Rapoport G, et al. Cardiovascular effects of pimobendan in healthy mature horses. Equine Vet J 2016;48:352–6.
29. Muir WW. The haemodynamic effects of milrinone HCl in halothane anaesthetised horses. Equine Vet J Suppl 1995;(19):108–13.
30. Sweeney RW, Reef VB, Reimer JM. Pharmacokinetics of digoxin administered to horses with congestive heart failure. Am J Vet Res 1993;54:1108–11.
31. Reef VB, Mcguirk SM. Diseases of the cardiovascular system. In: Smith BP, editor. Large animal internal medicine. 4th edition. St Louis (MO): Mosby Elsevier; 2009. p. 453–89.

32. Young L, Van Loon G. Editorial: atrial fibrillation in horses: new treatment choices for the new millennium? J Vet Intern Med 2005;19:631–2.
33. Reef VB, Levitan CW, Spencer PA. Factors affecting prognosis and conversion in equine atrial fibrillation. J Vet Intern Med 1988;2:1–6.
34. De Clercq D, Van Loon G, Tavernier R, et al. Atrial and ventricular electrical and contractile remodeling and reverse remodeling owing to short-term pacing-induced atrial fibrillation in horses. J Vet Intern Med 2008;22:1353–9.
35. Reef VB, Reimer JM, Spencer PA. Treatment of atrial fibrillation in horses: new perspectives. J Vet Intern Med 1995;9:57–67.
36. Morris DD, Fregin GF. Atrial fibrillation in horses: factors associated with response to quinidine sulfate in 77 clinical cases. Cornell Vet 1982;72:339–49.
37. Bertone JJ, Traub-Dargatz JL, Wingfield WE. Atrial fibrillation in a pregnant mare: treatment with quinidine sulfate. J Am Vet Med Assoc 1987;190:1565–6.
38. Parraga ME, Kittleson MD, Drake CM. Quinidine administration increases steady state serum digoxin concentration in horses. Equine Vet J Suppl 1995;19:114–9.
39. Baggot JD. The pharmacological basis of cardiac drug selection for use in horses. Equine Vet J Suppl 1995;(19):97–100.
40. Mcguirk SM, Muir WW, Sams RA. Pharmacokinetic analysis of intravenously and orally administered quinidine in horses. Am J Vet Res 1981;42:938–42.
41. De Clercq D, Van Loon G, Baert K, et al. Intravenous amiodarone treatment in horses with chronic atrial fibrillation. Vet J 2006;172:129–34.
42. Trachsel D, Tschudi P, Portier CJ, et al. Pharmacokinetics and pharmacodynamic effects of amiodarone in plasma of ponies after single intravenous administration. Toxicol Appl Pharmacol 2004;195:113–25.
43. De Clercq D, Van Loon G, Baert K, et al. Effects of an adapted intravenous amiodarone treatment protocol in horses with atrial fibrillation. Equine Vet J 2007;39:344–9.
44. Ohmura H, Nukada T, Mizuno Y, et al. Safe and efficacious dosage of flecainide acetate for treating equine atrial fibrillation. J Vet Med Sci 2000;62:711–5.
45. Van Loon G, Blissitt KJ, Keen JA, et al. Use of intravenous flecainide in horses with naturally-occurring atrial fibrillation. Equine Vet J 2004;36:609–14.
46. Dembek KA, Hurcombe SD, Schober KE, et al. Sudden death of a horse with supraventricular tachycardia following oral administration of flecainide acetate. J Vet Emerg Crit Care (San Antonio) 2014;24(6):759–63.
47. Ohmura H, Hiraga A, Aida H, et al. Determination of oral dosage and pharmacokinetic analysis of flecainide in horses. J Vet Med Sci 2001;63:511–4.
48. Risberg AI, Mcguirk SM. Successful conversion of equine atrial fibrillation using oral flecainide. J Vet Intern Med 2006;20:207–9.
49. Haugaard MM, Pehrson S, Carstensen H, et al. Antiarrhythmic and electrophysiologic effects of flecainide on acutely induced atrial fibrillation in healthy horses. J Vet Intern Med 2015;29:339–47.
50. De Clercq D, Van Loon G, Tavernier R, et al. Use of propafenone for conversion of chronic atrial fibrillation in horses. Am J Vet Res 2009;70:223–7.
51. Levy S, Lauribe P, Dolla E, et al. A randomized comparison of external and internal cardioversion of chronic atrial fibrillation. Circulation 1992;86:1415–20.
52. Mcgurrin MK, Physick-Sheard PW, Kenney DG, et al. Transvenous electrical cardioversion in equine atrial fibrillation: technique and successful treatment of 3 horses. J Vet Intern Med 2003;17:715–8.
53. Mcgurrin MK, Physick-Sheard PW, Kenney DG. Transvenous electrical cardioversion of equine atrial fibrillation: patient factors and clinical results in 72 treatment episodes. J Vet Intern Med 2008;22:609–15.

54. Bellei MH, Kerr C, Mcgurrin, et al. Management and complications of anesthesia for transvenous electrical cardioversion of atrial fibrillation in horses: 62 cases (2002-2006). J Am Vet Med Assoc 2007;231:1225–30.

55. Decloedt A, Verheyen T, Van Der Vekens N, et al. Long-term follow-up of atrial function after cardioversion of atrial fibrillation in horses. Vet J 2013;197:583–8.

56. Reimer JM, Reef VB, Sweeney RW. Ventricular arrhythmias in horses: 21 cases (1984-1989). J Am Vet Med Assoc 1992;201:1237–43.

57. Engelking LR, Blyden GT, Lofstedt J, et al. Pharmacokinetics of antipyrine, acetaminophen and lidocaine in fed and fasted horses. J Vet Pharmacol Ther 1987; 10:73–82.

58. Meyer GA, Lin HC, Hanson RR, et al. Effects of intravenous lidocaine overdose on cardiac electrical activity and blood pressure in the horse. Equine Vet J 2001;33: 434–7.

59. Milligan M, Kukanich B, Beard W, et al. The disposition of lidocaine during a 12-hour intravenous infusion to postoperative horses. J Vet Pharmacol Thera 2006;29:495–9.

60. Mullen KR, Gelzer AR, Kraus MS, et al. ECG of the month. Cardiac arrhythmias in a horse after lidocaine administration. J Am Vet Med Assoc 2009;235:1156–8.

61. Wijnberg ID, Van Der Kolk JH, Hiddink EG. Use of phenytoin to treat digitalis-induced cardiac arrhythmias in a miniature Shetland pony. Vet Rec 1999;144: 259–61.

62. Smith PA, Aldridge BM, Kittleson MD. Oleander toxicosis in a donkey. J Vet Intern Med 2003;17:111–4.

63. Wijnberg ID, Ververs FF. Phenytoin sodium as a treatment for ventricular dysrhythmia in horses. J Vet Intern Med 2004;18:350–3.

64. Tzivoni D, Banai S, Schuger C, et al. Treatment of torsade de points with magnesium sulfate. Circulation 1988;77:392–7.

65. Parikka H, Toivonen L, Naukkarinen V, et al. Decreases by magnesium of QT dispersion and ventricular arrhythmias in patients with acute myocardial infarction. Eur Heart J 1999;20:111–20.

66. Stern JA, Doreste YR, Barnett RD, et al. Resolution of sustained narrow complex ventricular tachycardia and tachycardia-induced cardiomyopathy in a quarter horse following quinidine therapy. J Vet Cardiol 2012;14:445–51.

67. Puigdemont A, Riu JL, Guitart R, et al. Propafenone kinetics in the horse. Comparative analysis of compartmental and noncompartmental models. J Pharmacol Methods 1990;23:79–85.

68. De Clercq D, Van Loon G, Baert K, et al. Treatment with amiodarone of refractory ventricular tachycardia in a horse. J Vet Intern Med 2007;21:878–80.

69. Geor RJ, Hinchcliff KW, Sams RA. β-adrenergic blockade augments glucose utilization in horses during graded exercise. J Appl Physiol (1985) 2000;89: 1086–98.

70. Goetz TE, Munsiff IJ, McKiernan BC. Pharmacokinetic disposition of an immediate release aminophylline and a sustained-release theophylline formulation in the horse. J Vet Pharmacol Ther 1989;12:369–77.

71. Goetz TE, Manohar M. Effects of age on isoproterenol-induced maximal heart rate in horses. Am J Vet Res 1990;51:1008–11.

72. Reef VB, Clark ES, Oliver JA, et al. Implantation of a permanent transvenous pacing catheter in a horse with complete heart block and syncope. J Am Vet Med Assoc 1986;189:449–52.

73. Van Loon G, Fonteyne W, Rottiers H, et al. Implantation of a dual-chamber, rate-adaptive pacemaker in a horse with suspected sick sinus syndrome. Vet Rec 2002;151:541–5.
74. Van Loon G, Fonteyne W, Rottiers H, et al. Dual-chamber pacemaker implantation via the cephalic vein in healthy equids. J Vet Intern Med 2001;15:564–71.
75. Taylor DH, Mero MA. The use of an internal pacemaker in a horse with Adams-Stokes syndrome. J Am Vet Med Assoc 1967;151:1172–6.

Pain Management in Horses

Alonso Guedes, DVM, MS, PhD

KEYWORDS

- Equine • Lameness • Inflammation • Visceral • Musculoskeletal

KEY POINTS

- Physiologic pain is a multidimensional experience (sensory and emotional) that is vital for survival, but becomes a problem when painful medical practices need to be performed.
- Tissue injury amplifies physiologic pain and can evolve to a state of pathologic pain if not appropriately managed.
- At the present time, monitoring changes in equine behavior and expression appears to be the best approach for assessing pain and response to analgesics.
- Surgery is one of the only situations in which the nature, location, and extent of tissue injury are precisely known in advance, and an appropriate analgesic protocol can be formulated and established.
- Pain therapy should focus on prevention as much as possible and include a multimodal approach with pharmacologic and nonpharmacologic strategies.

PAIN MANAGEMENT

Pain is an essential part of everyday life. It is necessary and helpful for the individual and the species to survive in a potentially hostile environment.[1] In this sense, pain is adaptive. In veterinary practice, however, many necessary interventions will cause pain as a byproduct. In this context, pain is maladaptive. Maladaptive pain can also be sequela of diseases, such as navicular syndrome, arthritis, laminitis, trigeminal nerve neuropathy, and others. Surgical trauma, especially in the presence of preoperative pain, may trigger a cascade of events that act to sensitize peripheral and central pain networks, resulting in long-lasting maladaptive pain.[2] Adaptive and maladaptive components often coexist in an individual animal (**Fig. 1**). The goal of pain management should be to eliminate the maladaptive portion while maintaining the adaptive component. Recognizing and understanding the differences between the adaptive and maladaptive aspects of pain are critical for effective pain management.

Department of Veterinary Clinical Sciences, College of Veterinary Medicine, University of Minnesota, 1352 Boyd Avenue, St Paul, MN 55108, USA
E-mail address: guede003@umn.edu

Vet Clin Equine 33 (2017) 181–211
http://dx.doi.org/10.1016/j.cveq.2016.11.006
0749-0739/17/© 2016 Elsevier Inc. All rights reserved.
vetequine.theclinics.com

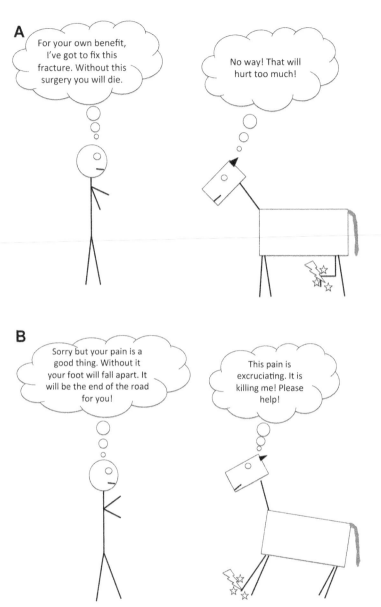

Fig. 1. (*A*) Pain can be adaptive or maladaptive. The normally protective functions of the nociceptive system become a problem when procedures aimed at restoring or improving health need to be performed. (*B*) Chemical, structural, and functional changes in the pain matrix associated with tissue injury secondary to surgery or disease can lead to exaggerated or maladaptive pain.

HOW PAIN HAPPENS

Integration between environmental noxious stimuli and the organism occurs as a series of events within the ascending nociceptive pathways of the somatosensory system (**Fig. 2**). Descending antinociceptive and pronociceptive pathways originating in several brain areas directly and indirectly influence incoming signals

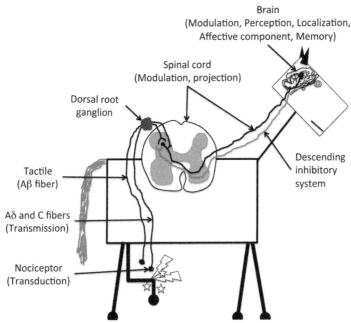

Fig. 2. Noxious environmental stimuli (chemical, mechanical, thermal) are recognized by unimodal (recognize a single type of stimulus) or polymodal (recognize multiple types of stimuli) nociceptors located on the terminals of primary afferent neurons (Ad and C) and transduce these stimuli into action potentials. The generated action potentials are transmitted to the dorsal horn of the spinal cord by the primary afferents via the dorsal nerve roots. In the dorsal horn, primary afferents synapse with local excitatory or inhibitory interneurons that modulate the sensory signal and with second-order projection neurons that project the stimulus to the brainstem and thalamus via the spinoreticulothalamic and spinothalamic tracts, respectively. From loci in the brainstem and thalamus, third-order projection neurons relay the signals to the somatosensory cortex, where location and intensity of the stimulus are identified. The Ad fibers provide a more discriminative localization of noxious stimuli and are responsible for the sharp qualities (primary pain) of some types of pain. The C-fibers provide a more generalized localization of noxious stimuli and transmit pain that is typically characterized by a burning, aching quality that occurs after the initial insult (secondary pain). From the brainstem and amygdala, projection neurons reach the cingulate and insular cortices, which are responsible for the affective/aversive component of the pain experience. Descending pain-modulatory systems (*dashed line*) encoded at several sites in the brainstem exert their modulatory effect predominantly via connections in the dorsal horn through release of neurotransmitters such as serotonin, norepinephrine, and dopamine. The neurotransmitter released and receptor subtype will essentially dictate an antinociceptive or pronociceptive effect. Dysregulation of this descending system may lead to persistent pain states.

primarily through synapses at the level of the spinal cord dorsal horn.[3–8] Under physiologic conditions, peripheral nociceptors have relatively high activation thresholds such that only noxious stimuli are able to generate and propagate action potentials.[9,10]

Following repeated injury or inflammation, both functional and structural changes effectively alter the function of these neural pathways in the periphery as well as centrally (**Table 1**). The changes can occur within microseconds to seconds (through activation of ligand-gated ion channels), seconds to minutes (through activation of G protein-coupled receptors), or minutes to hours (through activation of transcription

Table 1
Functional and structural changes in peripheral and central neural pathways that contribute to the development of pathologic pain

Phenotype	Change	Mechanism
Functional plasticity	Molecular	Activated kinases (PKC, PKA) sensitize ion channels and lower activation thresholds of peripheral nociceptors. Altered protein transcription and/or traffic lead to increased facilitated neurotransmission.
	Synaptic	Enhanced presynaptic neurotransmitter release and postsynaptic receptor density/sensitivity cause central amplification of afferent signals.
	Cellular	Spontaneous activity, after-discharges (ongoing activity after termination of stimulus), and/or expanded peripheral receptive fields (hyperalgesia that has spread to noninjured areas).
	Network	Widespread signal propagation in the central nervous system caused by changes in firing patterns and spread of calcium waves.
Structural plasticity	Synaptic spines	Increase in size or density of synaptic connectivity.
	Connectivity	Axons may sprout, leading to aberrant connectivity (connection between motor/tactile and nociceptive neurons, for example).
	Cell numbers	Axons may degenerate (interneuron loss, for example). Astrocytes and microglia, which release regulatory molecules that influence nociceptive processing, may proliferate.

factors).[9,10] In the sensitized state, innocuous stimuli may be perceived as painful (ie, allodynia); noxious stimuli may result in greater pain (ie, hyperalgesia), and spontaneous discharges may lead to spontaneous pain, indicating the presence of a pathologic pain state (**Fig. 3**).

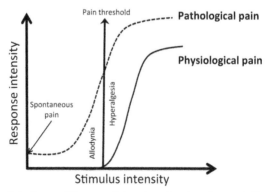

Fig. 3. Under physiologic conditions, peripheral nociceptors have relatively high activation thresholds as not to be triggered by innocuous stimuli, which would interfere with normal activities (but they are also low enough to be evoked before actual tissue damage occurs). Following tissue injury or inflammation, the normal physiologic pain response is shifted to the left. Depending on the conditions, neurons might develop ectopic discharges leading to spontaneous or ongoing pain; innocuous stimuli might produce pain (ie, allodynia), and noxious stimuli produce exaggerated pain (ie, hyperalgesia). This pathologic pain state needs to be managed.

PAIN ADJECTIVES AND CLASSIFICATION

Traditionally, pain has been classified according to duration (acute, chronic), anatomic location (superficial, deep, visceral, somatic, musculoskeletal), quality (dull, sharp, burning, stabbing, throbbing, persistent, recurrent), and intensity (mild, moderate, severe, excruciating, crippling). Although these definitions are helpful, they do not encompass any underlying mechanisms that would help with a rational treatment approach. A more mechanistic and helpful classification has been added and includes nociceptive pain, inflammatory pain, and neuropathic pain.[11]

Nociceptive Pain

Nociceptive pain is produced by activation of high-threshold Aδ- and C-fiber nociceptors (**Fig. 4**). It comprises an alarm system that is activated in response to impending injury, dominates attention, and elicits a strong motivational drive.[11] In veterinary medicine, nociceptive pain is usually not chronically or permanently disabled, but rather must be temporarily halted to allow for the humane performance of medical and surgical interventions. Occasionally, however, permanently or chronically disabling this

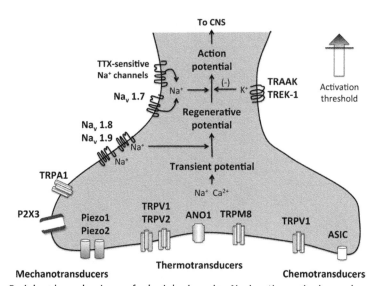

Fig. 4. Peripheral mechanisms of physiologic pain. Nociceptive pain is produced under physiologic conditions only by noxious stimuli acting on high-threshold nociceptors (mechanotransducers, thermotransducers, and chemotransducers). Physicochemical stimuli (pressure, temperature, chemicals) activate ion channels located on sensory nerve endings, creating a transient change in membrane potential that is amplified by sodium channels such as $Na_V1.8$ and $Na_V1.9$ to form a "regenerative potential." At this stage, endogenous inhibition may occur via activation of potassium channels, such as the 2-pore channels TRAAK1 and TREK-1, or further amplified by sodium channels such as $Na_V1.8$ and tetrodotoxin (TTX)-sensitive sodium channels to create an action potential that is propagated toward the central nervous system (CNS) where it will be modulated and finally perceived as an unpleasant physical and emotional sensation known as pain. ANO1, calcium-gated chloride channel (detect heat); ASIC, acid-sensing ion channels (detect protons); P2X3, ATP-gated purinergic ion channel (mediate mechanical hyperalgesia); Na_V 1.7/1.8/1.9, sodium channel subtypes (Na_V 1.7 required for nociception; Na_V 1.8/1.9 required for cold-associated pain); TRAAK, TREK-1, potassium channel subtypes (inhibit regenerative potential); TRP, transient potential channels (TRPV1, TRPM8, and TRPA1 detect heat, cold, and pressure, respectively).

pathway, with a neurectomy for example, may be the best or only option for quality of life of the patient.

Inflammatory Pain

Inflammatory pain is produced by activation of both low- and high-threshold Aδ- and C-fiber nociceptors. Chemical mediators released by damaged and inflammatory cells (aimed at restoring health to the injured tissue) may directly activate nociceptors and evoke pain or, more commonly, act together to sensitize and lower the activation thresholds in peripheral (**Fig. 5**) and/or central neurons (**Fig. 6**). In the periphery, nerve endings begin to secrete inflammatory molecules in a process termed neurogenic inflammation. The sensory system is more easily activated, encouraging a decrease

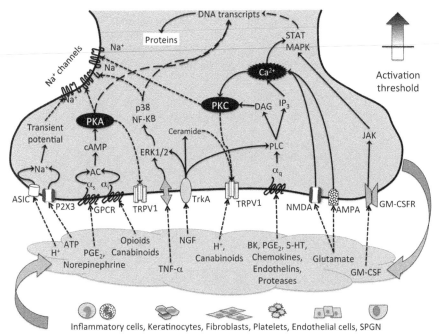

Fig. 5. Peripheral mechanism of pathologic pain. At the site of tissue injury, inflammatory mediators lead to sensitization of nociceptive (A-δελτα and C-fibers) as well as nonnociceptive (A-beta) sensory afferents. Upon injury, both inflammatory and noninflammatory cells release a host of signaling molecules. Mediators such as prostaglandin E$_2$ (PGE$_2$), bradykinin (BK), ATP, hydrogen ions (H$^+$), histamine, serotonin (5-HT), nerve growth factor (NGF), TNF-α, interleukin-6 (IL-6), and others activate ligand-gated ion channels and G protein-coupled receptors (GPCRs) leading to increases in intracellular ion concentration (Na$^+$, Ca^{2+}), activation of calcium-dependent and cyclic adenosine monophosphate (cAMP)-dependent protein kinases (PKC and PKA, respectively), which phosphorylate membrane ion channels and other GPCRs, lowering their activation threshold. Altered protein trafficking and activation of transcription factors (which translocate to the nucleus located in the cell bodies within the dorsal root ganglion) lead to decreased expression of potassium channels (TRAAK, TREK-1) and increased expression of sodium channels (Na$_v$ 1.8/1.9), contributing to lowering the activation threshold of peripheral nociceptors and increasing afferent excitability. With these changes, nerve endings begin to secrete vasoactive and proinflammatory substances, such as calcitonin gene-related peptide (CGRP), substance P, and others, in a process termed neurogenic inflammation, providing a positive feedback to the inflammatory process. GM-CSF, granulocyte-macrophage colony-stimulating factor.

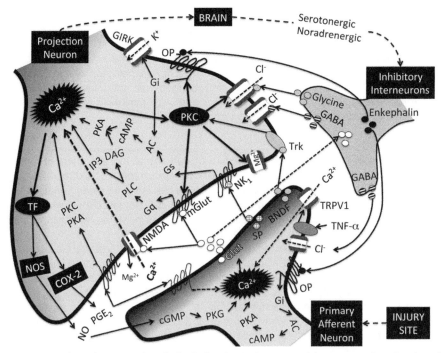

Fig. 6. Central mechanisms of pathological pain. Action potentials generated at the site of injury and propagated via primary afferents to the spinal cord dorsal horn lead to activation of voltage-gated calcium channels (VGCC), calcium-dependent pre-synaptic release of neurotransmitters such as glutamate (Glut), substance P (SP), calcitonin gene-related peptide (CGRP) and brain-derived neurotrophic factor (BNDF) and activation of post-synaptic projection neurons as well as of inhibitory interneurons. Glutamate is the primary mediator of excitatory neurotransmission, with modulatory influences from SP, CGRP and BNDF. Inhibitory neurotransmitters include glycine, γ-aminobutiric acid (GABA) and opioid peptides such as enkephalin released by inhibitory interneurons. They decrease pre-synaptic neurotransmitter release and post-synaptic neuronal excitability by activating chloride (Cl^-) influx (GABA, glycine), by inhibiting adenylyl cyclase (AC) and thus preventing activation of cAMP-dependent protein kinase (PKA). They also activate G protein-coupled inwardly rectifying potassium (GIRK) channels (enkephalin and other opioids). Glutamate transporters located on inhibitory interneurons control synaptic concentrations of glutamate. Glutamate released during persistent nociceptive activity activates N-methyl-D-aspartate (normally blocked by magnesium, Mg^{2+}) and metabotropic glutamate receptors (NMDA and mGlut, respectively), resulting in intracellular calcium (Ca^{2+}) responses with subsequent activation of calcium-dependent protein kinase (PKC), as well as activation of transcription factors (TF). PKC phosphorylates and change the functional properties of ion channels and receptors. Phosphorylation of excitatory receptors (NMDA, mGlut) decreases their activation threshold and increase excitability. Phosphorylation of inhibitory receptors (GABA, glycine, OR) leads to lack of responsiveness to respective ligands and decreased inhibition. Activation of transcription factors (TF) induce the synthesis of proteins such as nitric oxide synthase (NOS) and cyclooxygenase type 2 (COX-2), with production of nitric oxide (NO) and prostaglandin E2 (PGE2). Both NO and PGE_2 act pre-synaptically to potentiate neurotransmitter release, and PGE_2 also act post-synaptically at different prostanoid receptors to activate PKA- and PKC-dependent signaling mechanisms, which will contribute to excitability of projection neurons. Excessive uptake of glutamate leads to death of inhibitory interneurons, further contributing to disinhibition. Microglial release of several inflammatory mediators, including tumor necrosis factor (TNF)-α, lead to transcriptional changes in both pre- and post-synaptic neurons that contribute to increased excitability and long-term potentiation of central pain circuits. cGMP, DAG, diacylglycerol; guanosine 3',5'-cyclic monophosphate; Gs, Gi and Gq, heterotrimeric G protein-coupled receptors; IP3, inositol 1,4,5-trisphophate; NK1, neurokinin 1 receptor; OP, opioid receptors; PKG, protein kinase G; PLC, phospholipase C; TRPV1, transient receptor potential V1 or vanilloid receptor 1; TrK, tyrosine kinase receptor.

in mobility until the tissue heals (adaptive response). However, neuronal changes often result in spontaneous and excessive evoked pain, which is maladaptive and needs to be managed.[11–14] Inflammatory pain can be managed with anti-inflammatory therapies (pharmacologic and nonpharmacologic) and with minimally invasive surgical techniques to decrease extent of tissue trauma.

Neuropathic Pain

Neuropathic pain results from dysfunction of or damage to the peripheral or central nervous system with no discernible protective or reparative role.[11] It is often maladaptive and needs to be controlled. Conditions such as headshaking (ie, trigeminal nerve neuropathy), arthritis, laminitis, and surgical trauma can be associated with neuropathic changes and possibly neuropathic pain.[2,15–17] In humans, neuropathic pain has been identified months to years after surgery.[2]

The goal of this update on equine pain management is to summarize the latest developments in this field. It will also highlight the importance of understanding pain expression and mechanisms to enable a rational approach to pain assessment, prevention, and management in the equine patient. Detailed description of drug doses, techniques and procedures was not feasible in this update. Interested readers can consult a recently published review by Sanchez & Robertson[105] as well the cited references for detailed description of specific protocols and procedures.

OVERVIEW OF PATIENT EVALUATION

Verbally able humans can objectively report whether pain is present or not (which is easily understood by another verbally able human) and can offer descriptors of the magnitude, duration, and characteristics of the pain experience (these are subjective and more difficult to be comprehended by another person). Verbal expression is not an option to assess equine pain. Instead, behavior observations, coupled with evaluation of physiologic parameters, are the backbone for assessing pain and response to analgesics (**Box 1**).

The subject of pain assessment in equine patients has been reviewed in depth recently, albeit descriptively rather than systematically.[18] Different assessment tools may be needed for varying types of pain and painful conditions. Interindividual differences in pain expression and response to analgesics, as well as interevaluator differences in scoring pain, should be taken into account when assessing pain. It is important to recognize that exact recipes for pain assessment and pain management may not suit all horses, even those that have undergone a similar surgical procedure or have the same painful medical condition. Currently, there are no "gold-standard" methods for pain assessment in horses, but there are some "golden rules" that, if followed, should maximize the ability to recognize and treat pain in horses (**Box 2**).

FREQUENT PAIN ASSESSMENT

Systematic pain assessments encourage frequent evaluation of the horse's condition, enabling early detection of changes in pain levels. Early identification of pain not only

---

Box 1
Fundamentals of pain assessment in horses

In general, horses in pain will express new and unusual behaviors and stop expressing normal behaviors, spontaneously or evoked. These behaviors may or may not be accompanied by changes in physiologic parameters such as heart rate, respiratory rate, blood pressure, and gut motility. These parameters should be normalized by adequate analgesic strategies.

Box 2
Golden rules for pain assessment

1. Prevent: Whenever tissue trauma is predictable (ie, surgery), preemptive multimodal therapy should be established, to focus on minimizing the occurrence of neuroplasticity and heightened pain.[19]

2. Be proactive: Do not use rigid minimum pain scores to prompt therapy. If a painful situation/ condition is present, but it is not clear if the horse is painful, or if the pain score is low, consider treating for pain conservatively and observe the results. Individual animal behaviors suggestive of pain or distress should overrule results of pain scores. Critically ill or compromised horses may not be able to express behaviors required to prompt treatment using a pain scale. In these cases, consider a test dose of an analgesic (eg, low-dose opioid) and evaluate results. Increased awareness of surroundings and manifestation of normal behaviors by the affected horse, rather than agitation, suggest a beneficial effect.

3. Be observant: Frequently observe for signs of pain. The health status, extent of surgery or injuries, and anticipated duration of analgesic drugs determine the frequency and interval of evaluations. Expected duration of administered analgesics and how the horse responds to analgesics further help in determining frequency of evaluations.

---

makes it easier to manage but also contributes diagnostic and prognostic value regarding the course of healing. Early detection of problems maximizes the chances of treatment success. Recognition of subtle changes in pain levels may signal the need to review and adjust the analgesia plan. Pain assessment tools should never be used to deny analgesics to a horse that is likely to be in pain. Rather, the tools should be used to determine whether analgesics need to be increased, need to be modified, or can be tapered.

Although frequent pain assessments are important, horses should be allowed to rest and not be unduly disturbed by them. Frequent undisturbed observations of a horse's position within the stall, its body expression, and degree of awareness, coupled with periodic interactive observations, provide more information than the occasional observation of the horse through the stall door. Examples of stall position include whether the horse is in the front or back of the stall and whether it is facing toward the front or back of the stall. Examples of body expression include ear position and movement, relaxed or tense face, chin, and body, calm or agitated demeanor, and whether the horse is standing or lying down. The degree of awareness includes whether the horse is curious, dissociated, or annoyed. Examples of periodic interactive observations include how the horse responds to being talked to, to opening the stall door, and to palpation of wounds or painful areas. In general, the more frequent and attentive the observations, the more likely that subtle signs of pain will be detected and the patient will be better managed. In surgical patients, these observations should start before the procedure to capture what might constitute "normal" behaviors for that individual horse for comparison purposes.

Pain assessment tools are broadly categorized into "unidimensional" and "multidimensional." Unidimensional pain scoring systems are relatively simple, focusing primarily on pain intensity without much regard to sensory and emotional qualities of pain. Multidimensional pain scoring systems are more complex, examining the intensity as well as the sensory and affective (emotional) qualities of pain, to provide a more comprehensive assessment of a patient's pain. These tools have been reviewed in detail recently.[18] A brief description of each assessment tool is presented in **Table 2**.

GENERAL CONSIDERATIONS FOR PAIN THERAPY

1. Pain versus nociception: Pain requires activation of the entire neural pathway, concluding with awareness of a peripheral noxious stimulus. The neural processes

Table 2
Pain assessment tools available for use in horses

Category	Scale	Description	Reliability in Horses
Unidimensional	Preemptive Pain Scoring (PPS)	Relates the expected level of pain with the invasiveness of the procedure. A degree of pain (none, mild, moderate, severe) is assigned based on this criterion. Simple and useful for planning perioperative analgesic strategies. Does not take into account individual variation. Not useful in assessing response to therapy.	Not tested for reliability but useful for planning perioperative analgesic protocol.
Unidimensional	Simple Descriptive Scales (SDS)	The most basic pain scale. This usually includes 4 or 5 descriptors from which observers choose level (no pain, mild pain, moderate pain, severe pain, very severe pain). Simple to use, but extremely subjective and discontinuous. Heavily evaluator-dependent. Does not detect small changes in pain behavior.	Not tested for reliability.
Unidimensional	Numerical Rating Scales (NRS)	These can include simple descriptive scales with numbers assigned to each pain level for ease of tabulation and analyses (0 = no pain, 1 = mild pain, 2 = moderate pain, 3 = severe pain, 4 = very severe pain) or it may constitute numbers from 0 (no pain) to 10 (worst pain possible) placed at equal distances along a horizontal line. This implies equal difference or weighting between numbers, which is often not the case, and they are discontinuous scales.	Not tested for reliability.
Unidimensional	Visual Analog Scale (VAS)	Created in an attempt to improve on discontinuous scales. This scale has been widely used in veterinary medicine. Consists of a continuous line (usually 100 mm) anchored at either end with a description of the limits of the scale (no pain at one end and severe pain at the other end). The observer places a mark on this line corresponding to the perceived degree of pain in the horse under observation. The pain score is the distance (in mm) from zero to the mark.	Tested for reliability in laminitis,[139] colic,[140] and synovitis.[141] In general, it has fair (synovitis) to good (colic) to very good (laminitis) interobserver reliability.

Unidimensional or multidimensional	Dynamic and Interactive Visual Analog Scale (DIVAS)	An extension of the VAS. Horses are first observed for normal/abnormal behaviors (ie, expression, demeanor, posture, stance and mobility) from a distance undisturbed. They are then approached, handled, and encouraged to walk by offering food/treats or using a lead rope. The painful site and surrounding area are then palpated, and a final overall assessment of pain is made, usually using a 100-mm line as in the VAS.	Not tested for reliability but presumably at least as reliable as VAS. Used to assess laminitis pain.[86]
Multidimensional	Composite Pain Scales (CPS)	It is a further development of the simple descriptive and numerical rating systems. Certain behavior categories are chosen (ie, pawing, kicking at abdomen, appetite, appearance, sweating, posture) and assigned a value according to descriptors of intensity/frequency.	Many uses. Has been reliably used for assessing abdominal[140] and musculoskeletal pain.[85,142]
Multidimensional	Horse Grimace Scale/Pain Face	Focuses on changes in facial expression described as low or asymmetrical ears, angle appearance of the eyes, withdrawn or tense stare, mediolaterally dilated nostrils, and tension of lips, chin and certain facial muscles (Fig. 7).	Used to assess postcastration pain,[143] in 2 experimental models of acute pain (mechanical and chemical),[144] and in horses with acute laminitis.[145] Appears to be effective and reliable for assessing acute pain, but not yet formally validated.

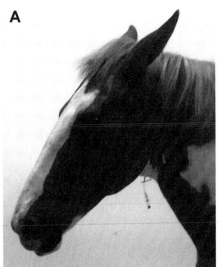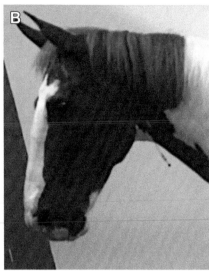

Fig. 7. Pain face. A 17-year-old Missouri Fox Trotter gelding with a 5-month history of right thoracic limb lameness due to ruptured superficial digital flexor tendon. (*A*) Approximately 4 hours after check ligament desmotomy under general anesthesia. Note facial expressions indicative of excessive pain: (1) stiffly backwards ears, (2) orbital tightening, and (3) strained nostrils and flattening of the profile of the nose with elongated lips (upper lip drawn back and lower lip causing pronounced chin). The horse was indifferent to human verbal interaction, positioned at the back of the stall and reluctant to bear weight on affected limb. (*B*) One hour after administration of 60 mg of morphine intravenously. Note changes in the facial expressions. Horse was less withdrawn, more responsive to human verbal interaction, and more willing to bear weight on affected limb. For the procedure, horse preemptively received phenylbutazone (2 g) and was sedated with xylazine (300 mg) and morphine (30 mg). Anesthesia was induced with midazolam (25 mg) and ketamine (1100 mg) and maintained with isoflurane. Additional morphine (30 mg) was given during the 2-hour surgery. Romifidine (10 mg) and morphine (30 mg) were administered to provide sedation and analgesia during recovery. All drugs were given intravenously.

encoding noxious stimuli, but without producing awareness, are termed nociception (**Fig. 8**). Modern inhalation anesthetics (eg, isoflurane, sevoflurane, desflurane) illustrate these differences, in that they are effective in preventing awareness of surgical trauma, but are usually not very effective in preventing encoding of noxious stimuli. In other words, they prevent pain, but not nociception. This distinction is important because activation of neural pathways during surgery, for example, can cause neuroplasticity and enhanced pain postoperatively.[2] This process can also arise if nonsurgical pain is poorly controlled.

2. Preemptive analgesia: This is considered the preventive medicine of pain. Instituting antinociceptive therapy before tissue injury may prevent or significantly reduce pathologic pain and the need for analgesics. Surgery is a unique circumstance in which the precise timing, extent, and nature of the physical insult and ensuing pain are reasonably known in advance, providing an opportunity to design a preventative antinociceptive protocol.

3. Multimodal analgesia: Although a particular type of pain may predominate in individual horses, most clinical scenarios involve more than one type of pain. Even a single type of pain involves multiple mechanisms. Combining pharmacologic and nonpharmacologic strategies with distinct structural and molecular targets provides the most effective pain control (see **Fig. 8**; **Fig. 9**).

Phenotype	Neural Pathway	Therapy	Clinical Relevance

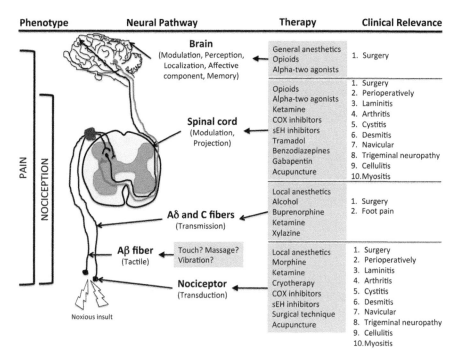

Fig. 8. Pain, nociception, and approaches to analgesic therapy. Pain involves activation of the entire neural pathway. The signal goes from the peripheral nociceptor to the somatosensory cortex in the brain, and the individual becomes aware of the peripheral noxious insult. Therefore, blocking awareness with general or local anesthetic techniques effectively controls pain. However, blocking only the awareness component at the level of the brain does not preclude neural coding to occur at other levels of the nociceptive pathways. This process is termed nociception and can trigger neuronal plasticity that leads to pathologic pain. Several therapeutic strategies targeting different mechanisms at multiple levels in the nociceptive pathways can be used for multimodal pain management of painful conditions or diseases.

PHARMACOLOGIC TREATMENT OPTIONS FOR NOCICEPTIVE PAIN

Nociceptive pain is caused by activation of high-threshold peripheral nociceptors. Response to nociception includes a behavioral response characterized by a motor withdrawal reflex or more complex nocifensive behaviors in conscious horses. Cardiovascular (heart rate, blood pressure) and respiratory (rate and depth) stimulation may also occur as a result of activation of the autonomic nervous system and may be all that is present in the unconscious (ie, anesthetized) horse.

The most effective and desirable method to control nociceptive pain is to interrupt neurotransmission near the site of injury with the use of local or regional blocks using sodium channel blockers (eg, lidocaine, mepivacaine, bupivacaine).[20] Nerve blocks and local analgesic techniques can easily be performed to control pain associated with procedures or conditions on the head, limbs, chest, abdomen, and testicles of horses (**Figs. 10–14**).[21–26] In surgical patients, nerve blocks can be performed in conjunction with sedation or general anesthesia.[27–29] Nociceptive pain can also be modulated with drugs such as alpha-2 agonists and opioids. Alpha-2 agonists decrease afferent activity and activate descending inhibitory neurons. Opioids decrease Aδ- and C-fibers neurotransmitter release and result in hyperpolarization and reduced responsiveness of projection neurons.[30–33] Greater sedative and analgesic effects are often obtained with a

Clinical scenario	Example of Analgesic Strategy	Neural Targets

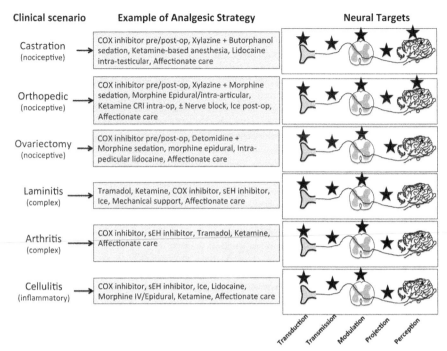

Castration (nociceptive) → COX inhibitor pre/post-op, Xylazine + Butorphanol sedation, Ketamine-based anesthesia, Lidocaine intra-testicular, Affectionate care

Orthopedic (nociceptive) → COX inhibitor pre/post-op, Xylazine + Morphine sedation, Morphine Epidural/intra-articular, Ketamine CRI intra-op, ± Nerve block, Ice post-op, Affectionate care

Ovariectomy (nociceptive) → COX inhibitor pre/post-op, Detomidine + Morphine sedation, morphine epidural, Intra-pedicular lidocaine, Affectionate care

Laminitis (complex) → Tramadol, Ketamine, COX inhibitor, sEH inhibitor, Ice, Mechanical support, Affectionate care

Arthritis (complex) → COX inhibitor, sEH inhibitor, Tramadol, Ketamine, Affectionate care

Cellulitis (inflammatory) → COX inhibitor, sEH inhibitor, Ice, Lidocaine, Morphine IV/Epidural, Ketamine, Affectionate care

Transduction   Transmission   Modulation   Projection   Perception

Fig. 9. Examples of multimodal approaches and neural targets (stars) to maximize the management of conditions characterized by nociceptive, inflammatory, or complex pain in horses.

combination of alpha-2 and opioid receptor agonists,[34,35] and these drug combinations are commonly used in equine practice for perioperative pain control.[36–39]

General anesthetics cause unconsciousness and thus are also effective in controlling nociceptive pain. However, they do not significantly modulate neural coding of noxious stimuli and therefore are not as effective in controlling nociception as local analgesic techniques. The dissociative anesthetics ketamine and tiletamine are probably the only general anesthetics that can also modulate mechanical nociceptive pain to some extent.[40,41] However, they are best at preventing or treating N-methyl-D-aspartate (NMDA) receptor–mediated central sensitization in providing analgesia, in improving response to other analgesics, and in the return to normal function.[42–44]

The most effective and frequently used methods to temporarily halt nociceptive pain involve combinations of general and local anesthetic techniques.[45] The benefits of this approach in surgical patients have been well recognized for more than a century.[20,46,47] These pain treatment options are listed in **Table 3**.

PHARMACOLOGIC TREATMENT OPTIONS FOR INFLAMMATORY PAIN

Inflammatory mediators sensitize and lower the activation threshold of peripheral nociceptors and cause changes in central neural pathways (see **Figs. 5** and **6**), meaning that pain will be elicited by activation of both low- and high-threshold nociceptors. With inflammation, non-noxious stimuli may be perceived as painful, and noxious stimuli cause exaggerated pain, which are referred to as allodynia and hyperalgesia, respectively (see **Fig. 3**).

Despite these changes induced by inflammation, neurotransmission can be effectively interrupted with sodium channel blockers administered perineurally or topically in most inflammatory painful conditions. Intra-articular administration of mepivacaine,[48]

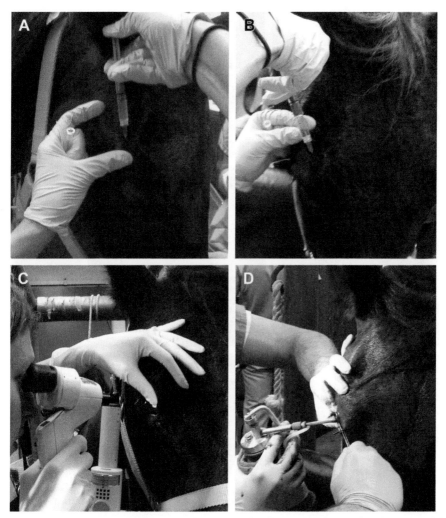

Fig. 10. Auriculopalpebral and supraorbital nerve block in a standing sedated 11-year-old Friesian mare to facilitate ophthalmologic examination and cryosurgery for a small upper eyelid mass.

or ropivacaine,[49] significantly decreased pain scores in horses with lipopolysaccharide (LPS)-induced synovitis, and no adverse reactions were reported. In inflamed joints, μ-opioid receptor expression is upregulated,[50,51] likely through prostaglandin signaling,[50] and intra-articular morphine produces slow-onset, but long-lasting analgesia ($\geq$24 hours).[49,52] Plasma concentrations of morphine were very low after intra-articular administration,[53] which should minimize the risks of adverse effects, such as ileus. Morphine (0.1 mg/kg) can also be added to intravenous regional limb perfusion because it penetrates joints[54,55] without affecting synovial fluid gentamicin concentrations,[55] anecdotally producing analgesia similar to the intra-articular route.[54]

Intra-articular injections of combinations of ropivacaine and morphine,[49] or mepivacaine and triamcinolone,[48] resulted in rapid onset and long-lasting analgesia in the LPS-induced synovitis model. Significant anti-inflammatory effects were

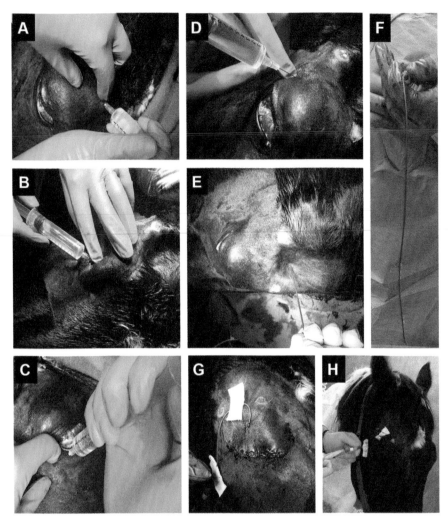

Fig. 11. Preemptive and postsurgical local anesthesia with 0.5% bupivacaine in a 27-year-old Paint horse gelding with ocular neoplasia (teratoid medulloepithelioma) and elevated creatinine secondary to administration of COX inhibitors. After induction of anesthesia, the supraorbital (A), infrathroclear (B), zigomatic (C), and lacrimal (D) nerves were blocked with 2 mL of 0.5% bupivacaine, and the optic nerve was blocked with 10 mL of 0.5% bupivacaine via a supraorbital approach (E). An infusion catheter was custom made by puncturing a red rubber catheter using a 25-gauge needle, sealing the end of the catheter with heat, and capping it with an infusion plug (F). The catheter was placed within the empty orbit and secured in place with Chinese finger-trap suture and butterfly tape (G) and used for postoperative administration of 6 mL of 0.5% bupivacaine twice a day (H). The catheter was left in place for 48 hours without complications and overt signs of either spontaneous or evoked (palpation) pain.

demonstrated with intra-articular triamcinolone[48] as well as with morphine and/or ropivacaine[49,52] but not with mepivacaine.[48] Triamcinolone administered in the distal interphalangeal joint or in the navicular bursa may be effective in reducing foot pain.[56,57]

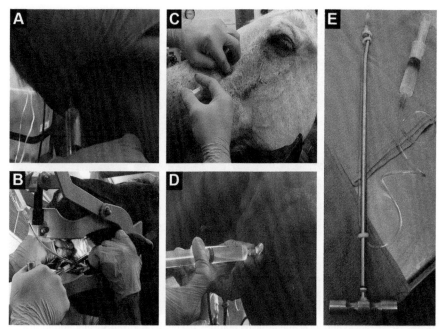

Fig. 12. Middle mental (*A*), inferior alveolar (*B*), infraorbital (*C*), and maxillary (*D*) nerve blocks with 2% mepivacaine in standing sedated horses for odontologic surgical procedures. The inferior alveolar nerve is blocked using an intraoral approach using a custom-made device (*E*), which consists of a metal handle, a regular Luer lock extension set, which is secured to the handle with elastrator rubber bands and connected to a 20-mL plastic syringe on one end and to a 1.5-inches 19-gauge needle on the other end. The needle is slightly curved (~20°) using the needle cap.

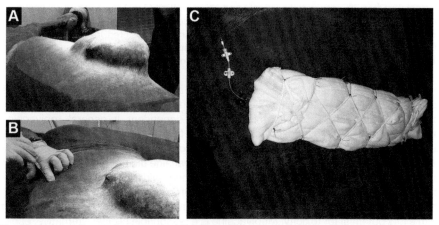

Fig. 13. Preemptive and postsurgical local anesthesia with 0.5% bupivacaine in a 17-year-old Arabian gelding undergoing excision of a noninfiltrative chest wall mass (lipoma; [*A*]). After induction of anesthesia and clipping of the surgical area, intercostal nerves T7 to T13 were blocked with 0.5% bupivacaine (5 mL/site; [*B*]). After mass excision, a commercially available infusion catheter was placed and the incision was closed (*C*). Postoperatively, 20 mL of 2% mepivacaine was infused via the catheter twice a day for 48 hours. Additional analgesics included morphine 45 mg once every 8 hours after surgery and flunixin meglumine (0.5–1 mg/kg) once a day for 7 days.

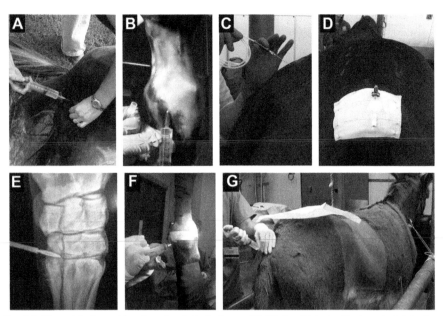

Fig. 14. Nerve blocks and local analgesic techniques. (*A*) Bilateral intratesticular administration of 2% lidocaine (20 mL/testicle in adult horses) helps control nociception and greatly facilitates anesthetic management. (*B*) An abaxial nerve block with 2% mepivacaine performed to facilitate palmar neurectomy. Other nerve blocks (digital palmar/plantar, low or high 4 points, and so forth) can be used to control nociception associated with surgery on the distal limbs. Loss of proprioception is not a major concern, especially if a cast, bandage, or splint is in place. Even very low inhalant anesthetic concentrations will interfere with proprioception, regardless of nerve blocks. (*C, D*) An epidural catheter is being placed for administration of preservative-free morphine 0.1 mg/kg to control pain associated with a P2 fracture. (*E, F*) Intra-articular administration of preservative-free 2% mepivacaine (10 mL) and 1% morphine (3 mL) for postsurgical analgesia in a horse with carpometacarpal osteoarthritis. (*G*) Preservative-free morphine (21 mg) diluted to 12 mL volume with preservative-free 0.9% NaCl and administered in the sacrococcygeal epidural space of a 6-year-old, 210-kg donkey before laparoscopic ovariectomy under standing sedation. Epidural morphine is a useful adjunct for postoperative analgesia in these procedures.

The potential for chondrocyte toxicity with intra-articular local anesthetics should be considered. Studies with cultured equine and human chondrocytes indicate that chondrotoxicity is drug, concentration, and time dependent. In general, ropivacaine appears to be the least cytotoxic local anesthetic, followed by mepivacaine, lidocaine, and bupivacaine.[58,59] In cultured human chondrocytes, concentrations up to 0.5% ropivacaine, 0.25% bupivacaine, and 0.5% mepivacaine did not cause any significant chondrotoxicity.[59] Altogether, the above-mentioned evidence suggests that ropivacaine might be the preferred local anesthetic for intra-articular administration in inflamed joints in horses, because of its analgesic and anti-inflammatory effects, along with a low potential for toxicity. Mepivacaine is a reasonable clinical alternative, especially if combined with morphine or triamcinolone.

In horses, intravenous infusions of lidocaine decrease inflammatory responses to intestinal ischemia and reperfusion.[60,61] Although lidocaine does not appear to change normal gastrointestinal transit time,[62] the incidence of reflux associated with ileus is reduced.[63] Intravenous lidocaine appears not to change visceral mechanical nociception of the healthy equine duodenum,[64] but responses of injured or inflamed viscera have not been evaluated. Conflicting results have been published regarding thermal

Table 3	
Treatment options for the different forms of pain	
Pain Phenotype	**Treatment Options**
Nociceptive	Local or general anesthetics
	Opioids
	Alpha-2 agonists
	Acupuncture
Inflammatory	COX inhibitors
	Soluble epoxide hydrolase inhibitors
	Local anesthetics
	Acupuncture
	Opioids
	Fish oil
	Cryotherapy
	Tiludronate
	Polyphenols (ie, resveratrol)
	Weight management
Neuropathic	Tramadol
	Ketamine
	Soluble epoxide hydrolase inhibitors
	Gabapentin
	Local anesthetics
	Fish oil
	Cyproheptadine
	Tiludronate
	Polyphenols (ie, resveratrol)
	Acupuncture

antinociception produced by intravenous infusions of lidocaine alone[62,64] or combined with ketamine and/or butorphanol[62] in nonpainful, healthy horses. In humans, this technique decreases postsurgical abdominal pain.[65] Considered together, these results support a role for systemic lidocaine in the management of horses with intestinal inflammation and possibly pain.

Several cyclooxygenase (COX) inhibitors are available for the treatment of painful inflammatory conditions in horses. Nonsteroidal anti-inflammatory drugs (NSAIDs) produce pain relief by blocking the generation of proinflammatory and pro-algesic lipids from the oxidative metabolism of arachidonic acid (**Fig. 15**). Despite these beneficial effects, NSAIDs carry a risk of gastrointestinal, renal, and coagulation adverse effects, especially in critically ill horses.[66] In ponies with LPS-induced synovitis, oral phenylbutazone significantly decreased lameness and pain scores without affecting cartilage catabolism, but possibly decreased collagen synthesis.[67] In horses surgically treated for strangulating small intestinal lesions, flunixin meglumine was associated with significantly lower postoperative pain scores compared with meloxicam, whereas there were no major differences in clinical outcomes.[68] In an open-label, single-arm study, a 2-week oral administration of the COX-2-specific inhibitor firocoxib improved signs of lameness in approximately 80% of a group of 390 horses with osteoarthritis. Adverse effects (colic, oral ulcers, edema of lips and gums, lethargy, sedation) were mild and resolved with discontinuation of therapy.[69]

Cytochrome P450 epoxygenases mediate another pathway of arachidonic and other polyunsaturated fatty acid metabolism (see **Fig. 15**). This pathway results in the production of endogenous bioactive lipids known as epoxy-fatty acids (EpFAs), which are subsequently inactivated by the action of the enzyme-soluble epoxide

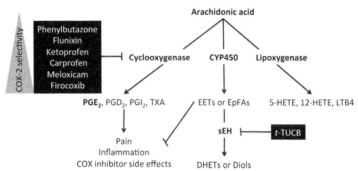

Fig. 15. The arachidonic acid cascade. Arachidonic acid is metabolized by cytochrome P450 enzymes into anti-inflammatory lipids known as EETs (epoxyeicosatrienoic acid) or EpFAs, whereas the COX and lipoxygenase (LOX) enzymes produce largely proinflammatory metabolites. The EETs are rapidly degraded by the sEH to their corresponding diols, the dihydroxyeicosatrienoic acids (DHETs). Inhibitors of sEH such as t-TUCB block this degradation and stabilize EET levels in vivo, leading to suppression of COX-2 transcription and thus affecting the arachidonic acid cascade in multiple ways. Several COX inhibitors, with different COX-2 selectivity, produce anti-inflammatory and antinociceptive effect, along with variable side effects, by blocking production of lipid metabolites such as prostaglandin E$_2$ (PGE$_2$), prostaglandin D$_2$ (PGD$_2$), prostaglandin I$_2$ (PGI$_2$ or prostacyclin), and thromboxane (TXA). Inhibitors of sEH produce antinociception by affecting peripheral and central nociceptive mechanisms and protect against the gastrointestinal side effects of COX inhibitors. COX and sEH inhibitors synergize in terms of antinociception. Key lipoxygenase metabolites include 5-hydroxyeicosatetraenoic acid (5-HETE), 12-hydroxyeicosatetraenoic acid (12-HETE), leukotriene B4 (LTB4). Other polyunsaturated fatty acids can enter this pathway, yielding a variety of EpFAs, with those derived from the ω-3 fatty acid docosahexaenoic acid (DHA) showing the strongest antihyperalgesic activity and being the preferred substrates for sEH.

hydrolase (sEH).[70–76] In rodent inflammatory and neuropathic pain models, pharmacologic inhibition of sEH stabilizes EpFAs and produces antinociception in both the peripheral and central nervous systems.[76–84] The most effective antihyperalgesic EpFAs are those derived from the omega-3 (ω-3) epoxy eicosapentaenoic acid (EPA).[76] Fish oil, a rich source of ω-3 fatty acids, has been included in laminitis and foot pain management,[85] and an sEH inhibitor was useful in managing refractory pain in one laminitic horse.[86] A recent study[87] revealed that digital laminae sEH activity is significantly increased in laminitic compared with nonlaminitic horses. Adjunct analgesic therapy with the sEH inhibitor trans-4-{4-[3-(4-Trifluoromethoxy-phenyl)-ureido]-cyclohexyloxy}-benzoic acid in 10 laminitic horses significantly improved subjectively assigned pain scores. It also improved objectively evaluated forelimb lifts, a pain-associated behavior of equine laminitis,[16] with negligible negative side effects. These results support additional investigations into the potential role of these molecules as a therapeutic approach for laminitis and other painful inflammatory conditions. These treatment options are listed in **Table 3**.

PHARMACOLOGIC TREATMENT OPTIONS FOR NEUROPATHIC PAIN

Neuropathic pain occurs after injury to peripheral or central nervous system neurons, secondary to trauma or chronic inflammatory diseases.[16] In horses, conditions that may be associated with neuropathic pain include idiopathic headshaking,[15,88] laminitis,[16,44] arthritis,[17,89] navicular syndrome,[90] and others. A common feature of the neuropathic pain phenotype is ongoing pain, hyperalgesia, and allodynia that is typically poorly responsive to many conventional analgesics.[9,10,16]

Electrophysiologic studies in horses with idiopathic headshaking have revealed functional changes in trigeminal nerve function, characterized by decreased activation threshold but normal conduction velocities.[15,88] Consistent with these findings, headshaking episodes are often triggered by nonnoxious mechanical stimuli such as touch.[15,91,92] The findings that headshaking episodes may also be triggered by exposure to sunlight and sound produced by clapping hands[91,92] suggest that there may also be changes in the central coding of nonnoxious afferent signals. Changes in sodium channels within primary afferents may be part of the pathophysiology of the disease; infusions of lidocaine or mepivacaine around the maxillary foramen may not block sensory conduction[15] or relieve clinical signs[93] in affected horses. Treatment with NSAIDs, gabapentin, acepromazine, surgical compression with platinum coils, acupuncture, chiropractic and diet modification often shows limited success in headshakers (typically <50%).[15,88,92,93] The success rate appears to be improved (~70%) with oral administration of cyproheptadine, a drug with multimodal mechanisms of action that include antihistaminic, anticholinergic, antiserotonergic, and local anesthetic properties.[15,91] Other treatments, such as phenobarbital, fluphenazine, sodium cromoglycate eye drops, melatonin, and magnesium supplementation, may be useful in individual cases. Readers may consult a recent publication for more details.[92]

A landmark study in laminitic horses revealed reduced numbers of both nonmyelinated (C-fibers) and myelinated (A-fibers) fibers in the digital nerve, upregulation of neuronal injury markers, and increased expression of neuropeptide Y compared with nonlaminitic horses. Laminitic horses also displayed behavioral changes (withdrawn appearance, positioned in back of stall, and increased weight shifts) suggestive of ongoing pain and a hyperalgesic state.[16] Laminitic horses also have increased circulating levels of tumor necrosis factor-α (TNF-α),[44,94] a cytokine that causes aberrant electrophysiologic activity independent of peripheral nociceptor involvement, and may lead to NMDA receptor–mediated central hyperalgesia.[9,95]

Multimodal analgesic strategies are therefore more effective than single-modality therapy in horses with laminitis.[44,96] Accordingly, drugs such as tramadol and the NMDA receptor antagonist ketamine might be beneficial in managing laminitis pain along with NSAIDs and other analgesics.[44]

Tramadol is an opioid receptor agonist, responsible for approximately 30% of its analgesic properties in humans, as well as a neuronal serotonin and norepinephrine reuptake antagonist.[97,98] It can also decrease plasma TNF-α concentrations in patients with neuropathic pain.[99] A study in horses with chronic laminitis showed that oral tramadol had only a transient antinociceptive effect, as assessed with off-loading frequency determined using a force plate system, and only minimal effects on plasma TNF-α concentrations.[44] Poor oral bioavailability[100–102] was not the reason for the limited analgesic efficacy; tramadol is consistently measured in plasma after oral administration, and it has also shown some degree of accumulation at the doses studied (5 and 10 mg/kg, orally every 12 hours).[103] Horses rapidly produce 2 main tramadol metabolites, M1 and M2, but M1 is rapidly and extensively (99%) conjugated such that the free fraction is relatively small. Results of a subsequent study in horses with chronic laminitis showed that off-loading frequency decreased significantly with 10-mg/kg, but not 5-mg/kg doses, and that plasma tramadol and metabolite concentrations were comparable to previous studies.[103] Tramadol has risks of gastrointestinal adverse effects, especially with the 10-mg/kg dose. One of 9 horses administered tramadol (10 mg/kg orally, every 12 hours for 5 days) developed mild colic.[104] Collectively, these results suggest that tramadol may have a place in laminitis pain management. However, it may not be satisfactory as monotherapy for chronic laminitis cases, despite its multimodal mechanisms of action.

A combination of ketamine and tramadol may have a role in treating chronic laminitis pain. At the level of the spinal cord, the molecular mechanisms that lead to neuronal hyperresponsiveness to afferent signals, both from sensitized nociceptors and from low-threshold mechanoreceptors, are highly dependent on activation of NMDA receptors.[104] Ketamine is an NMDA antagonist. A subanesthetic dose of ketamine (0.6 mg/kg/h for 6 h/d for the first 3 days of the study) significantly improved the antinociceptive effects of concurrently administered oral tramadol (5 mg/kg orally, every 12 hours for 7 days) in horses with chronic laminitis. The improvement was evident for an additional 3 days after discontinuation of tramadol. There was also a mild to moderate transient decrease in plasma TNF-α concentrations in these horses.[44] Collectively, these data support the notion that NMDA receptor activation plays a role in laminitis pain, and that ketamine may be a useful component of a multimodal approach for laminitis pain management.

Blocking the generation of proalgesic and proinflammatory lipids with COX inhibitors is a mechanistically sound and commonly used strategy for managing pain in horses, including pain associated with arthritis and laminitis.[96,105,106] However, both arthritis and laminitis pain can be refractory to NSAIDs and other analgesics,[16,44,105,107] suggesting the presence of additional pain mechanisms in these cases. Recent studies in laminitic horses[87] suggest that sEH inhibitors may prove to be an effective strategy to control the neuropathic component of laminitis pain.

Titration of a diluted local anesthetic solution (bupivacaine or ropivacaine 0.125%–0.25%) along the digital palmar nerves through percutaneously placed catheters has been suggested for use in chronically laminitic horses refractory to systemic analgesic therapy.[96] This technique was also successfully used for analgesia in an experimental model of laminitis,[108] but there have been no reports of its use in the clinical setting. Single or repeated epidural (through an epidural catheter) administration of analgesics, such as opioids, alpha-2 agonists, or their combination, is another option for pelvic limb pain management[96,109]; however, their use for laminitis pain has yet to be critically evaluated. Finally, limb amputation and prosthetics may be a palliative option in selected cases.[110]

Intravenous lidocaine may not suppress evoked pain in healthy horses[62,64] or decrease digital laminar inflammation in experimental laminitis.[111] However, it may be helpful in controlling spontaneous pain in clinical laminitis cases. It has resulted in suppression of ectopic activity in A- and C-fibers in rats with experimental nerve injury.[112] Anecdotally, lidocaine patches applied over the digital nerves may play a role in multimodal pain management of laminitis, but studies are needed to evaluate this objectively. In horses with multisite foot lesions and intractable pain,[56] intraneural injection of ethyl alcohol or formaldehyde may provide substantial pain relief for almost 4 months, but these are considered extreme measures.[113] Digital neurectomy may also be an option when other alternatives are not available and the horse can be cared for appropriately.[56]

Although not confirmed in horses, it is likely that arthritis-associated pain may also have a neuropathic component as it does in other species.[89,107] This notion is supported by aging- and obesity-related increases in the expression of proinflammatory and proalgesic cytokines such as interferon-γ (IFN-γ) and TNF-α.[114,115] Cytokines have a role in the pathogenesis of both osteoarthritis[116] and neuropathic pain.[3] A neuropathic component should be suspected in painful arthritic horses that do not respond favorably to COX inhibitors (ie, NSAIDs). In these cases, a multimodal analgesia approach including a COX inhibitor, such as firocoxib,[69] in combination with gabapentin[117] and/or tramadol,[118,119] may prove to be beneficial. Research studies are required to confirm this hypothesis.

Tiludronate, a drug with anti-inflammatory and anti–bone resorptive properties, may be a therapeutic option for horses with osteoarthritis or navicular syndrome.[120] It inhibits cytokine and nitric oxide release as well as osteoclast activity. The drug has been approved by the US Federal Drug Administration for the management of navicular syndrome in horses. Horses with refractory pain and lameness secondary to navicular syndrome responded favorably to a single systemic injection of tiludronate.[121] Similar results were obtained in horses with pain associated with spontaneous thoracolumbar osteoarthritis,[122] in horses with aseptic osteoarthritis of the distal tarsal joint,[120] and in dogs with experimentally induced knee osteoarthritis.[123]

Polyphenols such as resveratrol may become a novel anti-inflammatory and antinociceptive therapeutic option for chronic inflammatory conditions in horses in the future. In one study, these substances were as effective as COX inhibitors in decreasing in vitro production of IFN-γ and TNF-α by peripheral blood mononuclear cells obtained from geriatric horses.[124] Finally, the use of sEH inhibitors is another promising strategy to manage neuropathic pain and to minimize gastrointestinal adverse effects associated with NSAIDs as suggested by results of studies in laminitic horses[86,87] and in rodents.[125] These treatment options are listed in **Table 3**.

NONPHARMACOLOGIC TREATMENT OPTIONS

The role of manual therapies in equine pain management has been reviewed in depth.[126] Manual therapies are thought to affect pain physiology in the periphery (transduction, transmission) as well as centrally (modulation, projection), including an effect on the affective component.[126] Weight management may improve pain symptoms by decreasing load on joints and tissues as well as by reducing the systemic inflammation that to some extent develops with aging (ie, inflammaging) and is accentuated by increased body fat.[115]

Acupuncture can be effective in reducing nociceptive pain. A systematic review identified encouraging evidence on the effectiveness of veterinary acupuncture for cutaneous pain.[127] A recent report[128] described surgical procedures (skin wound closures, sinus trephination, mass removals on eye, chest and abdominal walls, castration, urethrostomy, herniorrhaphy, flank laparotomy, and colonotomy) successfully performed in horses and donkeys with the use of electroacupuncture alone. The investigators cited lack of pain, relaxed surgical conditions, reduced intraoperative hemorrhage, and improved healing as benefits. At least one mechanism of acupuncture-induced antinociception involves increases in cerebrospinal fluid concentrations of β-endorphin.[129] In experimental horses, electroacupuncture produced significant antinociception to rectal distension, as compared with saline,[130] but not to duodenal distension.[131] Positive results have also been reported in horses with chronic musculoskeletal pain.[132,133] Electroacupuncture could alter the gait of both sound and mildly lame horses,[134] but it did not change the lameness associated with palmar heel pain in a group of 9 horses.[135]

Except for diets supplemented with ω-3 fatty acids in dogs, the evidence of efficacy of nutraceuticals to alleviate clinical signs of osteoarthritis in horses, dogs, and cats is poor.[136] Interestingly, as discussed above, the most effective antihyperalgesic EpFAs are those derived from the ω-3 fatty acid EPA.[76] Preventing the breakdown of these EpFAs with sEH inhibitors might constitute a valuable strategy to improve the efficacy of nutraceuticals in horses.[86,87]

Physical agents used to manipulate temperature (ice, heat), magnetic fields, compression, and movement have been recommended as part of equine rehabilitation therapy,[137] but there continues to be a paucity of published studies evaluating these therapeutic modalities. Cryotherapy has received much attention in the prevention and treatment of laminitis in recent years, although this modality has yet to be evaluated as an analgesic in clinical studies. In the oligofructose laminitis model, cryotherapy combined with continuous peripheral nerve blocks with 0.25% bupivacaine and systemic phenylbutazone administration appeared to further decrease weight shifts and prevented lamellar separation.[108]

Although no comprehensive studies could be found, good nursing care and adequate welfare should be integral parts of pain management in horses. Anxiety and stress can enhance pain perception and vice versa[138] and should be proactively managed.

SUMMARY

Physiologic pain is a multidimensional sensory and emotional experience that is vital for survival, but becomes a problem when painful medical practices need to be performed. Tissue injury amplifies physiologic pain and can evolve to a pathologic pain state if not appropriately managed. Surgery is one of the only situations in which the nature, location, and extent of tissue injury are known in advance and an appropriate analgesic protocol can be formulated and established. At the present time, monitoring changes in equine behavior and expression appear to be the best method for assessing pain and response to analgesics. Pain therapy should focus on prevention as much as possible and include a multimodal approach with both pharmacologic and nonpharmacologic strategies.

REFERENCES

1. Cox JJ, Reimann F, Nicholas AK, et al. An SCN9A channelopathy causes congenital inability to experience pain. Nature 2006;444(7121):894–8.
2. Borsook D, Kussman BD, George E, et al. Surgically induced neuropathic pain: understanding the perioperative process. Ann Surg 2013;257(3):403–12.
3. Basbaum AI, Bautista DM, Scherrer G, et al. Cellular and molecular mechanisms of pain. Cell 2009;139(2):267–84.
4. Guo W, Robbins MT, Wei F, et al. Supraspinal brain-derived neurotrophic factor signaling: a novel mechanism for descending pain facilitation. J Neurosci 2006; 26(1):126–37.
5. Lau BK, Vaughan CW. Descending modulation of pain: the GABA disinhibition hypothesis of analgesia. Curr Opin Neurobiol 2014;29:159–64.
6. Yoshimura M, Furue H. Mechanisms for the anti-nociceptive actions of the descending noradrenergic and serotonergic systems in the spinal cord. J Pharmacol Sci 2006;101(2):107–17.
7. Julius D. TRP channels and pain. Annu Rev Cell Dev Biol 2013;29:355–84.
8. Bourne S, Machado AG, Nagel SJ. Basic anatomy and physiology of pain pathways. Neurosurg Clin N Am 2014;25(4):629–38.
9. Kuner R. Central mechanisms of pathological pain. Nat Med 2010;16(11):1258–66.
10. Gold MS, Gebhart GF. Nociceptor sensitization in pain pathogenesis. Nat Med 2010;16(11):1248–57.
11. Scholz J, Woolf CJ. Can we conquer pain? Nat Neurosci 2002;5(Suppl):1062–7.
12. Kassuya CA, Ferreira J, Claudino RF, et al. Intraplantar PGE2 causes nociceptive behaviour and mechanical allodynia: the role of prostanoid E receptors and protein kinases. Br J Pharmacol 2007;150(6):727–37.
13. Ferreira J, Triches KM, Medeiros R, et al. Mechanisms involved in the nociception produced by peripheral protein kinase c activation in mice. Pain 2005; 117(1–2):171–81.

14. Claudino RF, Kassuya CA, Ferreira J, et al. Pharmacological and molecular characterization of the mechanisms involved in prostaglandin E2-induced mouse paw edema. J Pharmacol Exp Ther 2006;318(2):611–8.

15. Aleman M, Rhodes D, Williams DC, et al. Sensory evoked potentials of the trigeminal nerve for the diagnosis of idiopathic headshaking in a horse. J Vet Intern Med 2014;28(1):250–3.

16. Jones E, Vinuela-Fernandez I, Eager RA, et al. Neuropathic changes in equine laminitis pain. Pain 2007;132(3):321–31.

17. Schaible HG. Mechanisms of chronic pain in osteoarthritis. Curr Rheumatol Rep 2012;14(6):549–56.

18. de Grauw JC, van Loon JP. Systematic pain assessment in horses. Vet J 2016; 209:14–22.

19. Deumens R, Grosu I, Thienpont E. Surgically induced neuropathic pain: understanding the perioperative process. Ann Surg 2015;261(6):E161–2.

20. McQuay HJ, Carroll D, Moore RA. Postoperative orthopaedic pain–the effect of opiate premedication and local anaesthetic blocks. Pain 1988;33(3):291–5.

21. Tremaine WH. Local analgesic techniques for the equine head. Equine Vet Educ 2007;19(9):495–503.

22. Henry T, Pusterla N, Guedes AG, et al. Evaluation and clinical use of an intraoral inferior alveolar nerve block in the horse. Equine Vet J 2014;46(6):706–10.

23. Zarucco L, Driessen B, Scandella M, et al. Sensory nerve conduction and nociception in the equine lower forelimb during perineural bupivacaine infusion along the palmar nerves. Can J Vet Res 2010;74(4):305–13.

24. Morath U, Luyet C, Spadavecchia C, et al. Ultrasound-guided retrobulbar nerve block in horses: a cadaveric study. Vet Anaesth Analg 2013;40(2):205–11.

25. O'Neill HD, Garcia-Pereira FL, Mohankumar PS. Ultrasound-guided injection of the maxillary nerve in the horse. Equine Vet J 2014;46(2):180–4.

26. Haga HA, Lykkjen S, Revold T, et al. Effect of intratesticular injection of lidocaine on cardiovascular responses to castration in isoflurane-anesthetized stallions. Am J Vet Res 2006;67(3):403–8.

27. Labelle AL, Metzler AG, Wilkie DA. Nictitating membrane resection in the horse: a comparison of long-term outcomes using local vs. general anaesthesia. Equine Vet J Suppl 2011;43(Suppl 40):42–5.

28. Pollock PJ, Russell T, Hughes TK, et al. Transpalpebral eye enucleation in 40 standing horses. Vet Surg 2008;37(3):306–9.

29. Oel C, Gerhards H, Gehlen H. Effect of retrobulbar nerve block on heart rate variability during enucleation in horses under general anesthesia. Vet Ophthalmol 2014;17(3):170–4.

30. Philipp M, Brede M, Hein L. Physiological significance of alpha(2)-adrenergic receptor subtype diversity: one receptor is not enough. Am J Physiol Regul Integr Comp Physiol 2002;283(2):R287–95.

31. Al-Hasani R, Bruchas MR. Molecular mechanisms of opioid receptor-dependent signaling and behavior. Anesthesiology 2011;115(6):1363–81.

32. Valverde A. Alpha-2 agonists as pain therapy in horses. Vet Clin North Am Equine Pract 2010;26(3):515–32.

33. Hofmeister EH, Mackey EB, Trim CM. Effect of butorphanol administration on cardiovascular parameters in isoflurane-anesthetized horses—a retrospective clinical evaluation. Vet Anaesth Analg 2008;35(1):38–44.

34. Chabot-Dore AJ, Schuster DJ, Stone LS, et al. Analgesic synergy between opioid and alpha2-adrenoceptors. Br J Pharmacol 2015;172(2):388–402.

35. Kruluc P, Nemec A. Electroencephalographic and electromyographic changes during the use of detomidine and detomidine-butorphanol combination in standing horses. Acta Vet Hung 2006;54(1):35–42.
36. Gozalo-Marcilla M, Gasthuys F, Schauvliege S. Partial intravenous anaesthesia in the horse: a review of intravenous agents used to supplement equine inhalation anaesthesia. Part 2: opioids and alpha-2 adrenoceptor agonists. Vet Anaesth Analg 2015;42(1):1–16.
37. Clarke KW, Paton BS. Combined use of detomidine with opiates in the horse. Equine Vet J 1988;20(5):331–4.
38. Love EJ, Taylor PM, Whay HR, et al. Postcastration analgesia in ponies using buprenorphine hydrochloride. Vet Rec 2013;172(24):635.
39. Sellon DC, Roberts MC, Blikslager AT, et al. Effects of continuous rate intravenous infusion of butorphanol on physiologic and outcome variables in horses after celiotomy. J Vet Intern Med 2004;18(4):555–63.
40. Wagner AE, Mama KR, Contino EK, et al. Evaluation of sedation and analgesia in standing horses after administration of xylazine, butorphanol, and subanesthetic doses of ketamine. J Am Vet Med Assoc 2011;238(12):1629–33.
41. Natalini CC, Alves SD, Guedes AG, et al. Epidural administration of tiletamine/zolazepam in horses. Vet Anaesth Analg 2004;31(2):79–85.
42. Muir WW. NMDA receptor antagonists and pain: ketamine. Vet Clin North Am Equine Pract 2010;26(3):565–78.
43. Guedes AG, Pluhar GE, Daubs BM, et al. Effects of preoperative epidural administration of racemic ketamine for analgesia in sheep undergoing surgery. Am J Vet Res 2006;67(2):222–9.
44. Guedes AG, Matthews NS, Hood DM. Effect of ketamine hydrochloride on the analgesic effects of tramadol hydrochloride in horses with signs of chronic laminitis-associated pain. Am J Vet Res 2012;73(5):610–9.
45. Valverde A. Balanced anesthesia and constant-rate infusions in horses. Vet Clin North Am Equine Pract 2013;29(1):89–122.
46. Crile GW, Lower WE. Anoci-association. Philadelphia: W. B. Sauders Company; 1914.
47. Katz J. George Washington Crile, anoci-association, and pre-emptive analgesia. Pain 1993;53(3):243–5.
48. Kay AT, Bolt DM, Ishihara A, et al. Anti-inflammatory and analgesic effects of intra-articular injection of triamcinolone acetonide, mepivacaine hydrochloride, or both on LPS-induced lameness in horses. Am J Vet Res 2008;69(12):1646–54.
49. Santos LC, de Moraes AN, Saito ME. Effects of intraarticular ropivacaine and morphine on lipopolysaccharide-induced synovitis in horses. Vet Anaesth Analg 2009;36(3):280–6.
50. van Loon JP, de Grauw JC, Brunott A, et al. Upregulation of articular synovial membrane mu-opioid-like receptors in an acute equine synovitis model. Vet J 2013;196(1):40–6.
51. Sheehy JG, Hellyer PW, Sammonds GE, et al. Evaluation of opioid receptors in synovial membranes of horses. Am J Vet Res 2001;62(9):1408–12.
52. van Loon JP, de Grauw JC, van Dierendonck M, et al. Intra-articular opioid analgesia is effective in reducing pain and inflammation in an equine LPS induced synovitis model. Equine Vet J 2010;42(5):412–9.
53. Lindegaard C, Frost AB, Thomsen MH, et al. Pharmacokinetics of intra-articular morphine in horses with lipopolysaccharide-induced synovitis. Vet Anaesth Analg 2010;37(2):186–95.

54. Valverde A, Cribb N, Arroyo L. Morphine concentrations in distal forelimb synovial fluid following intravenous regional perfusion in horses. Paper presented at: American College of Veterinary Anesthesia and Analgesia Annual Meeting. San Diego (CA), September 8th, 2013.
55. Hunter BG, Parker JE, Wehrman R, et al. Morphine synovial fluid concentrations after intravenous regional limb perfusion in standing horses. Vet Surg 2015; 44(6):679–86.
56. Gutierrez-Nibeyro SD, White Ii NA, Werpy NM. Outcome of medical treatment for horses with foot pain: 56 cases. Equine Vet J 2010;42(8):680–5.
57. Manfredi JM, Boyce M, Malone ED, et al. Steroid diffusion into the navicular bursa occurs in horses affected by palmar foot pain. Vet Rec 2012;171(25):642.
58. Park J, Sutradhar BC, Hong G, et al. Comparison of the cytotoxic effects of bupivacaine, lidocaine, and mepivacaine in equine articular chondrocytes. Vet Anaesth Analg 2011;38(2):127–33.
59. Breu A, Rosenmeier K, Kujat R, et al. The cytotoxicity of bupivacaine, ropivacaine, and mepivacaine on human chondrocytes and cartilage. Anesth Analg 2013;117(2):514–22.
60. Cook VL, Jones Shults J, McDowell M, et al. Attenuation of ischaemic injury in the equine jejunum by administration of systemic lidocaine. Equine Vet J 2008;40(4):353–7.
61. Cook VL, Jones Shults J, McDowell MR, et al. Anti-inflammatory effects of intravenously administered lidocaine hydrochloride on ischemia-injured jejunum in horses. Am J Vet Res 2009;70(10):1259–68.
62. Elfenbein JR, Robertson SA, MacKay RJ, et al. Systemic and anti-nociceptive effects of prolonged lidocaine, ketamine, and butorphanol infusions alone and in combination in healthy horses. BMC Vet Res 2014;10(Suppl 1):S6.
63. Malone E, Ensink J, Turner T, et al. Intravenous continuous infusion of lidocaine for treatment of equine ileus. Vet Surg 2006;35(1):60–6.
64. Robertson SA, Sanchez LC, Merritt AM, et al. Effect of systemic lidocaine on visceral and somatic nociception in conscious horses. Equine Vet J 2005; 37(2):122–7.
65. Tikuisis R, Miliauskas P, Samalavicius NE, et al. Intravenous lidocaine for post-operative pain relief after hand-assisted laparoscopic colon surgery: a randomized, placebo-controlled clinical trial. Tech Coloproctol 2014;18(4): 373–80.
66. Cook VL, Blikslager AT. The use of nonsteroidal anti-inflammatory drugs in critically ill horses. J Vet Emerg Crit Care (San Antonio) 2015;25(1):76–88.
67. de Grauw JC, van Loon JP, van de Lest CH, et al. In vivo effects of phenylbutazone on inflammation and cartilage-derived biomarkers in equine joints with acute synovitis. Vet J 2014;201(1):51–6.
68. Naylor RJ, Taylor AH, Knowles EJ, et al. Comparison of flunixin meglumine and meloxicam for post operative management of horses with strangulating small intestinal lesions. Equine Vet J 2014;46(4):427–34.
69. Orsini JA, Ryan WG, Carithers DS, et al. Evaluation of oral administration of firocoxib for the management of musculoskeletal pain and lameness associated with osteoarthritis in horses. Am J Vet Res 2012;73(5):664–71.
70. Wagner K, Inceoglu B, Hammock BD. Soluble epoxide hydrolase inhibition, epoxygenated fatty acids and nociception. Prostaglandins Other Lipid Mediat 2011;96(1–4):76–83.
71. Spector AA, Kim HY. Cytochrome P450 epoxygenase pathway of polyunsaturated fatty acid metabolism. Biochim Biophys Acta 2015;1851(4):356–65.

72. Wagner K, Inceoglu B, Gill SS, et al. Epoxygenated fatty acids and soluble epoxide hydrolase inhibition: novel mediators of pain reduction. J Agric Food Chem 2011;59(7):2816–24.
73. Hwang SH, Tsai HJ, Liu JY, et al. Orally bioavailable potent soluble epoxide hydrolase inhibitors. J Med Chem 2007;50(16):3825–40.
74. Morisseau C, Newman JW, Tsai HJ, et al. Peptidyl-urea based inhibitors of soluble epoxide hydrolases. Bioorg Med Chem Lett 2006;16(20):5439–44.
75. Chacos N, Capdevila J, Falck JR, et al. The reaction of arachidonic acid epoxides (epoxyeicosatrienoic acids) with a cytosolic epoxide hydrolase. Arch Biochem Biophys 1983;223(2):639–48.
76. Morisseau C, Inceoglu B, Schmelzer K, et al. Naturally occurring monoepoxides of eicosapentaenoic acid and docosahexaenoic acid are bioactive antihyperalgesic lipids. J Lipid Res 2010;51(12):3481–90.
77. Inceoglu B, Bettaieb A, Trindade da Silva CA, et al. Endoplasmic reticulum stress in the peripheral nervous system is a significant driver of neuropathic pain. Proc Natl Acad Sci U S A 2015;112(29):9082–7.
78. Inceoglu B, Wagner KM, Yang J, et al. Acute augmentation of epoxygenated fatty acid levels rapidly reduces pain-related behavior in a rat model of type I diabetes. Proc Natl Acad Sci U S A 2012;109(28):11390–5.
79. Inceoglu B, Wagner K, Schebb NH, et al. Analgesia mediated by soluble epoxide hydrolase inhibitors is dependent on cAMP. Proc Natl Acad Sci U S A 2011;108(12):5093–7.
80. Inceoglu B, Jinks SL, Schmelzer KR, et al. Inhibition of soluble epoxide hydrolase reduces LPS-induced thermal hyperalgesia and mechanical allodynia in a rat model of inflammatory pain. Life Sci 2006;79(24):2311–9.
81. Inceoglu B, Schmelzer KR, Morisseau C, et al. Soluble epoxide hydrolase inhibition reveals novel biological functions of epoxyeicosatrienoic acids (EETs). Prostaglandins Other Lipid Mediat 2007;82(1–4):42–9.
82. Inceoglu B, Jinks SL, Ulu A, et al. Soluble epoxide hydrolase and epoxyeicosatrienoic acids modulate two distinct analgesic pathways. Proc Natl Acad Sci U S A 2008;105(48):18901–6.
83. Wagner K, Inceoglu B, Dong H, et al. Comparative efficacy of 3 soluble epoxide hydrolase inhibitors in rat neuropathic and inflammatory pain models. Eur J Pharmacol 2013;700(1–3):93–101.
84. Terashvili M, Tseng LF, Wu HE, et al. Antinociception produced by 14,15-epoxyeicosatrienoic acid is mediated by the activation of beta-endorphin and met-enkephalin in the rat ventrolateral periaqueductal gray. J Pharmacol Exp Ther 2008;326(2):614–22.
85. Dutton DW, Lashnits KJ, Wegner K. Managing severe hoof pain in a horse using multimodal analgesia and a modified composite pain score. Equine Vet Educ 2009;21(1):37–43.
86. Guedes AG, Morisseau C, Sole A, et al. Use of a soluble epoxide hydrolase inhibitor as an adjunctive analgesic in a horse with laminitis. Vet Anaesth Analg 2013;40(4):440–8.
87. Guedes A, Galuppo L, Hood D, et al. Soluble epoxide hydrolase activity and pharmacologic inhibition in horses with chronic severe laminitis. Equine Vet J 2016. [Epub ahead of print].
88. Aleman M, Williams DC, Brosnan RJ, et al. Sensory nerve conduction and somatosensory evoked potentials of the trigeminal nerve in horses with idiopathic headshaking. J Vet Intern Med 2013;27(6):1571–80.

89. Ohtori S, Orita S, Yamashita M, et al. Existence of a neuropathic pain component in patients with osteoarthritis of the knee. Yonsei Med J 2012;53(4):801–5.
90. Leise BS, Faleiros RR, Watts M, et al. Hindlimb laminar inflammatory response is similar to that present in forelimbs after carbohydrate overload in horses. Equine Vet J 2012;44(6):633–9.
91. Madigan JE, Bell SA. Owner survey of headshaking in horses. J Am Vet Med Assoc 2001;219(3):334–7.
92. Pickles K, Madigan J, Aleman M. Idiopathic headshaking: is it still idiopathic? Vet J 2014;201(1):21–30.
93. Roberts VL, Perkins JD, Skarlina E, et al. Caudal anaesthesia of the infraorbital nerve for diagnosis of idiopathic headshaking and caudal compression of the infraorbital nerve for its treatment, in 58 horses. Equine Vet J 2013;45(1):107–10.
94. Treiber K, Carter R, Gay L, et al. Inflammatory and redox status of ponies with a history of pasture-associated laminitis. Vet Immunol Immunopathol 2009;129(3–4):216–20.
95. Sorkin LS, Xiao WH, Wagner R, et al. Tumour necrosis factor-alpha induces ectopic activity in nociceptive primary afferent fibres. Neuroscience 1997;81(1):255–62.
96. Driessen B, Bauquier SH, Zarucco L. Neuropathic pain management in chronic laminitis. Vet Clin North Am Equine Pract 2010;26(2):315–37.
97. Collart L, Luthy C, Favario-Constantin C, et al. Duality of the analgesic effect of tramadol in humans. Schweiz Med Wochenschr 1993;123(47):2241–3 [in French].
98. Desmeules JA, Piguet V, Collart L, et al. Contribution of monoaminergic modulation to the analgesic effect of tramadol. Br J Clin Pharmacol 1996;41(1):7–12.
99. Kraychete DC, Sakata RK, Issy AM, et al. Proinflammatory cytokines in patients with neuropathic pain treated with Tramadol. Rev Bras Anestesiol 2009;59(3):297–303.
100. Stewart AJ, Boothe DM, Cruz-Espindola C, et al. Pharmacokinetics of tramadol and metabolites O-desmethyltramadol and N-desmethyltramadol in adult horses. Am J Vet Res 2011;72(7):967–74.
101. Shilo Y, Britzi M, Eytan B, et al. Pharmacokinetics of tramadol in horses after intravenous, intramuscular and oral administration. J Vet Pharmacol Ther 2008;31(1):60–5.
102. Giorgi M, Soldani G, Manera C, et al. Pharmacokinetics of tramadol and its metabolites M1, M2 AND M5 in horses following intravenous, immediate release (fasted/fed) and sustained release single dose administration. J Equine Vet Sci 2007;27:481–8.
103. Guedes AG, Knych HK, Soares JH, et al. Pharmacokinetics and physiological effects of repeated oral administrations of tramadol in horses. J Vet Pharmacol Ther 2014;37(3):269–78.
104. Bennett GJ. Update on the neurophysiology of pain transmission and modulation: focus on the NMDA-receptor. J Pain Symptom Manage 2000;19(1 Suppl):S2–6.
105. Sanchez LC, Robertson SA. Pain control in horses: what do we really know? Equine Vet J 2014;46(4):517–23.
106. Owens JG, Kamerling SG, Stanton SR, et al. Effects of ketoprofen and phenylbutazone on chronic hoof pain and lameness in the horse. Equine Vet J 1995;27(4):296–300.
107. Christianson CA, Corr M, Firestein GS, et al. Characterization of the acute and persistent pain state present in K/BxN serum transfer arthritis. Pain 2010;151(2):394–403.

108. van Eps AW, Pollitt CC, Underwood C, et al. Continuous digital hypothermia initiated after the onset of lameness prevents lamellar failure in the oligofructose laminitis model. Equine Vet J 2014;46(5):625–30.
109. Natalini CC. Spinal anesthetics and analgesics in the horse. Vet Clin North Am Equine Pract 2010;26(3):551–64.
110. West CM. Supporting limb laminitis: learning how to save horses such as Barbaro. Available at: http://www.thehorse.com/articles/18109/supporting-limb-laminitis-learning-how-to-save-horses-such-as-barbaro. Accessed January 7, 2016
111. Williams JM, Lin YJ, Loftus JP, et al. Effect of intravenous lidocaine administration on laminar inflammation in the black walnut extract model of laminitis. Equine Vet J 2010;42(3):261–9.
112. Kirillova I, Teliban A, Gorodetskaya N, et al. Effect of local and intravenous lidocaine on ongoing activity in injured afferent nerve fibers. Pain 2011;152(7):1562–71.
113. Schneider CP, Ishihara A, Adams TP, et al. Analgesic effects of intraneural injection of ethyl alcohol or formaldehyde in the palmar digital nerves of horses. Am J Vet Res 2014;75(9):784–91.
114. Katepalli MP, Adams AA, Lear TL, et al. The effect of age and telomere length on immune function in the horse. Dev Comp Immunol 2008;32(12):1409–15.
115. Adams AA, Katepalli MP, Kohler K, et al. Effect of body condition, body weight and adiposity on inflammatory cytokine responses in old horses. Vet Immunol Immunopathol 2009;127(3–4):286–94.
116. Sutton S, Clutterbuck A, Harris P, et al. The contribution of the synovium, synovial derived inflammatory cytokines and neuropeptides to the pathogenesis of osteoarthritis. Vet J 2009;179(1):10–24.
117. Davis JL, Posner LP, Elce Y. Gabapentin for the treatment of neuropathic pain in a pregnant horse. J Am Vet Med Assoc 2007;231(5):755–8.
118. Guedes A, Knych H, Hood D. Plasma concentrations, analgesic and physiological assessments in horses with chronic laminitis treated with two doses of oral tramadol. Equine Vet J 2016;48(4):528–31.
119. Guedes A, Meadows J, Pypendop B, et al. Evaluation of tramadol in osteoarthritic geriatric cats. J Am Vet Med Assoc 2016.
120. Gough MR, Thibaud D, Smith RK. Tiludronate infusion in the treatment of bone spavin: a double blind placebo-controlled trial. Equine Vet J 2010;42(5):381–7.
121. Whitfield CT, Schoonover MJ, Holbrook TC, et al. Quantitative assessment of two methods of tiludronate administration for the treatment of lameness caused by navicular syndrome in horses. Am J Vet Res 2016;77(2):167–73.
122. Coudry V, Thibaud D, Riccio B, et al. Efficacy of tiludronate in the treatment of horses with signs of pain associated with osteoarthritic lesions of the thoracolumbar vertebral column. Am J Vet Res 2007;68(3):329–37.
123. Moreau M, Rialland P, Pelletier JP, et al. Tiludronate treatment improves structural changes and symptoms of osteoarthritis in the canine anterior cruciate ligament model. Arthritis Res Ther 2011;13(3):R98.
124. Siard MH, McMurry KE, Adams AA. Effects of polyphenols including curcuminoids, resveratrol, quercetin, pterostilbene, and hydroxypterostilbene on lymphocyte pro-inflammatory cytokine production of senior horses in vitro. Vet Immunol Immunopathol 2016;173:50–9.
125. Goswami SK, Wan D, Yang J, et al. Anti-ulcer efficacy of soluble epoxide hydrolase inhibitor TPPU on diclofenac-induced intestinal ulcers. J Pharmacol Exp Ther 2016;357(3):529–36.
126. Haussler KK. The role of manual therapies in equine pain management. Vet Clin North Am Equine Pract 2010;26(3):579–601.

127. Habacher G, Pittler MH, Ernst E. Effectiveness of acupuncture in veterinary medicine: systematic review. J Vet Intern Med 2006;20(3):480–8.
128. Sheta E, Ragab S, Farghali H, et al. Successful practice of electroacupuncture analgesia in equine surgery. J Acupunct Meridian Stud 2015;8(1):30–9.
129. Skarda RT, Tejwani GA, Muir WW 3rd. Cutaneous analgesia, hemodynamic and respiratory effects, and beta-endorphin concentration in spinal fluid and plasma of horses after acupuncture and electroacupuncture. Am J Vet Res 2002;63(10): 1435–42.
130. Skarda RT, Muir WW 3rd. Comparison of electroacupuncture and butorphanol on respiratory and cardiovascular effects and rectal pain threshold after controlled rectal distention in mares. Am J Vet Res 2003;64(2):137–44.
131. Merritt AM, Xie H, Lester GD, et al. Evaluation of a method to experimentally induce colic in horses and the effects of acupuncture applied at the Guan-yuan-shu (similar to BL-21) acupoint. Am J Vet Res 2002;63(7):1006–11.
132. Still J. Acupuncture treatment of pain along the gall bladder meridian in 15 horses. J Acupunct Meridian Stud 2015;8(5):259–63.
133. Xie H, Colahan P, Ott EA. Evaluation of electroacupuncture treatment of horses with signs of chronic thoracolumbar pain. J Am Vet Med Assoc 2005;227(2):281–6.
134. Dunkel B, Pfau T, Fiske-Jackson A, et al. A pilot study of the effects of acupuncture treatment on objective and subjective gait parameters in horses. Vet Anaesth Analg 2016. [Epub ahead of print].
135. Robinson KA, Manning ST. Efficacy of a single-formula acupuncture treatment for horses with palmar heel pain. Can Vet J 2015;56(12):1257–60.
136. Vandeweerd JM, Coisnon C, Clegg P, et al. Systematic review of efficacy of nutraceuticals to alleviate clinical signs of osteoarthritis. J Vet Intern Med 2012; 26(3):448–56.
137. Porter M. Equine rehabilitation therapy for joint disease. Vet Clin North Am Equine Pract 2005;21(3):599–607, vi.
138. Muir WW. Stress and pain: their relationship to health related quality of life (HRQL) for horses. Equine Vet J 2013;45(6):653–5.
139. Vinuela-Fernandez I, Jones E, Chase-Topping ME, et al. Comparison of subjective scoring systems used to evaluate equine laminitis. Vet J 2011;188(2):171–7.
140. Sutton GA, Dahan R, Turner D, et al. A behaviour-based pain scale for horses with acute colic: scale construction. Vet J 2013;196(3):394–401.
141. Lindegaard C, Thomsen MH, Larsen S, et al. Analgesic efficacy of intra-articular morphine in experimentally induced radiocarpal synovitis in horses. Vet Anaesth Analg 2010;37(2):171–85.
142. Bussieres G, Jacques C, Lainay O, et al. Development of a composite orthopaedic pain scale in horses. Res Vet Sci 2008;85(2):294–306.
143. Dalla Costa E, Minero M, Lebelt D, et al. Development of the Horse Grimace Scale (HGS) as a pain assessment tool in horses undergoing routine castration. PLoS One 2014;9(3):e92281.
144. Gleerup KB, Forkman B, Lindegaard C, et al. An equine pain face. Vet Anaesth Analg 2015;42(1):103–14.
145. Dalla Costa E, Stucke D, Dai F, et al. Using the horse grimace scale (HGS) to assess pain associated with acute laminitis in horses (Equus caballus). Animals (Basel) 2016;6(8).

Compounding of Veterinary Drugs for Equine Practitioners

Scott D. Stanley, PhD[a],*, Krysta Moffitt, PharmD[a],
Valerie Wiebe, PharmD, FSVHP[b]

KEYWORDS

- Compounding • Extralabel drug use • Drugs • Horses

KEY POINTS

- Food and Drug Administration (FDA)–approved drugs have undergone safety and efficacy studies in accordance with federal mandates for quality assurance.
- The Animal Medicinal Drug Use Clarification Act of 1994 (AMDUCA) permits equine practitioners to prescribe extralabel uses of certain approved new animal drugs and approved human drugs for horses under certain conditions.
- Compounded veterinary drugs are not approved for any use by the FDA and are considered unapproved new animal drugs.
- Because compounded veterinary drugs are commonly used in horses, it is vital that equine practitioners remain familiar with regulatory recommendations for the use of all compounded drugs.

BACKGROUND

In 2001, the wife of a United Parcel Service (UPS) driver arrived home from work in Walnut Creek, California, to find her 47-year-old husband clutching his head and screaming in pain. He had received a "cortisone" injection that morning for chronic pain. Less than 24 hours after his "cortisone" injection, he was dead. Doctors assumed he died from a burst blood vessel in his brain. His wife wanted to donate his organs but the doctors called her with shocking news; his organs were riddled with bacteria. An autopsy concluded that the seemingly healthy UPS driver died from Serratia meningitis due to a contaminated batch of compounded drug. As a result of the contaminated batch of sterile betamethasone injection, 11 patients were confirmed to have Serratia infection and 3 died.[1] Although this incident caused the

---

Disclosure Statement: The authors have nothing to disclose.
[a] K.L. Maddy Equine Analytical Chemistry Laboratory, School of Veterinary Medicine, University of California, Davis, 620 West Health Science Drive, Davis, CA 95616, USA; [b] Director of Pharmacy, Adjunct Professor of the Department of Medicine and Epidemiology, William R. Prichard Veterinary Medical Teaching Hospital, University of California, Davis, Davis, CA, USA
* Corresponding author.
E-mail address: sdstanley@ucdavis.edu

Vet Clin Equine 33 (2017) 213–225
http://dx.doi.org/10.1016/j.cveq.2016.12.003
0749-0739/17/© 2016 Elsevier Inc. All rights reserved.

State of California to institute new regulations and oversight over sterile compounding, deaths across the nation continue to rise.

Since 2001, numerous human deaths have been linked to contaminated compounded "sterile" medications. A few examples are discussed. In 2011, 9 people died in Alabama after receiving contaminated nutritional supplements traced to a contaminated water supply.[2] In 2012, 64 people died and more than 800 were infected as a result of a contaminated "sterile" compounded steroid made by New England Compounding Center.[3] In May 2015, a $200 million settlement plan was approved setting aside funds for the victims and their families. In Texas, 15 people were hospitalized after heart surgery where a compounded calcium gluconate solution was used that had been contaminated with Rhodococcus equi.[4] In addition to deaths, a vast number of patients have experienced significant morbidity from sterile compounded products. In 2012, an investigation by the Centers for Disease Control and Prevention and state health departments found 47 human patients who developed fungal endophthalmitis from compounded "sterile" ophthalmic products, some containing triamcinolone. Approximately 98% developed vision loss.[5] In 2016, a US District Court issued a permanent injunction against the owner/operator of this Florida compounding pharmacy. The permanent injunction included limits, however, with an exception for drugs for animal use.

Although the equine industry, which is a large consumer of compounded sterile products, might seem spared from the morbidity and mortality witnessed in human patients, this may reflect the lack of forensic documentation in equine patients after death. To date, only the acute deaths of multiple horses all receiving the same batch of compounded drugs have been evaluated toxicologically, eventually linking deaths to misformulated drugs. Well-known examples of these include the polo pony and pyrimethamine incidences (discussed later).

In 2009, 21 Venezuelan polo ponies, on their way to participate in the US Open Polo Championships, died within hours of receiving a compounded vitamin/mineral injection from a Florida compounding pharmacy. The supplement, made to replicate a European medication (Biodyl, Merial, Lyon, France), contained selenium, magnesium, vitamin B, and potassium. It had been incorrectly formulated with toxic levels of selenium.[6,7] Unfortunately, the supplement was used to treat fatigue in horses and not medically necessary.

In 2014, 4 horses died and 6 became ill after receiving a compounded oral product containing pyrimethamine and toltrazuril from a veterinary compounding pharmacy in Lexington, Kentucky. Two lots (one a paste and the other a suspension) were made that were believed to contain extremely high concentrations of pyrimethamine. One of the compounds was tested by the FDA and determined to contain 2380% of the pyrimethamine concentration stated on the label.[8] This drug combination is not approved for any use in the United States and was used to treat horses with equine protozoal myeloencephalitis (EPM). FDA-approved drugs (pyrimethamine/sulfadiazine, diclazuril, and ponazuril) are available in the United States and labeled for treatment of EPM, but an unapproved product compounded from bulk chemical was administered instead. Remarkably, the veterinary compounding pharmacy in this case filed a third-party complaint against the veterinarian who called in the prescription.[9]

Again, the limited number of reported deaths in equine patients is most likely due to significant under-reporting. Therefore, those reported incidences of compounded-associated equine deaths may only represent the tip of the iceberg. From human medicine, the use of compounded products, in particular "sterile" products, is understood to have the potential to carry a very high risk of contamination or of being wrongly formulated. Although new federal and state regulations may improve quality control, the cost of licensing and regulatory oversight may drive some compounding pharmacies out of business or vastly increase product costs. Compounding of sterile drugs is inherently difficult and carries a risk even if all regulations are followed. Unfortunately, the FDA has only recently begun to oversee compounding pharmacies and although new guidelines and regulations have been set (United States Pharmacopeia [USP] 797 and 795) problems with morbidity and mortality continue to be reported. Although compounding pharmacies continue to work toward Good Manufacturing Practice (GMP) standards, it is prudent that veterinarians use FDA-approved drugs whenever possible. Compounded drugs should only be used for those patients where no other options are available.

DEFINITIONS
Food and Drug Administration–Approved Drugs

FDA-approved drugs have undergone safety and efficacy studies in accordance with federal mandates for quality assurance. They must be formulated according to GMPs. Product quality, stability, absorption, storage conditions, therapeutic consistency, and proper labeling are all federally mandated. Labels should have a National Drug Code (NDC) or a New Animal Drug Application number on the label. The label, as well as a manufacturer's package insert, should include the species the product is approved for, dosing, storage information, potential adverse reactions, and manufacturer's information for reporting of adverse reactions.

Not all products that have an NDC number are FDA approved. Products, such as supplements, may have an NDC number but have not undergone the testing to ensure quality, safety, and efficacy. To verify if a product is FDA approved, refer to the FDA Orange Book for approved human medications and the FDA Green Book for approved animal medications.

Generic Drugs

Generic drugs are comparable to brand name drugs in that they have the same dosage form, strength, route of administration, quality, performance characteristics, and intended use. They have undergone testing to establish bioequivalence to the brand name product. Generic drugs may have different inactive ingredients (binding agents and others) but must demonstrate that absorption into the blood stream of the active ingredients is the same as for the brand name drug. An evaluation of 2070 human studies conducted between 1996 and 2007 suggested that the average difference in absorption between generic and brand named drugs in humans was 3.5%.[10] Aside from cost differences, all other manufacturing, packaging, and quality-assurance standards are the same as for brand name products.

Extralabel Drug Use

The AMDUCA permits veterinarians to prescribe extralabel uses of approved new animal drugs and approved human drugs for animals under certain conditions. Extralabel use refers to the use of an approved drug in a manner that is not in accordance with the approved label directions. Extralabel drug use (ELDU) of only FDA-approved drugs (brand name or generic) in animals is considered legal if all AMDUCA regulations and other federal regulations are followed. Veterinary drug compounding is allowed under ELDU. Section 21 Code of Federal Regulations (CFR) 530.13[11] of AMDUCA provides specific conditions under which ELDU from compounding of approved animal drugs or approved human drugs is permitted. The ELDU regulation does not permit animal drug compounding from active pharmaceutical ingredients, also known as bulk drugs. A draft guidance document prepared by the Center for Veterinary Medicine in consultation with the Center for Drug Evaluation and Research and the Office of Regulatory Affairs has been distributed for comments, but as of this writing it has not been finalized.[12]

Adulterated Drugs

A drug or device is deemed adulterated if it consists in whole or in part of any filthy, putrid, or decomposed substance or has been prepared, packed, or held under unsanitary conditions whereby it may have been contaminated with filth. The drug or device may also be deemed adulterated if it may have been rendered injurious to health or if the facilities or controls used for its manufacture, processing, packaging, or holding do not conform to, are not operated under, or are not administered in conformity with current GMP. For compounding purposes, a drug may be adulterated even if it is pure, because a drug is deemed adulterated if it is (1) prepared, packaged, or held in conditions where it may have been contaminated; (2) exposed to a container that may have contaminated it; or (3) manufactured under conditions that do not conform to current GMP.

Misbranded Drugs

Whereas adulteration deals with a drug's strength, purity, and quantity, misbranding focuses on representations made by the manufacturer's label. A drug is considered misbranded if the labeling is false or misleading. Labeling must include (1) the established name of the drug or active ingredients; (2) the proportion of active and inactive ingredients; (3) the name and place of business of the manufacturer, packer, or distributor; (4) an accurate statement of the quantity of the contents; (5) required information to render it likely to be read and understood by the user; (6) adequate directions for use; and (7) adequate warnings against use in pathologic conditions or by children (eg, "Keep out of reach of children"). For FDA-approved drugs, the FDA must approve, as part of the drug approval process, the exact wording of a drug's label and labeling.

Compounded Drugs

The American Veterinary Medical Association (AVMA) statement on Veterinary Compounding[13] states that compounding, consistent with the FDA ELDU regulations, is the customized manipulation of an FDA-approved drug(s) by a veterinarian or by a pharmacist on the prescription of a veterinarian to meet the needs of a particular patient. Compounded medications are often made by compounding pharmacies, outsourcing facilities, laboratories, and veterinarians. Drugs diluted according to the manufacturer's directions or that have added flavoring are currently not considered compounded. Any other manipulation of a chemical or commercial dosage form is considered compounding. Compounded preparations are required to be prepared from FDA-approved animal or human drugs. Common examples in equine medicine include mixing of 2 or more injectable drugs into a syringe or preparing an oral suspension or paste from crushed tablets or capsules.

Compounded drugs are not approved for any use by the FDA and are considered unapproved new animal drugs. Under strict interpretation of the federal Food, Drug, and Cosmetic Act (FDCA), the preparation, sale, distribution, and use of unapproved new animal drugs is in violation of the FDCA. The FDA and federal courts have held that federal drug laws prohibit compounding from bulk chemicals or raw pharmaceutical ingredients; as such, compounds are unapproved new animal drugs. The AVMA has established policies on "Compounding from unapproved (bulk) substances in non-food animals."[14] Preparation of compounded drugs from bulk chemicals is only permissible if medically necessary and when there is no approved product available.

REGULATION OVER COMPOUNDED DRUGS
History

Prior to the evolution of modern pharmaceutical companies, pharmacists and veterinarians prepared medications from bulk chemical ingredients that did not have to meet any standards for purity or safety. Drug labels did not reflect the ingredients, and the lack of any quality assurance resulted in morbidity and mortality of consumers. In 1906, public outcry for safe food and medication resulted in Congress enacting The first Pure Food and Drug Act. This prohibited adulterated or misbranded drugs from interstate commerce. In 1931, the FDA was formally established as the regulatory agency to monitor the safety of all commercial preparations of food and drugs.

After this enactment, pharmacy compounding was legal simply because it was practiced on a small-scale basis by pharmacists who prepared medications based on an individual prescription. Compounded products used FDA-approved dosage forms (commercial tablets, capsules, solutions, and so forth) as their chemical source to formulate a more dilute or palatable product. These were often mixed with USP sources of diluents or chemicals. Regulatory oversight of compounded drugs has been significantly less rigorous in the past than that for FDA-approved drugs and, as such, has proved a much greater risk to patients. There is typically no stability, safety, efficacy, standardized labeling, or product information for safe use.

With the advent of large health care insurance plans for humans in the early 1990s, there was a significant loss in profits to pharmacies because prescription plan copays no longer covered the cost of most drugs. Cash-paying customers and products not covered by insurance (compounded drugs) were the only source of profit. With the limited profits made by pharmacists dispensing FDA-approved drugs, compounding pharmacists quickly identified a new cash-based consumer group. Compounding pharmacies then became engaged in activities that extended beyond the boundaries of traditional pharmacy compounding, including large-scale production of compounded medications not pursuant to an individual prescription and the use of bulk chemical products to circumvent costs.

Current Compounding Oversight

As a result of increasing reports of morbidity and mortality in human medicine resulting from compounded drugs, current regulations overseeing compounding for humans patients have become very strict. Federal law now mandates that all sterile products are made according to USP 797[15] standards and nonsterile products must be made according to USP 795[16] standards. The FDA has traditionally been more lenient concerning compounding for veterinary patients unless it involves food animals. In general, they defer to state authorities regarding the day-to-day regulation of compounding by veterinarians and pharmacists of drugs intended for use in animals. The AMDUCA does apply to compounding of animal drugs and has its own set of regulations that should also be followed. The FDCA does not distinguish between compounded versus manufactured drugs. Thus, the position of the FDA is that the FDCA does not exempt veterinarians or pharmacists from approval requirements in the new animal drug provisions of the FDCA (21 USC Section 360b).

If compounding activities by veterinarians or pharmacists result in significant violations of the new animal drug adulteration or misbranding provisions of the FDCA, the

FDA seriously considers enforcement action. The FDA has determined that it will take into consideration whether a veterinarian or pharmacist has engaged in any of the following:

1. Compounding of the drugs for use in situations where the health of the animal is not threatened
2. Compounding of drugs where suffering or death of the animal is not likely to result from failure to treat
3. Compounding of drugs for third parties who resell to individual patients
4. Offering compounded drug products at wholesale to other state licensed persons or commercial entities for resale
5. Failing to operate in conformance with applicable state law regulating the practice of pharmacy
6. Compounding of drugs for use in animals where an approved new animal drug or approved new human drug used as labeled or in conformity with 21 CFR part 530 will, in the available dosage form and concentration, appropriately treat the condition diagnosed

When to Use Compounded Products

The AVMA recommends the following when deciding to use compounded medications:

1. The decision to use a compounded product must be veterinary driven, based on a valid veterinarian-client-patient relationship, and should be based on evidence-based medicine.
2. Compounding should be implemented in compliance with AMDUCA. Use of compounded preparations in food animals may have food safety concerns that preclude their use unless information exists to assure avoidance of violative drug residues.
3. Use of a compounded preparation should be limited to
   a. Those individual patients for which no other method or route of drug delivery is practical
   b. Those drugs for which safety, efficacy, and stability have been demonstrated in the specific compounded form in the target species
   c. Disease conditions for which a quantifiable response to therapy or drug concentration can be monitored

PREPARATION OF COMPOUNDED PRODUCTS
Quality and Practice Standards

Compounding is divided into 2 categories, sterile versus nonsterile, with each category having its own set of guidelines to follow in its preparation. Nonsterile compounding includes medications, such as tablets, capsules, suspensions, solutions, and topical preparations. Sterile compounding in equine medicine most commonly includes products used for injections and ophthalmic preparations. The USP chapters 795 and 797 provide guidance on good practices for preparing nonsterile and sterile preparations, respectively. It is important to be familiar with these guidelines as a practitioner. USP 797 for sterile compounding establishes quality and practice standards to minimize harm to human and animal patients. It details the importance of the compounding area location, clean rooms, the use of International Organization for Standardization (ISO) hoods, aseptic technique, proper garbing, and guidelines for sterility and bacterial endotoxin testing.

Sterile Compounding

In 2014, the California State Board of Pharmacy found 49% of inspected sterile compounding sites to have 1 or more violations. Failure to meet or maintain facility and equipment standards, such as regular cleaning and disinfecting, were among the top violations.[17] With sterile compounding having a higher risk for potential harm to a patient, it is essential to have proper training, technique, equipment, and protocols in place.

A clean room is required in most states to perform sterile compounding. Current USP 797 requirements suggest that the clean room must be a separate area with walls and doors; there should be high-efficiency particulate air (HEPA)-filtered air that provides at least ISO class 7 or better air quality where the primary engineering control (PEC) is physically located. For nonhazardous compounding, a minimum positive pressure differential of 0.02-in to 0.05-in water column relative to all adjacent spaces is required. For hazardous drug compounding, at least 30 air changes per hour of HEPA-filtered supply air are required. In addition, the clean room must have a negative pressure of 0.01-in to 0.03-in water column relative to all adjacent spaces. In lieu of a clean room, a compounding aseptic containment isolator designed to provide worker protection from exposure to undesirable levels of airborne drugs may be used for nonhazardous preparations; the air must be exhausted to the outside for hazardous drugs. A compounding aseptic isolator specifically designed for nonhazardous compounding with a unidirectional HEPA-filtered air may also be used.

A segregated sterile compounding area means there is a designated space for sterile-to-sterile compounding. In this space, a PEC is located within either a demarcated area (with at least a 3-ft perimeter) or the PEC may be located in a separate room. The area should be free of traffic and materials extraneous to the compounding process. The area should not have a sink or other running water. All sterile products made in a segregated sterile compounding area must be administered to the patient within 12 hours or less.

Compounding from Bulk Drugs

The FDA recognizes that there are circumstances where no drug is available to treat a horse with a particular condition, because there either is not an approved drug or no drug is available under the ELDU provisions. In those limited circumstances, an animal drug compounded from bulk drug substances may be an appropriate treatment option. The FDA further suggests that "the unrestricted compounding of animal drugs from bulk drug substances has the potential to compromise food safety, place animals or humans at undue risk from unsafe or ineffective treatment, and undermine the incentives to develop and submit new animal drug applications to the FDA containing data and information to demonstrate that the product is safe, effective, properly manufactured, and accurately labeled."

In the FDA Guidance for Industry: Compounding Animal Drugs from Bulk Drug Substance[12] suggests the following guidelines.

Animal Drugs Compounded in a Licensed Pharmacy from Bulk Chemicals

1. The drug must be compounded by or under the direct supervision of a licensed pharmacist.[12]
2. "The drug is dispensed after receipt of a valid prescription from a veterinarian for an *individual animal patient* that comes directly from the prescribing veterinarian or from the patient's owner or caretaker to the compounding pharmacy. A drug may be compounded in advance of receipt of a prescription in a quantity that

does not exceed the amount of drug compounded pursuant to patient-specific prescriptions based on a history of receipt of such patient specific prescriptions for that drug product over any consecutive 14-day period within the previous 6 months."[12]

3. "The drug is not intended for use in food-producing animals and the prescription or documentation accompanying the prescription contains the statement "This patient is not a food-producing animal.""[12]

4. If the drug contains a bulk drug substance that is a component of any marketed FDA-approved animal or human drug, there must be a clinical difference for the patient as determined by the veterinarian, and the change between the compounded drug and FDA-approved drug must be documented.[12]

5. "If there is an FDA-approved animal or human drug with the same active ingredient(s) the pharmacy determines that the compounded drug cannot be made from the FDA-approved drug(s), and documents that determination."[12]

6. The pharmacy receives from the veterinarian (either directly or through the patients owner/caretaker), in addition to any other required by state law, the following, which can be documented on the prescription or documentation accompanying the prescription: (1) identification of the species and (2) the statement, "There are no FDA-approved animal or human drugs that can be used as labeled or in an extralabel manner under section 512(a) (4) or (5) and 21 CFR part 530 to appropriately treat the disease, symptom, or condition for which this drug is being prescribed."[12]

7. "Any bulk drug substance used to compound the drug is manufactured by an establishment that is registered under section 510 of the Federal Food, Drug and Cosmetic Act (21 U.S.C. 360) (including a foreign establishment that is registered under section 510) and is accompanied by a valid certificate-of-analysis."[12]

8. The drug is compounded in accordance with chapters 795 and 797 of the USP and National Formulary (USP-NF).[12]

9. "The drug is not sold or transferred by an entity other than the entity that compounded such drug. For purposes of this condition, a sale or transfer does not include administration of a compounded drug by a veterinarian to a patient under his or her care."[12]

10. "Within 15 days of becoming aware of any product defect or serious adverse event associated with animal drugs if compounded from bulk drug substances, the pharmacy reports it to FDA on Form FDA 1932a. FDA Form 1932a can be downloaded at http://www.fda.gov/downloads/aboutfda/reportsmanualsforms/forms/animaldrugforms/ucm048817.pdf."[12]

11. "The label of any compounded drug indicates the species of the intended animal patient, the name of the animal patient and the name of the owner or caretaker of the animal patient."[12]

Animal Drugs Compounded by a Licensed Veterinarian from Bulk Chemicals

1. The drug is compounded and dispensed by a veterinarian to treat an individual animal patient under his or her care.[12]

2. The drug is not intended for use in food-producing animals.[12]

3. If the drug contains a bulk drug substance that is a component of any marketed FDA-approved animal or human drug, the change between the compounded drug and the comparable FDA-approved animal or human drug must produce a clinical difference for the patient as determined by the veterinarian.[12]

4. "There are no FDA-approved animal or human drugs that can be used as labeled or in an extralabel manner under section 512(a)(4) or (5) of the FD&C Act and 21 CFR

part 530 to appropriately treat the disease, symptom, or condition for which this drug is being prescribed."[12]

5. The drug is compounded in accordance with USP-NF chapters 795 and 797.[12]

6. Any bulk drug substance used to compound the drug is manufactured by an establishment that is registered under section 510 of the FD&C Act (21 U.S.C. 360) (including a foreign establishment that is registered under section 510) and is accompanied by a valid certificate-of-analysis.[12]

7. "The drug is not sold or transferred by the veterinarian compounding the drug. For the purposes of this condition, a sale or transfer does not include the administration of a compounded drug by the veterinarian to a patient under his or her care, or the dispensing of a compounded animal drug by the veterinarian to the owner or caretaker of an animal under his or her care."[12]

8. "Within 15 days of becoming aware of any product defect or serious adverse event associated with animal drugs the veterinarian compounded from bulk drug substances, he or she reports it to FDA on Form FDA 1932a. FDA Form 1932a can be downloaded at http://www.fda.gov/downloads/aboutfda/reportsmanualsforms/forms/animaldrugforms/ucm048817.pdf."[12]

9. "The label of any compounded drug indicates the species of the intended animal patient, the name of the animal patient and the name of the owner or caretaker of the animal patient."[12]

Requirements

Prescriptions

A valid prescription written by a licensed veterinarian is needed for a compounded medication. For more information on the requirements of a prescription, refer to "Guidelines for Veterinary Prescription Drugs" from the AVMA.[18]

Record keeping/labeling

Veterinarians should comply with all aspects of the federal ELDU regulations, including record-keeping and labeling requirements and urge compounding pharmacies to do the same. In addition to state and federally required information for prescription labels, compounded prescription labels should specifically state that the product is not FDA approved and include a lot number, assigned beyond use date (BUD), generic name, quantity or concentration of each active ingredient, and storage conditions. For compounding, there are 2 types of records that need to be prepared: the Master Formulation Record and the compounding record. The Master Formulation Record is similar to a recipe; it is a document that outlines the exact details in how to prepare the compound, including calculations to verify quantities to be used, references used for development of the product, and established BUD. The compounding record is a document that is prepared each time a compound is made outlining the ingredients used, any deviations from the master formula, and final product description and verification.

The Master Formulation Record needs to include the following information:

- Assigned name, strength, and dosage form of the compound
- Calculations needed to determine and verify quantities of components and doses of active pharmaceutical ingredients
- Description of all ingredients and their quantities
- Compatibility and stability information, including references when available
- Equipment needed to prepare the preparation, when appropriate
- Detailed mixing instructions
- Sample labeling information

- Container used in dispensing
- Packaging and storage requirements
- Description of final compound
- Quality-control procedures and expected results

Compounding records need to include the following information:

- Name, strength, and dosage form of the compound
- Date, and time if sterile product, of preparation
- Assigned internal identification number, such as a lot number
- Signature or initials of individuals involved in each step of preparation or verification
- Name, weight/measurement, manufacturer, lot number, and expiration date of each ingredient
- Total quantity compounded
- Assigned BUD
- Documentation of the calculations made to determine and verify quantities and/or concentrations of components
- Documentation of quality control procedures (pH, visual inspection, and so forth)
- Description of final preparation
- Any deviations from the Master Formulation Record, if used, and any problems or errors experienced during the compounding

Consultation

Use of a compounded preparation should be accompanied by the same precautions followed when using an approved drug, which includes counseling of the client regarding potential adverse reactions, including therapeutic failure, and attention to the potential for unintended human or animal exposure to the drug. By law, clients must now be informed that compounded preparations have not been evaluated by the FDA for potency, stability, efficacy, or safety, and client consent should also be obtained. Consultation may be in writing or verbally given. Veterinarians should report suspected adverse events, including therapeutic failure and quality defects involving compounded preparations to the compounding pharmacy, state board of pharmacy, and the FDA Center for Veterinary Medicine.[19]

DISPENSATION OF COMPOUNDED PRODUCTS

The AVMA asserts that veterinarians should be able to legally maintain sufficient quantities of compounded preparations for their office for urgent administration needs or emergency situations. State laws and regulations vary, however, concerning the administration and dispensation of compounded products and the veterinarian should make themselves aware of the laws in their states. Currently states that do not allow administration or dispensation of compounded drugs for office use include New York and New Mexico.[20] States that currently permit both the administration and dispensation of compounded products for Office Use include California, Florida, Maine, Michigan, Minnesota, Nebraska, Tennessee, Texas, and Virginia.[19] In most states there are limitations on the quantities that can be dispensed to clients. For instance, in California there is currently a 72-hour limit of compounded drug for Office Use that can be sent home with a client. The idea here is that this duration permits enough time for a compounding facility to make further drug pursuant to a prescription. The drug can be sent directly to the client by the compounding facility. This law is currently under review in the State of California and may be expanded to a 120 day supply or limits may be lifted entirely for veterinary patients.

States that currently allow veterinary offices to administer compounded products but prohibit them from dispensing or reselling products compounded by a pharmacy include Alabama, Alaska, Arizona, Arkansas, Connecticut, Georgia, Iowa, Kentucky, Louisiana, Maryland, Missouri, North Carolina, North Dakota, Ohio, Oklahoma, Rhode Island, Utah, Vermont, Washington, West Virginia, and Wyoming.[19] Other states typically allow administration but are not clear regarding dispensation of compounded products. Verification should be obtained with each state board of pharmacy for any changes on their regulation for use and dispensation of compounded products.

It is illegal to compound large quantities of compounded products to be sold to third parties (including veterinarians and companies) or wholesalers for resale to individual patients.

RECOMMENDATIONS ON SELECTION OF COMPOUNDING PHARMACIES

Consider the following when deciding how to choose a compounding pharmacy:

- Is the compounding pharmacy licensed with the state board of pharmacy?
  - The pharmacy needs to be licensed with the board of pharmacy in the state that the medication is prepared in.
  - Most states also require the compounding pharmacy to be licensed with the board of pharmacy in each state that it ships prescriptions to.
- Do the pharmacist and compounding personnel have specialized training in veterinary pharmacy and compounding?
  - There are differences in the utilization and metabolism of medications in animals and veterinary pharmacology is not standardized in the pharmacy school curriculum. Thus, it is important that the compounding pharmacy has knowledge of these differences.
- Is the pharmacy accredited by an independent organization?
  - Independent accrediting organizations, such as the Pharmacy Compounding Accreditation Board (PCAB), highlight pharmacies that adhere to standards and best practices, such as those published by the USP, to help provide the highest quality in their compounding process and products.
- How does the pharmacy establish BUDs?
  - The BUD, as defined by USP, is the date after which a compounded preparation should not be used; this is determined from the date the preparation is compounded. The compounding pharmacist is responsible for establishing the BUD and should use stability information, if available, on the drug and preparation in question. When stability information is not available, the USP has guidelines for setting a maximum BUD.
- Have there been any disciplinary actions taken against the pharmacy?
  - Check with the state board of pharmacy to see if any citations have been made against the pharmacy.
  - Check with the state FDA Web site to see if any warning letters have been made against the pharmacy.
- Will the pharmacy compound a similar product to one that is commercially available for a cheaper price?
  - If so, this is a red flag that the pharmacy is likely not following regulations and inappropriately using bulk chemicals from a non–FDA-approved source.

SUGGESTED WEB SITES

1. USP: www.usp.org

2. The Ins and Outs of Extra-Label Drug Use in Animals: A Resource for Veterinarians www.fda.gov/AnimalVeterinary/ResourcesforYou/ucm380135.htm
3. PCAB: www.achc.org/pcab
4. FDA-approved human drugs (FDA Orange Book): www.accessdata.fda.gov/scripts/cder/ob/
5. FDA-approved animal drugs (FDA Green Book): www.accessdata.fda.gov/scripts/animaldrugsatfda/
6. Form to report adverse event for animal drugs, including compounded drugs: www.fda.gov/downloads/AboutFDA/ReportsManualsForms/Forms/AnimalDrugForms/UCM048817.pdf

REFERENCES

1. Civen R. Outbreak of *Serratia marcescens* infections following injection of betamethasone compounded at a community pharmacy. Clin Infect Dis 2006;43(7):831–7.
2. Gupts N. Outbreak of *Serratia marcescens* bloodstream infections in patients receiving parenteral nutrition prepared by a compounding pharmacy. Clin Infect Dis 2014;59(1):1–8.
3. Multistate outbreak of fungal meningitis and other infections. Available at: http://www.cdc.gov/hai/outbreaks/meningitis.html. Accessed March 7, 2016.
4. FDA announces nationwide voluntary recall of all products for sterile use from Specialty Compounding. Available at: http://www.fda.gov/NewsEvents/Newsroom/PressAnnouncements/ucm364644.htm. Accessed March 7, 2016.
5. Mikosz CA, Smith RM, Kim M, et al. Fungal endophthalmitis associated with compounded products. Emerg Infect Dis 2014;20(2). Available at: http://wwwnc.cdc.gov/eid/article/20/2/13-1257_article. Accessed June 2, 2016.
6. Desta B, Maldonado G, Reid H, et al. Acute selenium toxicosis in polo ponies. J Vet Diagn Invest 2011;23(3):623–8.
7. Osborne M. Compounding issues resurface in wake of ponies' deaths. JAVMA News 2009. Available at: https://www.avma.org/News/JAVMANews/Pages/090615r.aspx. Accessed March 6, 2016.
8. FDA Warning Letter. Available at: http://www.fda.gov/ICECI/EnforcementActions/WarningLetters/2014/ucm410141.htm. Accessed March 6, 2016.
9. AVMA PLIT: Risk awareness alert. Available at: http://www.avmaplit.com/Risk-Awareness-Alert/. Accessed June 2, 2016.
10. Davit BM, Nwakama PE, Buehler GJ, et al. Comparing generic and innovator drugs: a review of 12 years of bioequivalence data from the United States Food and Drug Administration. Ann Pharmacother 2009;43(10):1583–97.
11. 21 CFR 530.13 Extra Label Use From Compounding of Approved New Animal and Approved Human Drugs. Available at: http://www.ecfr.gov/cgi-bin/text-idx?SID=e260b8ac1a597285e44396032d59ab3a&mc=true&node=pt21.6.530&rgn=div5#se21.6.530_113. Accessed June 2, 2016.
12. Guidance for Industry Compounding Animal Drugs from Bulk Drug Substances (Draft). Available at: http://www.fda.gov/downloads/AnimalVeterinary/GuidanceComplianceEnforcement/GuidanceforIndustry/UCM446862.pdf. Accessed May 20, 2016.
13. AVMA: Veterinary Compounding. Available at: https://www.avma.org/KB/Policies/Pages/Compounding.aspx. Accessed June 2, 2016.
14. AVMA: Compounding from Unapproved (Bulk) Substances in Non-Food Animals. Available at: https://www.avma.org/KB/Policies/Pages/Compounding-from-Unapproved-Bulk-Substances-in-Non-Food-Animals.aspx. Accessed June 2, 2016.

15. USP <797> Pharmaceutical Compounding- Sterile Preparations.
16. USP <795> Pharmaceutical Compounding- Nonsterile Preparations.
17. California Board of Pharmacy, Department of Consumer Affairs, Enforcement and Compounding Committee Meeting Minutes, June 24, 2015.
18. Guidelines for Veterinary Prescription Drugs. Available at: https://www.avma.org/KB/Policies/Pages/Guidelines-for-Veterinary-Prescription-Drugs.aspx. Accessed June 2, 2016.
19. Form to report adverse event for animal drugs, including compounded drugs. Available at: www.fda.gov/downloads/AboutFDA/ReportsManualsForms/Forms/AnimalDrugForms/UCM048817.pdf. Accessed June 2, 2016.
20. AVMA: Administration and dispensing of compounded veterinary drugs. Available at: https://www.avma.org/Advocacy/StateAndLocal/Pages/compoundinglaws.aspx. Accessed June 2, 2016.

Special Review
by Consulting Editor
Thomas J. Divers

Literature Review

Recent Equine Scientific Publications of Interest—"Just in Case You Missed Them"

The equine publications I have listed and commented on are certainly not the only important equine publications this year but, instead, comprise a mixture of medicine, surgery, ophthalmology, reproduction, and anesthesia publications that I wanted to make sure you have read. Each of these publications either provides new information that might be directly applicable to clinical practice, previously unknown information about a disorder, or points out a new idea/concept for consideration. I hope that I have accurately summarized each article and that the comments I have added do not detract from the articles.

The Equine Movement Disorder "Shivers" Is Associated With Selective Cerebellar Purkinje Cell Axonal Degeneration. Valberg SJ, Lewis SS, Shivers JL, Barnes NE, Konczak J, Draper AC, Armién AG. Vet Pathol 2015;52(6):1087–98.

"Shivers," a progressive movement disorder that most commonly affects Draft, Thoroughbred, or Warmblood horses, has been recognized for more than a century. The disorder most often manifests as hypertonia of the hind limbs and tail upon backing or manually lifting a hind limb but may also be observed during slow forward motion. A neurophysiologic and pathologic mechanism for the syndrome has been elusive. In the report by Valberg and colleagues, a detailed neuroanatomic and neuropathologic analysis of the sensorimotor system in affected (N = 5) and control (breed, height at withers, and age matched) horses was performed. Primary muscle and peripheral nerve disease was not found in horses with shivers. Instead, in the deep cerebellar nuclei, spheroids were found in the lateralis and interpositus nuclei and present to a lesser degree in the nucleus fastigii in shivers horses but rarely were found in control horses. There was more than an 80-fold increase in spheroids in Purkinje cell axons focally within the deep cerebellar nuclei of shivers compared with control horses. On electron microscopy, unilateral lamellar or membranous structures resembling marked myelin decompaction were present between myelin sheaths of presumed Purkinje cell axons in the deep cerebellar nuclei of the horses with shivers but not in controls. The dorsal portion of the lateral cerebellar nuclei has a key role in modulating voluntary movement of the extremities. There was an increased ratio of type 2A to 2B muscle fibers (hind limb and triceps muscles) in shivers horses, which was hypothesized to be a result of constant muscle fiber recruitment induced by myoclonus. The findings of this study indicate, for the first time, that shivers is caused by neuroaxonal degeneration in the deep cerebellar nuclei.

"I guess this explains why my attempted treatment with dietary changes, steroid epidurals, etc, have been unsuccessful in the past."

Vet Clin Equine 33 (2017) 227–237
http://dx.doi.org/10.1016/j.cveq.2016.10.001
0749-0739/17/© 2016 Published by Elsevier Inc.

vetequine.theclinics.com

There have been several outstanding publications on equine metabolic disorders. The intent of these publications is to improve our understanding of pathophysiology of equine metabolic syndrome, including insulin resistance or insulin dysregulation, and diagnostic testing for early detection of both equine metabolic syndrome (EMS) and pituitary pars intermedia dysfunction (PPID, Cushing disease).

Use of the Oral Sugar Test in Ponies When Performed with or Without Prior Fasting. Knowles EJ, Harris PA, Elliott J, Menzies-Gow NJ. Equine Vet J. 2016.
Knowles and colleagues evaluated the differences between insulin responses to an oral sugar test (OST; 0.15 mL/kg light Karo syrup) in a crossover study either in healthy ponies fasted overnight with morning testing or in those same ponies at a later date without fasting but kept continually at pasture. The authors rightfully point out a purpose for the study: overnight fasting is not always feasible in some management situations. Results showed that serum insulin was higher between 60 (T_{60}) and 90 (T_{90}) minutes following overnight fasting than when ponies were not fasted but kept on pasture. Mean serum differences between fasted and fed ponies were 23.5, 27.1, and 41.8 μiu/mL at T_{60}, T_{75}, and T_{90}, respectively. This was not surprising because absorption of glucose might be expected to be more rapid when performed on an "empty" stomach. The authors conclude that it is inadvisable to use results of fed versus fasted protocols interchangeably. However, results obtained under FED conditions had similar reliability (ie, discriminatory power) to those obtained under FASTING conditions and produced similar results, when interpreted on a dichotomous (samples tested at T_{30} and T_{60}) basis using alternative criteria for insulin resistance; >51 μiu/mL fed and >60 μiu/mL fasted. Therefore, when fasting is impractical, similar basic OST interpretation may be obtained without prior fasting as under standardized fasted conditions. The authors point out that a limitation of the fed aspect of the study was that different pastures may cause very different test results.

An interesting finding in the study was that the most commonly recorded T_{max} for serum insulin was at 30 minutes, faster than reported in horses and a previous pony study. The time of post-OST sample collection should, therefore, be considered as another variable that might decrease predictive value of the test. Importantly, the authors performed the OST 4 times (twice fasted and twice fed) on the same ponies, thus providing important information on repeatability of the OST for insulin dysregulation. Repeatability of the OST was poor regardless of ponies being fasted or fed, and the authors point out that clinicians should therefore be cautious in interpreting a single OST result!

Equine Hyperinsulinemia: Investigation of the Enteroinsular Axis During Insulin Dysregulation. de Laat MA, McGree JM, Sillence MN. Am J Physiol Endocrinol Metab. 2016;310(1):E61–72.
de Laat and colleagues used insulin dysregulated ponies fasted and administered oral glucose and intravenous dextrose in a crossover study and found that all 22 ponies had abnormally high serum insulin after oral glucose challenge, but 7 of those had normal insulin and glucose responses following intravenous (IV) glucose administration. This suggested that these 7 ponies had insulin dysregulation but not insulin resistance. This would support recent thoughts that peripheral insulin resistance is not the sole cause of equine metabolic syndrome, that insulin dysregulation in horses/ponies can occur independently of tissue resistance to insulin, and thus, the term insulin dysregulation may be a preferred term to describe EMS.

In a second experiment in the publication using 9 additional ponies, a marked hyperglycemic response to oral dextrose was noted in 5 of 9 ponies, hyperinsulinemic and hyperglycemic responses to intravenously administered dextrose had been similar among all ponies. The insulin responsiveness to oral glucose was strongly associated with markedly increased blood glucose concentrations. Further evaluation revealed no difference in glucose clearance rates in the 2 pony groups, suggesting the marked hyperglycemia may have been due to enhanced glucose absorption or differences in glucose "first-pass" effects in the liver, causing a corresponding increase in serum insulin. An incretin hormone, α-glucagon-like peptide (aGLP-1), had a higher under the curve value in those 5 ponies with marked hyperglycemia than in the other 4 ponies following the oral glucose test. GLP-1 contributes to insulin secretion and in an additive manner, to hyperglycemia. Using all 9 ponies, it was calculated that the contributions of glucose and a aGLP-1 to the variability in insulin secretion following the oral test were 75.5 and 22.7%, respectively. Similar results in glucose, insulin, and GLP-1 dynamics were found in these 9 ponies when oats or a commercial grain mixture was fed.

In summary, this study demonstrated that

1. Insulin resistance might not be a prerequisite for, nor a necessary precursor to the hyperinsulinemia that may predispose horses to laminitis.
2. Insulin dysregulation may have a gastrointestinal cause due, in part, to incretin hormone release, and ponies with excessive hyperglycemic responses to oral nonstructured carbohydrates either absorb more glucose or metabolize less during first pass in the liver.

The study is highlighted because it provides information that further suggests that EMS is much more complex than simply peripheral insulin resistance. Both of the above studies on EMS suggest to me that we do not have a uniformly accepted standardized test to detect insulin dysregulation in horses and ponies.

Lamellar Pathology in Horses with Pituitary Pars Intermedia Dysfunction. Karikoski NP, Patterson-Kane JC, Singer ER, McFarlane D, McGowan CM. Equine Vet J. 2016;48(4):472–8.

In a prospective case control study, histomorphometric and pathologic lesions were described in hoof lamellar tissue of 16 horses that had PPID (Cushing disease). Six of the 16 horses had clinically apparent laminitis and 10 did not. Fasting-serum insulin, plasma, adrenocorticotropin (ACTH), and blood glucose were measured before euthanasia in all horses. All of the PPID horses with laminitis had fasting hyperinsulinemia, whereas PPID horses without laminitis had normal serum insulin. Plasma ACTH concentrations and ages of the 2 PPID groups were similar. Only PPID horses with clinically apparent laminitis and hyperinsulinemia had laminar pathology different from other horses in the study. Although the number of horses in the study was relatively small, these findings suggest that hyperinsulinemia (insulin dysregulation) is causal of laminitis in horses with PPID. Measurement of serum insulin and blood glucose would seem to be important for therapeutic and prognostic reasons in horses with PPID.

Electrophysiologic Study of a Method of Euthanasia Using Intrathecal Lidocaine Hydrochloride Administered During Intravenous Anesthesia in Horses. Aleman M, Davis E, Williams DC, Madigan JE, Smith F, Guedes A. J Vet Intern Med. 2015;29(6):1676–82.

This recent publication by Aleman and colleagues evaluated electrophysiologic findings, including electroencephalogram, electro-oculogram, brainstem-evoked response, and electrocardiogram, in horses anesthetized with the combination of xylazine, midazolam, and ketamine, and then euthanized with intrathecal (atlanto-occipital puncture) administration of lidocaine. Intrathecal administration of lidocaine was shown to be an effective alternative to the barbiturate overdose method of euthanasia in adult horses. Brain death occurred within 4 minutes before cardiac death (300-1279 seconds) following lidocaine administration. In a separate article (J Vet Intern Med. 2016;30(4):1322-6), the same authors investigated drug residues in the horses receiving xylazine, midazolam, ketamine, and lidocaine–induced euthanasia. Blood skeletal muscle and cerebrospinal fluid were tested for drug residue. Although drug residues were found in the tissue of all horses, the concentrations were extremely low and would pose low risk of toxicity to carnivores and scavengers who might consume a carcass.

I chose to include the above article in my "In Case You Missed it List" because of continued alarming reports on the death of eagles, other birds of prey and other animals that may feed on improperly disposed of animals euthanized with barbiturates (*Secondary Pentobarbital Poisoning of Wildlife. US Fish and Wildlife Service Fact Sheet*). Equine veterinarians have the responsibility to humanely and properly euthanize horses and with a reasonable certainty that the carcass will be disposed of properly. This study provides an alternative method of euthanasia when pentobarbital is unavailable, a bullet method cannot be used, or for some reason the body may not be properly disposed of.

A Comparison of Three Doses of Omeprazole in the Treatment of Equine Gastric Ulcer Syndrome: A Blinded, Randomised, Dose-Response Clinical Trial. Sykes BW, Sykes KM, Hallowell GD. Equine Vet J. 2015;47(3):285–90.

An omeprazole dose-related response for the treatment of gastric ulcers in horses was reported by Sykes and colleagues in 2015. This was a blinded, randomized dose-response clinical trial using 60 Thoroughbred racehorses with at least grade 2 squamous ulcers and/or glandular ulcers. Horses received either 1.0, 2.0, or 4.0 mg/kg of an enteric-coated omeprazole orally 1-4 hours before exercise. It should be pointed out that this particular omeprazole product is not GastroGuard®, but it has been shown to have similar bioavailability and healing effect in previous studies. The authors diligently pointed out that this study was performed in horses following a brief fast, and this may have improved bioavailability. Confirming previous observations of many practitioners that although healing of squamous ulcers was good, healing of glandular ulcers with omeprazole treatment was poor. In fact, 36% of treated horses had worsening glandular ulcers following treatment. The study suggests that omeprazole should not be relied on as the sole daily treatment for glandular ulcers. Other drugs, such as misoprostol, which is both cytoprotective and increases gastric pH (*Res Vet Sci.* 1989;47(3):350–4) in horses, should be considered for glandular ulcers.

Macrolide-induced Hyperthermia in Foals: Role of Impaired Sweat Responses. Stieler AL, Sanchez LC, Mallicote MF, Martabano BB, Burrow JA, MacKay RJ. Equine Vet J. 2016;48(5):590–4.

In this erythromycin-induced hyperthermia study in foals, Stieler and colleagues suggested a mechanism for hyperthermia in 2- to 3-month-old foals treated with macrolides. This drug-related problem has been discussed for more than a decade, but until Stieler's publication, no mechanistic reason for the macrolide/hyperthermia association was shown. In this blinded, crossover study, 10 foals were given either erythromycin (25 mg/kg every 8 hours orally) or no macrolide placebo treatment for 10 days. Quantitative intradermal terbutaline (a beta-adrenergic agonist) sweat tests were performed on or before treatment and on days 3, 10, and 30. Sweating was significantly reduced from baseline in erythromycin-treated foals at 3, 10, and 30 days, and peak rectal temperature of erythromycin-treated foals was higher than controls. Only the erythromycin-treated foals required treatment for hyperthermia when turned out in the Florida heat. Ten days following the last erythromycin treatment, sweating responses had only partially recovered. The authors' belief is that drug-induced anhidrosis is the likely cause of hyperthermia in foals treated with erythromycin. It would now be of interest to repeat this study using azithromycin and clarithromycin in foals because these newer macrolides have mostly replaced erythromycin for treatment of *Rhodococcus* pneumonia in foals.

Environmental Heat and Airborne Pollen Concentration are Associated with Increased Asthma Severity in Horses. Bullone M, Murcia RY, Lavoie JP. Equine Vet J. 2016;48(4):479–84.

This publication by Bullone and colleagues on environmental heat and airborne-pollen concentrations in asthmatic horses provides some explanation for seasonal exacerbation of asthma in horses. I should add here that equine pulmonologists now recommend the term "equine asthma" to replace recurrent airway obstruction and chronic obstructive pulmonary disease in horses. The term "heaves" may be acceptable again? In this excellent study, the objectives were to investigate the association between environmental temperature and humidity and clinical signs of asthma in horses previously shown to have severe asthma. Fourteen asthmatic horses that had been kept at pasture for 4 months were used in this study. In midspring, the horses were moved to a stable for 18 or more hours per day and fed hay for 6 weeks (antigen exposure). A clinical scoring system was used to assess respiratory effort the first 5 weeks of the study, and pulmonary function testing to detect transpulmonary pressure were measured 4 days apart during the sixth week on both a hot (25°C) and a warm day (18°C). Temperature and relative humidity were recorded during the study, and air enthalpy (a measure of heat and humidity) was calculated. The concentration of outside airborne pollen and spores during the study period was obtained from an aerobiology research laboratory. Significant positive correlations were observed between clinical score and air enthalpy. Maximal daily temperatures correlated with airborne pollen concentration. Higher barn temperature and air enthalpy values were associated with increased pulmonary pressure, pulmonary resistance, and elastance values. The authors conclude that variations in environmental heat and associated pollen concentrations should be taken into account when evaluating equine asthma and response to treatment.

Although those of us in so-called cooler climates generally consider winter stabling to be a time of greatest allergen exposure in horses with asthma, we also recognize that late spring or summer exacerbations of the disease are common, whereby horses are spending more time outdoors. This study may help explain the reason for those observations.

Intra-articular Treatment with Triamcinolone Compared with Triamcinolone with Hyaluronate: A Randomised Open-Label Multicentre Clinical Trial in 80 Lame Horses. de Grauw JC, Visser-Meijer MC, Lashley F, Meeus P, van Weeren PR. Equine Vet J. 2016;48(2):152–8.

A publication by de Grauw and colleagues compared the intra-articular injection of triamcinolone acetate (12 mg) with or without high-molecular-weight hyaluronate (HA, 20 mg) in horses with clinical joint disease. This was a prospective, randomized multicentric but not blinded clinical trial. Eighty horses were included with lameness and joint effusion scores assessed by the attending veterinarian at baseline and 3 weeks after intra-articular therapies. Clinical success was defined as a 2 grade or greater lameness reduction (0-5 scale). The success rate of intra-articular triamcinolone at 3 weeks was 87.8%, whereas that of triamcinolone plus HA was 64.1%. A 3-month posttreatment follow-up with owners found that one-half of the horses in each group had returned to their previous level of performance. This study is to be applauded because prospective, randomized studies on treatment efficacy are not as common in equine as in human medicine. This study provides short-term objective data to help base our decision to treat synovitis or osteoarthritis with triamcinolone, HA, or both. Longer-term studies would be helpful, especially in light of a recent report by Knych and colleagues in Equine Vet J. 2016 (Epub ahead of print) demonstrating downregulation of collagen gene expression following intra-articular injection of 9 mg triamcinolone in healthy horses. It should also be remembered that in an older study (French et al. J Vet Pharmacol Ther. 2000;23(5):287–92) the administration of triamcinolone acetonide at 0.05 mg/kg intramuscularly to horses induced a prolonged hyperglycemia and hyperinsulinemia.

Evaluation of 10-Minute Versus 60-Minute Tourniquet Time for Intravenous Limb Perfusion with Amikacin Sulfate in Standing Sedated Horses. Kilcoyne I, Dechant JE, Nieto JE. Vet Rec. 2016 4;178(23):585.

Intravenous regional limb perfusion (IVRLP) with antibiotics will often result in micro-biologically acceptable drug concentrations locally, with minimal chance of systemic affects. Previous studies have identified the most effective tourniquets for the infusion, site of injection, and most appropriate volume to administer, but no previous studies have determined the most appropriate time to maintain the tourniquet in place. In this study by Kilcoyne and colleagues, synovial fluid and systemic concentrations of amikacin were measured following IVRLP with tourniquet maintained for either 10 or 30 minutes in 7 horses. IVRLP of the cephalic veins with a washout period between 10- and 30-minute tourniquet time was used for the infusion (2 g amikacin in 60 mL 0.9% saline). Synovial fluid was collected from the radiocarpal and metatarsophalangeal joints at 4 minutes and 24 hours after the tourniquet was removed, and amikacin concentration was measured. There was no significant different between synovial fluid amikacin concentration in the 2 study groups. Systemic venous blood concentration of amikacin was higher when the tourniquet was released at 10 minutes. Although the 10-minute tourniquet allowed a mean amikacin concentration of 48 µg/mL in the metacarpophalangeal joint and 54 µg/mL in the RC joint (therapeutic target concentration is considered to be 40 µg/mL), the higher systemic concentration in the 10-minute tourniquet group could indicate insufficient time for diffusion of the antibiotic into the soft tissue and synovial structures of the limb. A 10-minute tourniquet could be appropriate for IVRP amikacin, a concentration-dependent drug, although the wide variability between horses and changes in blood flow dynamics due to disease should be considered.

Outcome of Palmar/Plantar Digital Neurectomy in Horses with Foot Pain Evaluated with Magnetic Resonance Imaging: 50 Cases (2005-2011). Gutierrez-Nibeyro SD, Werpy NM, White NA 2nd, Mitchell MA, Edwards RB 3rd, Mitchell RD, Gold SJ, Allen AK. Equine Vet J. 2015;47(2):160–4.

Palmar or plantar digital neurectomy (PDN) has been performed for several decades in horses with chronic and usually incurable foot pain in order to alleviate pain and/or permit the horse to return to athletic use. Complications can occur, and proper case selection for the procedure is important. In the publication by Gutierrez-Nibeyro and colleagues, the authors point out that there is limited knowledge on foot lesions that influence the outcome of digital neurectomy, and in their article, a retrospective evaluation of MRI findings were performed in imaged horses that had a neurectomy in order to determine factors that may influence outcome following PDN. The medical records of 50 horses subjected to PDN were reviewed. Significant, athletic use, duration of lameness, response to anesthesia of palmar/plantar nerves, low-field MRI findings, and surgical techniques were analyzed with follow-up data to identify factors that influenced long-term outcomes. Forty-six of 50 horses responded favorably to surgery, and 40 were able to return to athletic use for 12 to 72 months. Age, breed, sex, athletic use, and choice of surgical technique were not associated with postoperative lameness. Residual lameness immediately after anesthesia of the palmar/plantar digital nerves was associated with increased rate of prolonged postoperative lameness. The authors, therefore, state that if the expectation of PDN is to render the horse sound for at least 30 months after surgery, anesthesia of the palmar/plantar digital nerves should completely resolve lameness.

Equine Odontoclastic Tooth Resorption and Hypercementosis: Histopathologic Features. Smedley RC, Earley ET, Galloway SS, Baratt RM, Rawlinson JE. Vet Pathol. 2015;52(5):903–9.

Equine odontoclastic tooth resorption and hypercementosis (EOTRH) has become a commonly recognized dental disorder in horses. I am still at loss for an explanation as to why this disease was not widely recognized before 2004. In the article by Smedley and colleagues, histologic features of this painful progressive condition of the incisors and sometimes canine teeth of older horses were described. All affected teeth exhibited cemental hyperplasia and lysis. The marked proliferation of cementum in severe cases caused bulbous enlargement of the intra-alveolar portions of affected teeth, and there were large regions of inflammatory resorption. In addition, periodontal disease characterized primarily by lymphoplasmacytic inflammation and fibrosis of the periodontal ligament was a common feature. In some cases, these lesions extended through the dentition into the pulp cavity, but resorption with secondary hypercementosis appears to begin on the external surface of the teeth rather than within the pulp cavity. The age of the 17 affected horses in this study ranged from 10 to 32 years with an average age of 21.7 years. The authors point out that a complete oral examination and dental radiographs are needed for diagnosis, especially when lesions are early and mild.

Clinical Treatment and Prognosis of Equine Odontoclastic Tooth Resorption and Hypercementosis. Lorello O, Foster DL, Levine DG, Boyle A, Engiles J, Orsini JA. Equine Vet J. 2016;48(2):188–94.

In a separate study, Lorello and colleagues report on the clinical treatment and prognosis for EOTRH. In this study, it was also reported that mild or early cases of the disease may have only radiographic changes and no gross clinical evidence of disease. Radiographs often reveal that the disease is more extensive than clinical examination had revealed. The mandibular incisors were generally affected earlier than the maxillary incisors. The 03s, the youngest of the incisor teeth, were most commonly affected. Treatment consisted of surgical extraction of some or all of the clinically affected teeth, and in some cases, extraction of affected teeth that were radiographically abnormal but clinically normal. One of the 18 horses had already lost its affected teeth! Dental extractions were performed under general anesthesia in 14 horses and under sedation with perineural or local anesthetic in other cases. Alveolar cavities were packed with plaster of Paris, mixed with antimicrobial/antiseptic agents. Within 1 week after surgery, all 14 horses having extraction performed under general anesthesia were eating a sweet feed mix or pelleted feed and hay. Grazing was restricted for 6 to 8 weeks. Horses that had extractions performed while standing appeared to be uncomfortable for the first 2 weeks following extraction with reportedly a decreased appetite. Follow-up reports were available on 12 horses; 9 horses that had all 12 incisors extracted (or lost) were healthy, eating hay, and grazing. Three horses that had 2, 4, and 7 incisors extracted were reported to be eating without difficulty and had improved body condition scores. Some horses were reported to "play with their tongue" and/or hang the tongue out of the mouth.

When the horses in both studies are combined, it should be noted that 34 of the 35 horses were males! The etiopathology of the disease is unknown, but this obvious sex difference in incidence of disease could provide an important clue in solving the mystery of EOTRH.

Effect of Topical Ophthalmic Dorzolamide (2%)-Timolol (0.5%) Solution and Ointment on Intraocular Pressure in Normal Horses. Tofflemire KL, Whitley EM, Flinn AM, Dufour VL, Ben-Shlomo G, Allbaugh RA, Griggs AN, Peterson CS, Whitley DR. Vet Ophthalmol. 2015;18(6):457–61.

In this study, a randomized, masked prospective design was used, with horses divided into 2 equal groups. One eye of each horse was selected for topical ophthalmic treatment with either 0.2 mL dorzolamide (2%)-timolol (0.5%) solution or 0.2 g dorzolamide(2%)-timolol (0.5%) ointment every 12 hours for 5 days. The contralateral eye of horses in both groups was untreated. Rebound tonometry was performed every 6 hours starting 2 days before and ending 2 days after the treatment period. The mean intraocular pressure (IOP) reduction in eyes treated with the solution or ointment formulations was 13%. Untreated eyes in both groups experienced a lesser but still statistically significant reduction in IOP. The IOP values did not return to baseline within 48 hours of the last treatment. The commercially available solution and compounded ointment formulations of ophthalmic dorzolamide (2%)-timolol (0.5%) had similar effects on IOP in normal horses. Persistent IOP reduction following cessation of treatment may indicate prolonged drug effect or acclimation of horses to tonometry. This information is especially helpful for owners of horses with equine glaucoma because a compounded ointment preparation is generally easier and more precisely administered than the commercially available drops.

Limbal Squamous Cell Carcinoma in Haflinger Horses. Lassaline M, Cranford TL, Latimer CA, Bellone RR. Vet Ophthalmol. 2015;18(5):404–8.

This was a retrospective medical record review of 19 Haflinger horses with limbal squamous cell carcinomas (LSCC). The average age at diagnosis with LSCC was 8.7 years. Eleven horses were males and eight were females. Four-generation pedigrees available for 15 of the horses were used to perform pedigree analysis and showed 13 of 15 affected horses for whom pedigrees were available shared a common ancestor within 5 generations, and all 15 shared a common ancestor from the A stallion line in the breed pedigree. Pedigree analysis identified a common sire of 2 of the affected male horses. Clinical examination of this sire that had no history of LSCC showed no current clinical signs of LSCC, suggesting an autosomal-recessive mode of inheritance. The conclusion of the study was that Haflingers may be overrepresented among horses with LSCC and may be diagnosed at a younger age than other breeds. Affected Haflingers appear closely related, suggesting a possible heritable basis for LSCC.

L-carnitine and Pyruvate are Prosurvival Factors During the Storage of Stallion Spermatozoa at Room Temperature. Gibb Z, Lambourne SR, Quadrelli J, Smith ND, Aitken RJ. Biol Reprod. 2015;93(4):104.

There were several potentially important articles on evaluating methods of preserving or storing equine sperm and the effect on fertility. Previous publications have shown that spermatozoa of many stallions do not tolerate being cooled (cold shock), thus restricting the commercial viability of these animals and necessitating the development of a chemically defined room temperature storage medium. The major advantage of chilling semen is a reduction in sperm metabolic rate that results in improved longevity during transport and storage. This is of particular importance in the case of stallion spermatozoa, which are almost entirely dependent on oxidative phosphorylation for ATP production for motility.

A study by Gibb and colleagues examined the impact of 2 major modulators of oxidative phosphorylation, pyruvate (Pyr) and L-carnitine (L-C), on the storage of stallion spermatozoa at room temperature. To investigate the effects of L-C as an osmolyte, comparisons were made between media that were osmotically balanced with NaCl, choline chloride, or L-C. This analysis demonstrated that spermatozoa stored in the L-C balanced medium had significantly higher total motility, rapid motility, and ATP levels (70.9 vs 12.8 ng/mL) following storage compared with the NaCl treatment, whereas choline chloride did not significantly improve these parameters compared with the control. Finally, mass spectrometry was used to demonstrate that a combination of Pyr and L-C produced significantly higher acetyl-L-C production than any other treatment (6.7 pg/10^6 spermatozoa versus control at 4.0 pg/10^6 spermatozoa). These findings suggest that Pyr and L-C could form the basis of a novel, effective room temperature storage medium for equine spermatozoa. The addition of Pyr and L-C was able to support mitochondrial ATP production while minimizing both ATP depletion and the damaging effects of metabolic byproducts, such as free radicals, and maintain progressive motility of sperm at room temperature for up to 3 days. Fertility trials are now needed to confirm the clinical importance, but the in vitro findings are certainly encouraging.

Leptospira abortions are in the news, especially since there is a recently approved equine vaccine labeled to prevent *Leptospira* bacteremia.

Multiple Specificities of Immunoglobulin M in Equine Fetuses Infected with Leptospira interrogans Indicate a Competent Immune Response. Velineni S, Timoney JF, Artiushin SC, Donahue JM, Steinman M. Equine Vet J. 2016;43(6):704–9.

In an article by Velineni and colleagues, interesting and clinically important information is provided from a farm investigation of an outbreak of *Leptospira* abortions in combination with a case control study of a larger set of fetal fluid samples from *Leptospira*-positive and -negative aborted fetuses. In the farm outbreak, either fetuses of 6 mares in the outbreak were either aborted or the foals died soon after birth. Rising and markedly high antibody titers in the mares to *Leptospira pomona* suggested the mares' infections had occurred 2 to 3 weeks before the first abortion. Five fetuses of 11 infected mares survived in utero in the presence of persistent placental infection and were healthy at foaling. Persistence of *L pomona kennewicki* in the amnion was not inevitably associated with clinical disease or death of the foal. Seven of the infected mares had urine samples tested by polymerase chain reaction for *Leptospira* for up to 1 to 3 months following the presumed infection date, and 6 were still shedding *Leptospira* in the urine. Significantly greater immunoglobulin M

(IgM) reactivity with all recombinant *Leptospira* proteins and with *L pomona kenne-wicki* sonicate was observed in 54 archived fluids from *Leptospira*-infected fetuses than in fluids of 30 of non-*Leptospira*-infected fetuses. The presence of specific antibodies in the fetal fluid, e.g., heart blood, suggests that aborted fetuses survived in utero for 2 weeks or longer following infection. Although mainly mediated by IgM, a high level of immune competence in aborted fetuses was evidenced by the multiplicity of *Leptospira* proteins targeted. This is likely to contribute to survival of foals in mares with evidence of placental infection at foaling.

This article has several important and clinically relevant findings: mares that suffer abortion from leptospirosis have high titers of *Leptospira* at the time of abortion; aborted fetuses have likely been infected for at least 1 week before being aborted and have antibody in fetal fluids/heart blood; some infected fetuses can survive and be born healthy; and *L pomona*-type *kenniwicki* is by far the most important pathogenic *Leptospira* strain in Kentucky.

Accuracy and Precision of Noninvasive Blood Pressure in Normo-, Hyper-, and Hypotensive Standing and Anesthetized Adult Horses. Heliczer N, Lorello O, Casoni D, Navas de Solis C. J Vet Intern Med. 2016;30(3):866–72.

Monitoring the critically ill horse is often based on clinical findings, response to treatments, and laboratory findings. The increasing use of point-of-care equipment for immediate determination of electrolytes, glucose, creatinine, acid-base, and lactate measurements in addition to cardiovascular ultrasound examination has greatly improved our ability to monitor the critically ill horse. Routine measurement of blood pressure (BP) in critically ill horses would be advisable, especially in horses that appear hypotensive, have blood and other fluid loss, or are in heart failure, and in some laminitic or chronically painful horses where there may be a concern about hypertension. Noninvasive, indirect oscillometric BP readings are easily obtained using tail cuff measurements in most standing horses, but due to the significant height difference between the base of the heart and coccygeal artery, there is generally an underestimation of BP in the standing horse and overestimation when the same location is used with a horse in dorsal recumbency. The accuracy of noninvasive, indirect BP measurements in adult standing horses in hypotensive and hypertensive ranges has not been evaluated.

In this study by Heliczer and colleagues, the accuracy of an oscillometric BP monitor was evaluated in standing horses by simultaneously measuring invasive (direct) and noninvasive (indirect) BP both before and during pharmacologically induced hypertension and hypotension with comparison of results in standing and anesthetized horses. Eight presumably healthy mares were used for standing measurements along with 8 different hospitalized horses undergoing general anesthesia. A cuff bladder width-to-tail girth ratio of 0.4–0.6 (manufacturer's recommendations) was used over the coccygeal artery on the base of the tail for measurement of indirect pressure measurements; for direct BP measurements, a 20- or 22-G over-the-needle catheter was placed in the facial or transversal facial artery. Direct and indirect BP, which was corrected to heart level, was measured simultaneously in all horses. In the standing horses, hypertension and hypotension were induced by administration of phenylephrine (3 μg/kg/min IV for 15 minutes) and acepromazine (0.05 mg/kg IV), respectively. In the standing horses, BP was obtained at 4 different time points: before pharmacological intervention, immediately after phenylephrine infusion, 35 minutes after phenylephrine infusion, and 30 minutes after acepromazine. Multiple consecutive readings were performed at each time period, and averages at each time point were used for analysis. If any pulse rate obtained by the oscillometric device differed by more than 20% of the heart rate obtained electrocardiographically, the value was excluded. In the anesthetized group, direct and indirect BP was recorded during regular hospital procedures. There was a significant correlation between mean direct and indirect BP measurements in both standing and anesthetized horses. The mean bias (lower, upper limit of agreement) was 16.4 (−16.1, 48.9) mmHg for mean BP in the standing horses and 0.5 (−22.3, 23.2) mmHg in the anesthetized horses. The noninvasive oscillometric device was capable of identifying the increase and decrease in BP in all horses, but in the standing horses, significant correlation between indirect and direct BP was only detected for the normotensive phase. Although the evaluated oscillometric BP device allowed estimation of BP and adequately differentiated marked trends, the accuracy and precision were low in standing horses.

Noninvasive BP should be used more when monitoring/treating critically ill horses, realizing that it provides a trend for changes in BP and likely underestimates the actual BP. Auscultated heart rate and BP monitor-calculated heart rate should be similar if BP results are to be considered valid.

Thomas J. Divers, DVM
Section of Large Animal Medicine
Cornell University
College of Veterinary Medicine
Ithaca, NY 14853, USA

E-mail address:
tjd8@cornell.edu

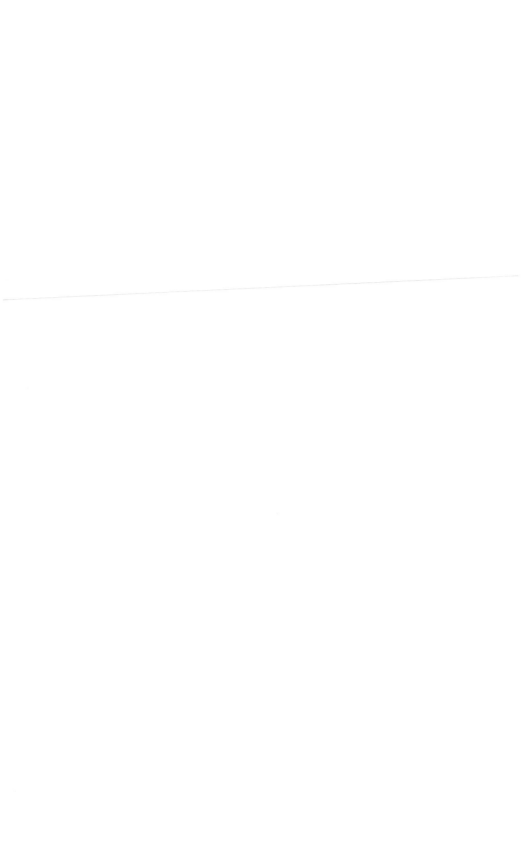

Index

Note: Page numbers of article titles are in **boldface** type.

A

Acyclovir
    for herpesviruses, 104–113
Adrenocortical disease, 134
Adulterated drugs
    compounding of
        for equine practitioners, 216
Aerosol(s)
    delivery of
        in inhalation therapy, 31–36 *See also* Inhalation therapy, aerosol delivery in
AF. *See* Atrial fibrillation (AF)
Aminoglycoside(s)
    in neonatal foals
        continuous infusions of, 55–57
Amiodarone
    in AF management, 171
Amoxicillin
    pharmacology of
        in neonatal foals, 47–48
Ampicillin
    pharmacology of
        in neonatal foals, 47–48
Analgesia
    NSAIDs for, 6
Antacids
    in EGUS management, 151–152
Antibiotics. *See* Antimicrobial agents
Antiherpetic drugs, **99–125**. *See also* Equine herpesvirus (EHV); Herpesvirus(es)
    acyclovir, 104–113
    cidofivir, 114–115
    for EHV-1, 115–116
    for EHV-2, 117
    for EHV-5, 116
    ganciclovir/valganciclovir, 113–114
    idoxuridine, 115
    introduction, 99–103
    long-term recommendations, 118–119
    outcome effects of, 118–119
    penciclovir/famciclovir, 113
    resistance to, 117–118
    trifluridine, 115
    types of, 104–117

Vet Clin Equine 33 (2017) 239–251
http://dx.doi.org/10.1016/S0749-0739(17)30013-5
0749-0739/17

vetequine.theclinics.com

Moving?

Make sure your subscription moves with you!

To notify us of your new address, find your **Clinics Account Number** (located on your mailing label above your name), and contact customer service at:

Email: journalscustomerservice-usa@elsevier.com

800-654-2452 (subscribers in the U.S. & Canada)
314-447-8871 (subscribers outside of the U.S. & Canada)

Fax number: 314-447-8029

Elsevier Health Sciences Division
Subscription Customer Service
3251 Riverport Lane
Maryland Heights, MO 63043

*To ensure uninterrupted delivery of your subscription, please notify us at least 4 weeks in advance of move.